# Principles and Practice of Toxicology in Public Health

## Ira S. Richards, PhD

Associate Professor
Environmental and Occupational Health
College of Public Health
University of South Florida

**JONES AND BARTLETT PUBLISHERS**
*Sudbury, Massachusetts*
BOSTON    TORONTO    LONDON    SINGAPORE

*World Headquarters*

Jones and Bartlett Publishers
40 Tall Pine Drive
Sudbury, MA 01776
978-443-5000
info@jbpub.com
www.jbpub.com

Jones and Bartlett Publishers Canada
6339 Ormindale Way
Mississauga, Ontario L5V 1J2
CANADA

Jones and Bartlett Publishers International
Barb House, Barb Mews
London W6 7PA
UK

Jones and Bartlett's books and products are available through most bookstores and online booksellers. To contact Jones and Bartlett Publishers directly, call 800-832-0034, fax 978-443-8000, or visit our Web site, www.jbpub.com.

Substantial discounts on bulk quantities of Jones and Bartlett's publications are available to corporations, professional associations, and other qualified organizations. For details and specific discount information, contact the special sales department at Jones and Bartlett via the above contact information or send an e-mail to specialsales@jbpub.com.

This publication is designed to provide accurate and authoritative information in regard to the Subject Matter covered. It is sold with the understanding that the publisher is not engaged in rendering legal, accounting, or other professional service. If legal advice or other expert assistance is required, the service of a competent professional person should be sought.

**Library of Congress Cataloging-in-Publication Data**
Richards, Ira S. (Ira Steven), 1948-
  Principles and practice of toxicology in public health / Ira S. Richards.
      p. ; cm.
  Includes bibliographical references and index.
  ISBN-13: 978-0-7637-3823-5 (pbk.)
  ISBN-10: 0-7637-3823-9 (pbk.)
  1. Toxicology. I. Title.
  [DNLM: 1. Toxicology. 2. Health Policy. 3. Public Health Practice. 4. Risk Assessment. QV 600 R515p
2007]
  RA1211.R52 2007
  615.9--dc22
                                            2007014175

6048

**Production Credits**
Publisher: Michael Brown
Associate Editor: Katey Birtcher
Production Director: Amy Rose
Production Editor: Tracey Chapman
Marketing Manager: Sophie Fleck
Manufacturing Buyer: Therese Connell
Composition: Arlene Apone

Cover Design: Kristin Ohlin
Photo Research Manager and Photographer: Kimberly Potvin
Associate Photo Researcher and Photographer: Christine McKeen
Cover Image: © Stephen Strathdee/ShutterStock, Inc.
Printing and Binding: Malloy, Inc.
Cover Printing: Malloy, Inc.

Printed in the United States of America
12  11  10  09  08    10  9  8  7  6  5  4  3  2

# Dedication

This book is dedicated to the memory of my parents
for all that they have done for me and to
Arun Kulkarni, teacher, scholar, and friend.

# Contents

# Preface

Toxicology deals with the harmful effects that may potentially result from exposures to chemical agents in humans and other organisms. Before 1970, there were virtually no academic programs of study in toxicology. Today, there are hundreds of colleges and universities with programs at the bachelor's level through the doctoral level, providing the requisite education for the student of toxicology. Recognition of the important role that the discipline plays in the protection of health and environment has also led to the development of programs in the interdisciplinary academic setting provided to students at schools and colleges of public health. A beginning course in toxicology here is typically graduate-level and attended by individuals with interests as diverse as environmental health, industrial hygiene, epidemiology, biostatistics, medicine, nursing, law, engineering, biology, and chemistry, as well as toxicology. Clearly, this is a very heterogeneous population of students, each viewing the practice of public health and dealing with public health issues from different perspectives.

Although recognizing that the study of toxicology, at a level commensurate with earning a graduate degree in this concentration, may be beyond the scope of perhaps most students of public health, we should also recognize that most, and perhaps all, public health students should be at least exposed to some of its content. The content selected in *Principles and Practice of Toxicology in Public Health* is intended to provide to both groups of students an understanding of the nature and scope of the discipline. This is necessary to participate in a meaningful way in the often highly visible problem-solving and decision-making processes required of public health professionals. Whether we are dealing with issues as diverse as a workers' compensation claim for a job-related exposure and injury or the removal of toxic wastes from an urban community, we must be able to communicate with each other, the public, and our political leaders concerning how chemicals can, and the conditions under which they may, realistically produce harm. Understanding is a requirement for establishing rational and better ways of protection and management for individuals, populations, communities, and our environment from the potentially harmful effects of chemical exposures. A required introduction to the scope and content of toxicology for public health students should therefore be viewed as not a punishment, but rather as an important part of a general education.

Public health professionals working in municipal departments of public health are generally very well informed about biological agents and perhaps less informed about chemical exposures and toxicity. In our "preparedness" for the general public, and especially in these troubled times, we recognize that both biological and chemical agents constitute an important concern, and it is anticipated that this book will provide some additional background and information for you as well.

# Acknowledgments

The author wishes to acknowledge his family for their understanding and enormous patience during the time of this writing. Thank you Barbara, Charles, Jeffrey, and Elizabeth for all of the hours that otherwise would have been devoted to you.

A very special thanks to Marie Bourgeois, for her enormous efforts in assisting me with this book. Without her planning, insight, and ability to deal with, at times, a cantankerous professor, it was doubtful that the book would have been completed within the allocated time. Thank you for ensuring that all went well.

# Toxicology and Its Roots as a Science

It is clear that we "live, work, and play" in environments where we are exposed to chemical agents. We justify their use to maintain and improve our own well-being and that of society in general. Unfortunately, we have seen, and may continue to see, incidents of chemical-induced adverse events in humans and other species with which we share our planet. Bhopal, India was the site of one of the largest industrial accidents of the 20th century. In 1984 an accidental discharge of methyl isocyanate into the air from a Union Carbide pesticide manufacturing facility resulted in the overnight deaths of approximately 4,000 individuals and over 100,000 sustained injuries, some of which were so severe that many thousands later died. The primary cause of death was pulmonary edema; many survivors showed signs of compromised respiration (e.g., bronchoalveolar lesions and decreased lung function) and impaired vision (e.g., loss of vision, loss of visual acuity, and cataracts).

Recognizing the benefits of chemicals in general, we accept the potential risks from their use until some undesirable event or additional information about any particular chemical forces us to reevaluate its benefit in light of the risk posed. As public health professionals, we further recognize that sometimes large numbers of individuals may be exposed to certain chemicals where there is often only limited information available on human health effects. This is especially true for chronic "low level" exposures. As we will see later, human safety is often inferred only from laboratory data in animals as the source of toxicity information as, for example, in the case of satisfying the regulatory requirement for the safety of a new food additive by the Federal Food and Drug Administration.

A simple yet comprehensive definition of toxicology is the study of the adverse effects of chemicals in biological systems. A biological system can be as complex as an entire organism or can be a less complicated *in vitro* cell culture system. As public health professionals, we direct most of our attention to human health effects; however, we must also recognize that we share our planet with other organisms, both plants and animals, that are also affected by chemical agents.

## Toxic Chemicals

Terms commonly used to refer to toxic chemicals are as follows:

- Toxic chemical
- Toxic substance
- Toxic agent
- Poison
- Toxin
- Toxicant
- Xenobiotic

Although the terms *toxicant* and *toxin* are frequently used interchangeably, they are different. A term to denote any chemical that can potentially produce harm is *toxicant*. Toxicants may affect specific tissues or organs (target tissues, target organs), such as benzene, which affects the blood and blood-forming tissues. Toxicants may also be relatively nonspecific, thus affecting the entire body. Sodium cyanide is an example of a systemic toxicant that has the ability to interfere with all body cell utilization of oxygen. A toxicant may be a heavy metal such as lead, a pesticide, an organic solvent, or even a toxin. The term *toxin*, however, *must* be reserved for those chemicals that are produced by living organisms. Rattlesnake venom or poisonous mushrooms contain toxins. Many toxins are extremely hazardous chemicals and can produce severe injury to tissues and organs, often to the extent that death may result from body system failure (Table 1.1).

A poison is generally defined as any substance that when ingested, inhaled, or absorbed or when applied to, injected into, or developed within the body in *relatively small amounts* may, by its chemical action, cause death or injury. A poison therefore could be any of the numerous synthetic chemicals or a chemical produced by a living organism (toxin). The commonly used term *toxic substance* does not describe whether one is speaking about a particular chemical or a mixture of chemicals that collectively have toxic properties. So whereas lead chloride is a discrete chemical that has toxic properties, asbestos is not a discrete chemical but is rather a mixture of various chemicals whose composition may vary.

**Table 1.1    Examples of Toxins**

| Toxin and Source | Example of Tissue/System Affected |
|---|---|
| Aflatoxin B (*Aspergillus flavus*) | Liver Necrosis and Cancer |
| α-Amanitin (*Amanita phalloides*) | Gastrointestinal Tract and Liver Cancer |
| Anatoxin (*Anabaena* spp) | Nervous System (anticholinesterase) |
| Sodium fluoroacetate (*Dichapetalum cymosum*) | Cardiac, Skeletal Muscle, Nervous |
| Ochratoxin A (*Aspergillus ocraceus*) | Kidney |
| Pyrethrin I (*Pyrethrum cinariaefolium*) | Nervous |
| Tetrodotoxin (*Puffer fish, Amphibians*) | Nervous |

The term *xenobiotic* literally means foreign to the body and can refer to any chemical that is not a natural component of the body (e.g., a synthetic antibiotic). The term, however, is typically used in the context of any synthetic chemical that has *no* beneficial effect on the body (Table 1.2).

The degree and nature of toxicity is not only related to which chemical one is exposed (the hazard) but to the conditions of exposure as well. So although ethanol can acutely produce its effects on the central nervous system, over the long term it produces chronic toxicity to the liver as well.

The practice of toxicology involves the application of toxicological principles that are focused on environmental, regulatory, industrial, clinical, or forensic issues, to name several. Indeed, any issue about the health risks from chemicals would be of concern to toxicologists. Toxicology is an applied science that has assimilated the theoretical and technical advances of disciplines such as

**Table 1.2    Examples of Xenobiotics**

| Toxicant and Source | Example of Tissue/System Affected |
|---|---|
| Deltamethrin (*insecticide*) | Nervous System |
| Ethylene glycol monomethylether (*solvent*) | Testis |
| n-Hexane (*solvent*) | Nervous System |
| Methyl isocyanate (*used in insecticide manufacture*) | Lung and Eye |
| 1-methyl 4-phenyl 1,2,3,6-tetrahydropyridine (MPTP) (*impurity in demerol*) | Nervous |
| Paraquat (*herbicide*) | Lung |
| Soman (*nerve gas*) | Nervous System |

chemistry, biology, physiology, pharmacology, pathology, epidemiology, and biostatistics. The duality of toxicology requires gathered and applied science. For this reason toxicology is often described as a "borrowing" science, and, indeed, this utilization of information from other disciplines is one of toxicology's greatest strengths. Toxicology can be considered as one of the most interdisciplinary sciences of the modern age.

## The Roots of Toxicology

Toxicology, from the ancient world and biblical times through medieval alchemy and the Renaissance, is a science that is rooted in a rich and interesting history. Reference to "poisonous" substances can be traced back to the use of natural poisons in hunting, "medicines," assassination, warfare, or for other purposes. Early records show that humans did indeed use poisons rather effectively. The Ebers Papyrus (circa 1500 B.C.) contains the recipes of more than 800 "medicinal" and poisonous preparations. It describes poisons known at that time, including hemlock, later to be used as the state poison of the Greeks ("Socrates' nightcap") as well as opium, aconite (a Chinese arrow poison), and heavy metals such as lead, copper, and antimony (Figure 1.1).

History has shown that it was not uncommon to retain the services of a poisoner to rid oneself of an inconvenient spouse or political rival or the services of a poison "taster" to ensure that the food and drink to be consumed would not result in one's own demise!

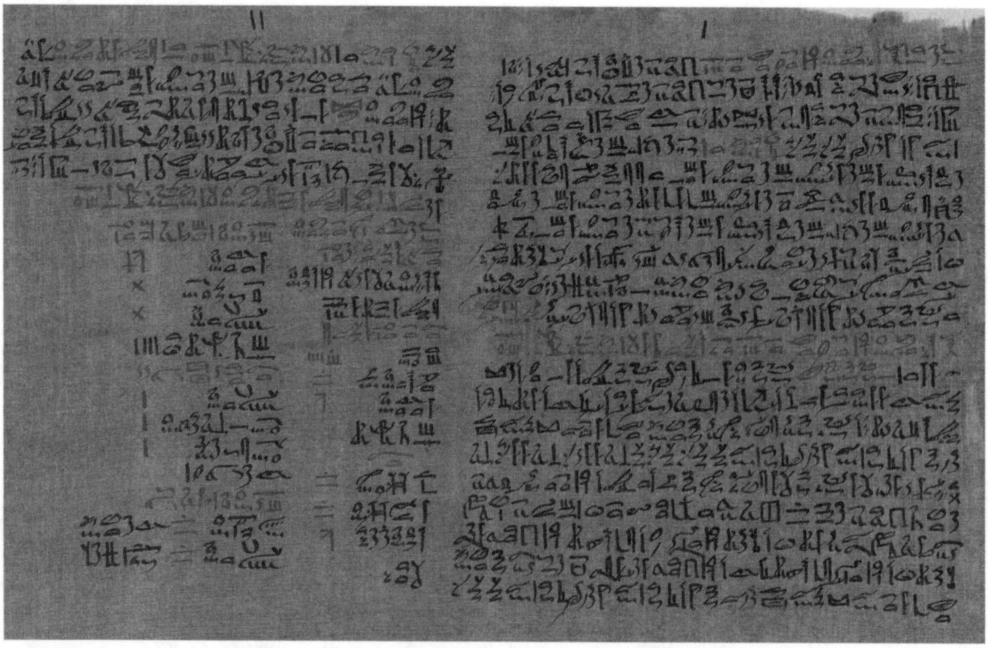

FIGURE 1.1    The Ebers Papyrus. Kol I-II. *Source:* Courtesy of the Leipzig University Library.

Fortunately, the science has expanded well beyond only the poisoner's perspective, although poisoning (whether intentional or accidental) still remains an important focus area for the modern specialties of clinical and forensic toxicology. As toxicology began to more fully develop, it shed the unsupported superstitions of the past. The use of more objective methodologies and experimentation to produce or challenge ideas or to question unsupported but long-held views about causality and nature became more firmly rooted as the best way to learn and advance the science.

Contributors to the developing discipline of toxicology are numerous. The physician Hippocrates (circa 400 B.C.) is credited with being one of the first physicians to apply basic pharmacology and toxicology principles to the practice of medicine, including concepts of bioavailability and overdose.

Several early toxicological treatises stand out as noteworthy. In his *De Historia Plantarum*, Theophrastus (371–287 B.C.) described numerous poisonous plants. Dioscorides (40–90 A.D.), a Greek pharmacist, physician, and botanist who served in the court of Roman emperor Nero, produced a pharmacopoeia to classify poisons according to their origin as animal, vegetable, or mineral. His *De Material Medica* is a five-volume systematic description of approximately 600 different plants and 1,000 different medications and has served as an important standard reference for almost 16 centuries. It is still considered a useful treatise even by today's standards.

The contributions of Moses ben Maimon, or Maimonides (1135–1204), to toxicology have survived through the years (Figure 1.2). He recognized that the bioavailability of many consumed toxins could be influenced by certain foods such as milk, butter, and cream, which appeared to impair their absorption. In addition to being a competent and well-respected physician, he was also a prolific writer. Of particular significance was his volume entitled *Poisons and Their Antidotes*, which was a guide to the treatment of accidental or intentional poisonings and animal bites. Maimonides recommended that suction be applied to insect stings or animal bites as a means of extracting the poison. He rejected numerous popular remedies of the day after testing them and finding them to be ineffective (e.g., the use of unleavened bread in the treatment of scorpion stings).

Philippus Aureolus Theophrastus Bombastus von Hohenheim (1493–1541) was a physician alchemist in the late Middle Ages who pioneered changes in the biomedical sciences. The importance of his contributions to the field cannot be underestimated; indeed, he changed his name later in life to Paracelsus (combining "para," or superior to, with Celsus) to reflect his own feeling that he should be regarded as superior to Aulus Cornelius Celsus, an early Roman physician. Paracelsus stated "What is there that is not poison? All things are poison and there is nothing without poison. Soley the dose determines that a thing is not a poison." Today, every student taking a first class in toxicology will hear his name and recognize the concept in one form or another, whether it is "The dose makes the poison," "All substances are poisons; there is none which is not

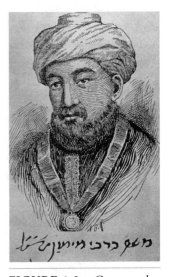

**FIGURE 1.2** Commonly used image indicating one artist's conception of Maimonides's appearance. *Source:* © National Library of Medicine.

a poison," or "The right dose differentiates a poison from a remedy." Although he was an alchemist by trade, Paracelsus advanced several principles that formed the basis of the modern dose–response relationship:

- Experimentation is essential in the examination of the response to chemicals.
- One should make the distinction between the therapeutic and toxic properties of a chemical.
- One can ascertain a degree of specificity of chemicals and their therapeutic or toxic effects.
- Therapeutic and toxic properties are sometimes only distinguishable by dose.

Paracelsus recognized, for example, that although mercury is a poison, it could also be used to treat syphilis. Paracelsus additionally wrote a treatise *"On the Miners' Sickness and Other Diseases of Miners,"* which appears to have been one of the first major works of occupational toxicology (Figure 1.3).

Toxicological specialties began to emerge in the 18th and 19th centuries. In 1700 Dr. Bernardino Ramazzini (1633–1714) published the first edition of his most famous book, the *De Morbis Artificum Diatriba* (*Diseases of Workers*), the first comprehensive work on occupational diseases outlining the health hazards of irritating chemicals, metals, dusts, and so forth that were encountered by workers in 52 occupations. This work became a standard reading in occupational medicine for the next 200 years.

As communities began to shift from more sparsely populated agricultural to more densely populated town-centered societies, the incidence of some diseases was more easily detected. Some diseases could be causally linked to specific occupations. As an example, a higher incidence of scrotal cancer in chimney sweeps was observed by Percival Pott (1714–1788), who recognized the relationship between the development of this disease through exposure to large amounts of soot and poor personal hygiene. Here we can see how perhaps a specific aspect of personal lifestyle in these individuals was an important contributing factor in the development of this disease. Had these workers better attended to their personal hygiene, advances in the area of chemical carcinogenesis may have been significantly delayed!

Mathieu Orfila (1787–1853), a Spanish physician serving in the French court during the 1800s, essentially established the discipline of forensic toxicology. He used chemical analysis and autopsy-related materials as proof of poisoning in legal proceedings. He developed a method for the analysis of arsenic that became the legal standard of the time. His book, *Traité des Poisons* (1814), went through several editions and is considered to be one of the most outstanding treatises in toxicology (Figure 1.4).

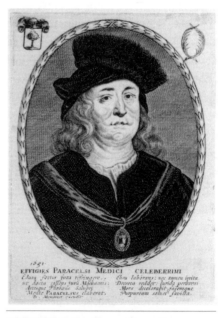

EFFIGIES PARACELSI MEDICI CELEBERRIMI

**FIGURE 1.3**   Paracelsus. *Source:* © National Library of Medicine.

The early history of toxicology, as previously mentioned, contains numerous references to intentional poisonings. The "execution" of Socrates (470–399 B.C.) by drinking hemlock is one of the best-known cases of suicide by poisoning, which was common practice in early Greek politics. Fear of being poisoned allegedly led Mithridates VI of Pontus (120–63 B.C.) to protect himself by consuming small doses of as many as 36 popular poisons of the day. As the story goes, his "self-inoculation" was apparently successful, because a later attempt at suicide by poisoning was completely ineffective and he was reduced to using a sword to accomplish his end. The term "mithridate" has been used to describe a concoction that possesses antidotal properties.

A contemporary of Paracelsus, Catherine de Medici (1519–1589), queen of France from 1547 to 1559, brought her poisoning skills from Italy to France where she practiced her trade by "treating" poor sick people with poisons, carefully evaluating their responses, the effectiveness of the dose, the parts of the body affected, and the signs and symptoms of her victims. She was quite the descriptive toxicologist, and one must wonder if she was familiar with some of the principles of Paracelsus.

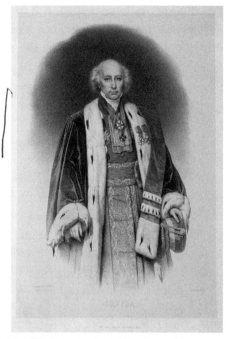

**FIGURE 1.4** Mathieu Joseph Bonaventure Orfila. *Source:* Courtesy of National Library of Medicine.

An Italian woman of the 17th century named Madame Giulia Toffana (1635–1719) developed a poisonous mixture and is reputed to have been responsible for greater than 500 killings. Her poisonous concoction containing arsenic was referred to as "Agua Toffana" ("the water of Toffana") or sometimes as "the Elixir of St. Nicholas of Bari," Bari being a town whose water was alleged to have healing properties. She sold it to individuals along with instructions concerning its proper use to get the job done. In 1719 she was executed in Naples; however, her "profession" was carried on by Heironyma Spara, a Roman contemporary who continued the training of young women in the art of how to murder their husbands by poisoning. She is said to have formed a local club of young wealthy married women, which soon became a club of eligible young wealthy widows. She was hanged along with other women, suspected to have been her aides.

In France, comparable activity was carried out by Catherine Deshayes (1638–1680), popularly known as La Voisin, who was also in the business of selling poisons to wives who wished to be rid of their husbands. The number of deaths that she may actually have been responsible for has been claimed to be in the thousands. She was burned at the stake in 1680.

Not all poisonings are intentional, and, indeed, a lack of knowledge concerning the toxicity of even commonly used substances may contribute to the development of health problems. The early Romans, as an example, boiled wines to make them sweeter and thicker. Unfortunately, the pots that they used were made from copper and lead. The early Roman body burden of lead may have been higher in the more affluent Romans who had the financial means to obtain as much wine as their social and political position demanded. Today, of course, we all recognize the association between the body's accumulation of lead and the neurotoxicity that it can produce and even may be tempted, as have others, to speculate on the role that lead may have played in the decline of ancient Rome.

The development of toxicology as a science has been, like most other disciplines, a long process of slow and steady growth from the work and deeds of the good and the not-so-good as referenced above. A growth spurt in its development has occurred over the past century that has been remarkable and stimulated by the widespread use of dangerous "patent remedies," environmental pollution, adulteration of foods, occupational injuries, consumer illness, surge of pesticide use, and chemical production, just to name a few. The confluence of public concern, legislative action, and research has produced a flurry of legislation, journals, professional organizations, and regulatory agencies.

The first professional organization for toxicologists, the Society of Toxicology, held its first formal meeting on April 15, 1962 in Atlantic City, New Jersey. The official journal of the Society, *Toxicology and Applied Pharmacology*, was probably the first dedicated publication for the dissemination of toxicology research. Today, toxicology is well rooted with numerous professional organizations, journals, and thousands of toxicologists internationally. The International Congress of Toxicology, composed of toxicology societies from the United States, Europe, Africa, Asia, South America, and Australia, provides an international forum through its meetings and publications to bring toxicologists together from all over the world.

## Bibliography

*History of toxicology*. (Undated). Retrieved May 2005 from http://courses.tox.ncsu.edu/tox401demo/Tutor/Content/history_toxicology.htm.

Klaassen, C. D. (2001). *Casarett & Doull's toxicology. The basic science of poisons*. New York: McGraw-Hill.

Klaassen, C. D., & Watkins, J. B. (2003). *Casarett & Doull's essentials of toxicology*. New York: McGraw-Hill.

National Toxicology Program. (Undated). Retrieved May 2005 from http://ntp-server.niehs.nih.gov/.

U.S. National Library of Medicine, National Institutes of Health, Environmental Health and Toxicology Specialized Information Services (SIS). (2005). *Toxicology tutorial I*. Retrieved May 2005 from http://www.sis.nlm.nih.gov/enviro/toxtutor.html.

# Chemical Properties and Information Resources on Hazardous Chemicals

## Elements, Atoms, and Compounds

All matter, whether a solid, liquid, or gas, is made up of *elements*. Thus far we have identified approximately 115 different elements. Many of these are familiar to us (e.g., aluminum, iron, lead, sulfur, carbon, silicon), whereas many others may not be (e.g., rhenium, thulium, terbium). An atom is the smallest unit of an element that retains the properties of that element. When an atom of one element chemically combines with atoms of the same element, a *molecule* is formed during this chemical reaction. When the atoms of different elements combine during a chemical reaction, a *compound* is formed. Our bodies are made up of elements that form inorganic and organic compounds. Of the greater than 90 naturally occurring elements, approximately 99% of our body weight is made up of compounds containing the elements carbon, hydrogen, nitrogen, oxygen, calcium, phosphorus, and sulfur. Simple inorganic compounds such as water and sodium chloride contribute to the larger portion of the mass of our bodies when compared with organic compounds, which are of much greater molecular weight than inorganic compounds. We are all familiar with many of the important compounds that make up the body (Figure 2.1).

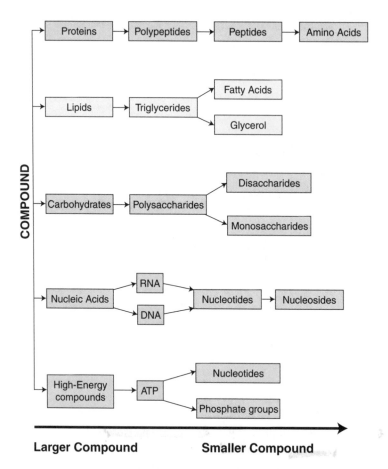

**FIGURE 2.1**    Important compounds of the body. *Source:* Courtesy of the Toxicology and Environmental Health Information Program of the National Library of Medicine, U.S. Department of Health and Human Services.

There are also millions of chemical compounds that have no physiological role in the body. There are greater than 6 million different chemical compounds that are known, with about 80,000 that are in common industrial and household use. Many thousands of new organic chemicals are synthesized yearly. With just carbon, nitrogen, hydrogen, oxygen, and sulfur, for example, numerous compounds can be formed, including some aromatic (=ring form) ones of toxicological importance (Figure 2.2).

## Mixtures, Suspensions, and Aerosols

The term *mixture* refers to any substance that contains more than one chemical compound or ~~e~~lement that has retained its individual properties. A mixture of alcohols, for example, may con- ~~~~ ethanol, isopropanol, and butanol all "mixed" together, giving the appearance of a single ~~~~ce. Each of the three components of this mixture is a *pure substance*, and each can be

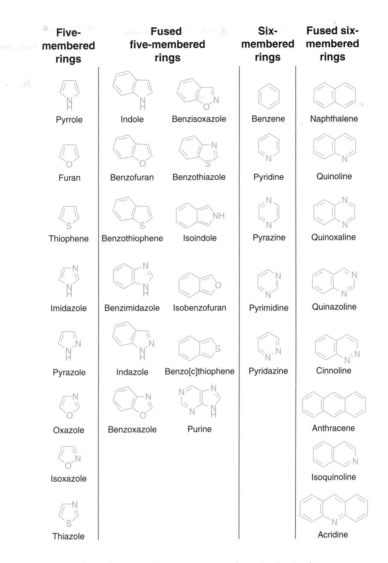

**FIGURE 2.2**    Examples of aromatic structures of toxicological importance.

individually recovered from the mixture using appropriate methods. The term *suspension* refers to a mixture of liquid and small solid substances, whereas an aerosol (mist) is a mixture of tiny droplets of a liquid or tiny particles of a solid in a gas.

## Identifying Chemicals

Chemicals have common names, trade names, technical names, and chemical formulas associated with them, which can often be confusing. Manufacturers frequently choose commercial names for their products. This is done for obvious marketing purposes because it is easier to remember a product by a simple trade name than a complex chemical name. The chemical formula uses the appropriate abbreviations for the elements that are contained in the molecules of the chemical question, for example, sodium = Na, hydrogen = H, carbon = C, and oxygen = O. What I refer to as bicarbonate of soda may be called sodium bicarbonate by another person or sodium hydrogen carbonate by a third. We are all referring, however, to a substance that contains these four elements that are chemically combined into a compound containing the chemical formula $NaHCO_3$. In this example, one atom each of sodium, hydrogen, and carbon and three atoms of oxygen combine to produce the compound. The chemical formula, however, may not be enough to indicate what the actual chemical is because several chemicals may share the same formula. Although the chemical formula tells us how many atoms of each element are contained within a compound, it does not specify the arrangement of these atoms. Different arrangements of the same types and numbers of atoms result in different compounds. Each compound, as we will see below, is identified by a different Chemical Abstracts Service (CAS) registry number. For example, $C_6H_8O_3$ is a formula that is shared by several different chemicals as shown in Figure 2.3.

The chemical structure is therefore important because it shows the arrangement of atoms within a compound, allowing us to identify the compound. The chemical structure is vitally important because it can provide important clues about the potential health effects from exposure to that chemical. Organic chemicals contain functional groups that can often indicate the type of toxicity one could predict from their exposure. Examples of common functional groups in toxicants are shown in Table 2.1.

- 2,3-Dihydro-4-hydroxy-2,5-dimethyl-3-furanone
  (CAS Registry Number: 3658-77-3)

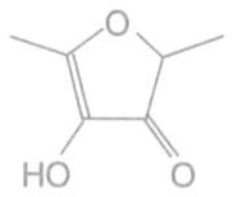

- 2-Propenoic acid, oxiranylmethyl ester
  (CAS Registry Number: 106-90-1)

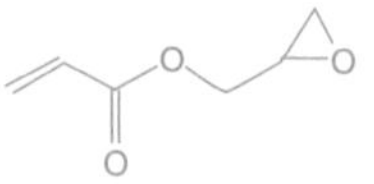

- 3-Methylglutaric anhydride
  (CAS Registry Number: 4166-53-4 )

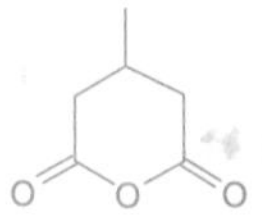

- 7-Oxy-6, 8-dioxabicyclo-(3,2,1) - octane
  (CAS Registry Number: 5257-20-5)

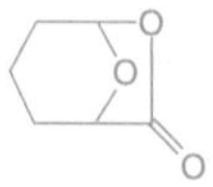

.ions of the formula $C_6H_8O_3$.

**Table 2.1    Common Functional Groups\***

| Functional Group | General Formula | Suffix/Examples |
|---|---|---|
| Hydroxyl | R–OH<br>Carbon–oxygen bond | -ol<br>(e.g., methanol, ethanol, propanol) |
| Methyl | R–CH$_3$<br>Carbon–carbon single bond | -ane<br>Methane (CH$_4$)<br>Ethane (C$_2$H$_6$)<br>Propane (C$_3$H$_8$)<br>Butane (C$_4$H$_{10}$) |
| Alkene | R–CH=CH–R' | -ene<br>Ethene (C$_2$H$_4$)<br>Propene (C$_3$H$_6$) |
| Alkyne | R–C≡C–R' | -yne<br>Ethyne (C$_2$H$_2$)<br>Propyne (C$_3$H$_4$)<br>Butyne (C$_4$H$_6$) |
| Amide | R–C(=O)N(–H)–R' | Ethanamide (CH$_3$CONH$_2$) |
| Primary amine | R–NH$_2$ | -amine<br>Ethylamine (C$_2$H$_5$NH$_2$)<br>Diethylamine (C$_2$H$_5$)$_2$NH<br>Triethylamine (C$_2$H$_5$)$_3$N |
| Secondary amine | R–N(–H)–R' | -amine<br>Dimethylamine (C$_2$H$_6$NH)<br>Diethylamine (C$_4$H$_{10}$NH) |
| Tertiary amine | R–N(–R')–R | -amine<br>Trimethylamine (CH$_3$)$_3$N |
| Azo | R–N=N–R' | Diazoacetamide |
| Nitrile | R–C≡N | Ethanenitrile (C$_2$H$_5$CN) |
| Pyridyl | R–C$_5$H$_4$N | |
| Carboxyl | R–C(=O)OH<br>*Non-ionized*<br>R–C(=O)O$^-$<br>*ionized* | -oic acid<br>Formic acid (CHCOOH)<br>Acetic acid (CCH$_3$COOH) |
| Aldehyde | R–C(=O)H | -al<br>(ethanal: CH$_3$CHO) |
| Ketone | R–C(=O)–R' | -one<br>Propanone (CH$_3$COCH$_3$) |
| Primary imine | R–C(=NH)–R' | -imine<br>*N*-methylimine |
| Secondary imine | R–C(–H)=N–R' | -imine |
| Ether | R–O–R' | Ethyl ether<br>CH$_3$OCH$_3$ |

(continue

**Table 2.1    Common Functional Groups (continued)**

| Functional Group | General Formula | Suffix/Examples |
|---|---|---|
| Ester | R–C(=O)O–R' | Ethyl acetate $CH_3OOCH_3$ |
| Halogen | F, Cl, Br, etc. Carbon–halogen bonding | Chloromethane ($CH_3Cl$) Iodobutane ($C_4H_9I$) |
| Isocyanate | R–N=C=O | Methyl isocyanate $CH_3NCO$ |
| Isothiocyanate | R–N=C=S | Methyl isothiocyanate $NCH_3S$ |
| Phenyl | R–$C_6H_5$ | Phenylethane (=ethylbenzene) $CH_3C_6H_5$ |
| Benzyl | R–$CH_2$–$C_6H_5$ | Benzyl acetate $C_9H_{10}O_2$ |
| Phosphodiester | R–OP(=O)$_2$O–R' | Nucleic acids |
| Sulfhydryl | R–SH | -thiol Methanethiol (= methyl mercaptan) $CH_3SH$ |
| Thioether | R–S–R' | Ethylthioether (=diethylsulfide) $CH_3SCH_3$ |

*R and R' can denote any group of atoms.

## Assigning Identification

Perhaps the best way to identify a chemical is by its CAS registry number. This is similar to the way a social security number identifies individuals as uniquely different. The CAS number does not provide information concerning the properties of the chemical. The use of the number is important in overcoming any confusion about the identity of the chemical due to multiple common, trade, and technical names. Use of the CAS number is observed in scientific literature and product information, including material safety data sheets. Another way that chemicals can be identified is through the Registry of Toxic Effects of Chemical Substances, or RTECS, number. This registry, operated by the National Institute for Occupational Safety and Health (NIOSH), contains technical information about commonly industrial chemicals. There are other systems that are in use for numbering and classifying, including the IUPAC (International Union for Pure and Applied Chemistry), (the European Community), and UN numbers, or UN IDs, which are four-identify hazardous substances and products (such as poisonous materials commercial importance. This numbering scheme is widely used in international commerce, for instance to label the contents of shipping containers for transportation of hazardous substances.

# Physical Properties of Chemicals

## Water Solubility

Water solubility is defined as the weight (generally in grams or milligrams) of a substance that can be completely dissolved in 1 liter of water to form a solution. The solubility in water may give some idea of what maximum concentrations might occur in water, whether we are referring to the body water of an organism or to an environmental body of water such as a lake.

## pH

A pH refers to how acid or basic (caustic) a substance is. A pH of 7 is considered neutral, whereas numbers below 7 are on the acid side of chemical neutrality and numbers above 7 are on the basic side. A pH of 1 is a very strong acid and a pH of 13 is very caustic.

## Relative Molecular Mass

This refers to the relative weight of a molecule of a chemical compared with the relative weight of an atom of the lightest element, hydrogen.

## Octanol-to-Water Partition Coefficient

This ratio indicates how readily any chemical dissolves in a fatty or oily medium compared with water. A very water-soluble chemical has a greater affinity for water than for octanol; thus it would have a low partition coefficient. A pesticide with the partition coefficient of 7, for example, indicates that it is much more lipophilic (fat loving) and thus accumulates in body fat where it may be stored for a relatively long time. The octanol-to-water partition coefficient is therefore an indicator of bioaccumulation. Chemicals that have relatively high octanol-to-water partition coefficients are usually absorbed quickly through the skin and enter into the blood.

## Boiling Point, Melting Point, and Vapor Pressure

The boiling point is the temperature at which the chemical changes from a liquid state to the gaseous state. The melting point of the chemical is the temperature at which there is a change from a solid to a liquid. The vapor pressure is the pressure at which the chemical in the liquid or solid state turns into the gaseous state even at temperatures below the boiling point. Chemicals with a high vapor pressure tend to "evaporate" more readily than others with a low vapor pressure and are therefore of more concern with respect to respiratory exposure.

## Flash Point

The flash point is the temperature at which a substance gives off enough vapor in the air to form an ignitable mixture. The lower the flash point, the greater the risk for explosion and fire.

## Autoignition Temperature and Flammability

The autoignition temperature is that temperature at which a substance spontaneously burns, that is, catches fire in the absence of a flame or a spark. A flammable material can be a solid, liquid, or gas. Something that is not flammable is not given the term *inflammable*. Inflammable is an older term for flammable and to avoid confusion should not be used.

## Flammability (Explosive) Limits

This represents a range of concentrations for a flammable vapor or gas in air at which an explosion may occur in the presence of a flame or spark. The lower explosive limit (LEL)is a level below which there is not enough chemical present to burn (i.e., the mixture is too lean). The upper explosive limit (UEL) is a level above which there is too much chemical to burn (i.e., the mixture is too rich).

## Relative Density or Specific Gravity

This is commonly defined as the weight of a specific volume of a liquid or solid chemical substance compared with the weight of the same volume of water. More correctly, specific gravity is the ratio of the density of a material to the density of water. The density of water is approximately 1 gram per cubic centimeter. Substances with a specific gravity of less than 1 are lighter than water and therefore float, whereas those that have specific gravities exceeding 1 are heavier than water and thus sink. Knowing the specific gravity is important for planning spill cleanup and fire-fighting procedures.

## Relative Vapor Density

The relative vapor density refers to the weight of a specific volume of a chemical substance in the gaseous state compared with the weight of the same volume of air. From exposure viewpoint, if the relative vapor density is less than 1, the gas collects at the ceiling level indoors or disperses into the atmosphere outdoors. On the other hand, if the gas is heavier than air (that is, it has a relative vapor density of a gas greater than 1), then the gas tends to collect at floor level indoors or in depressions outside. The possibility exists that gases having relative vapor densities greater than 1 may displace air in the breathing zone of confined spaces, thus leading to asphyxiation.

## Odor Threshold

Some chemicals when present in the air can be smelled, and this can serve as a warning. The *odor threshold* represents the smallest concentration of the chemical in the air that can be smelled and is usually expressed in parts per million or parts per billion. Some odor thresholds are sufficiently low enough to provide adequate warning properties (e.g., sulfur dioxide), but others are not. It is important to realize, however, that many chemicals have no smell associated with them and thus there are no warning properties associated with odor. Other important physical properties include the boiling point, vapor pressure, and melting point.

# Appendix
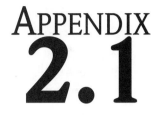

## 2.1

## Some Web-Based Resources

A vast amount of information about chemicals and their hazardous properties can be found on the WorldWideWeb. Information ranging from adverse reactions to clinical drugs to the physical chemical properties of industrial chemicals may be accessed with relative ease. Examples of these types of resources are provided as examples. Websites do change from time to time; however, at the time of this writing the websites as provided were current.

- **Adverse Reactions to Drug Reports:** Reports that are voluntarily submitted by physicians to the U.S. Food and Drug Administration (FDA) after a drug has been approved and in use. Adverse reactions to drugs in clinical trials are subject to mandatory report.

  http://www.fda.gov/medwatch/report/hcp.htm

- **Agency for Toxic Substances and Disease Registry (ATSDR):** The principal federal public health agency involved with hazardous waste issues. ATSDR helps to prevent or reduce the harmful effects of exposure to hazardous substances on human health. Information about ATSDR, a database containing all information where ATSDR has worked, fact sheets on 60 of the most common contaminants at Superfund sites, and links to related sites.

  http://www.atsdr.cdc.gov/

- **American Association of Poison Control Centers:** Brochures on preventing poisonings in the home, emergency action cards for poisoning, poisoning fact sheets, lists of Poison Centers, and so forth.

  http://www.aapcc.org

- **American College of Medical Toxicology:** Professional nonprofit association of physicians with recognized expertise in medical toxicology. Their mission is to ensure that patients exposed to poisons and toxic substances receive optimal care by direct contact with qualified medical toxicologists. Their publication, *Internet Journal of Medical Toxicology,* can be accessed from this site.

  http://www.acmt.net/main/

- **Carcinogenic Potency Project:** The Carcinogenic Potency Database (CPDB) covers results of long-term animal cancer tests.

  http://potency.berkeley.edu/cpdb.html

- **Centers for Disease Control and Prevention (CDC):** The CDC is one of the 13 major operating components of the Department of Health and Human Services (HHS), which is the principal agency in the U.S. government for protecting the health and safety of all Americans.

  http://www.cdc.gov/

- **ChemFinder:** A chemical database that provides basic chemical data, including CAS numbers, and also provides other information, including physical property data and two-dimensional chemical structures. It is the largest single list of chemical information sites. Individual access to ChemFinder is complimentary on a limited basis. Access by corporations, academic institutions, and government organizations is granted on an enterprise subscription basis.

  http://chemfinder.cambridgesoft.com/

- **Chemical Carcinogenesis Research Information System (CCRIS):** Carcinogenicity and mutagenicity test results for over 8,000 chemicals.

  http://toxnet.nlm.nih.gov/cgi-bin/sis/htmlgen?CCRIS

- **ClinicalTrials:** ClinicalTrials.gov provides regularly updated information about federally and privately supported clinical research in human volunteers.

  http://www.clinicaltrials.gov/

- **Developmental & Reproductive Toxicology (DART/ETIC):** References to developmental and reproductive toxicology literature.

  http://toxnet.nlm.nih.gov/cgi-bin/sis/htmlgen?DARTETIC

- **Environmental Protection Agency (EPA):** The mission of the EPA is to protect human health and the environment.

  http://www.epa.gov/

- **EXTOXNET:** Extension Toxicology Network. Information about pesticides and other toxicology issues from the consortium formed by University of California, Davis, Oregon State University, Michigan State University, Cornell University, and the University of Idaho.

  http://extoxnet.orst.edu/

- **Extremely Hazardous Substances (EHS):** Chemical profiles and emergency first aid guides.

  http://yosemite.epa.gov/oswer/ceppoehs.nsf/EHS_Profile?openform

- **Food and Drug Administration (FDA):** The FDA is responsible for protecting the public health by ensuring the safety, efficacy, and security of human and veterinary drugs, biological products, medical devices, our nation's food supply, cosmetics, and products that emit radiation.

  http://www.fda.gov/

- **Genetic Toxicology (Mutagenicity) (GENE-TOX):** Peer-reviewed genetic toxicology test data for over 3,000 chemicals.

  http://toxnet.nlm.nih.gov/cgi-bin/sis/htmlgen?GENETOX

- **Hazardous Materials:** U.S. Fire Administration. Guide for first responders.

  http://www.usfa.fema.gov/subjects/hazmat/

- **Hazardous Substances Data Bank (HSDB):** Comprehensive peer-reviewed toxicology data for about 5,000 chemicals.

  http://toxnet.nlm.nih.gov/cgi-bin/sis/htmlgen?HSDB

- **Integrated Risk Information System (IRIS):** Hazard identification and dose–response assessments for over 500 chemicals.

  http://toxnet.nlm.nih.gov/cgi-bin/sis/htmlgen?IRIS

- **Healthy People 2010:** Healthy People 2010 challenges individuals, communities, and professionals—indeed, all of us—to take specific steps to ensure that good health, as well as long life, are enjoyed by all.

  http://www.health.gov/healthypeople

- **International Toxicity Estimates for Risk (ITER):** Risk information for over 600 chemicals from authoritative groups worldwide.

  http://toxnet.nlm.nih.gov/cgi-bin/sis/htmlgen?iter

- **The Library of the Karolinska Institute of Sweden:** Collection of links to causes of poisoning, including food poisoning, bites and stings, drug toxicities, and lead poisoning.

  http://www.mic.ki.se/Diseases/C21.613.html

- **Material Safety Data Sheets Online**

  http://www.ilpi.com/msds/index.html

- **MEDLINEplus:** Comprehensive medical information and literature searches.

  http://medlineplus.gov

- **National Institute of Environmental Health Sciences (NIEHS):** Focuses on basic science, disease-oriented research, global environmental health, and multidisciplinary training for researchers.

  http://www.niehs.nih.gov/

- **National Institutes of Health (NIH):** The NIH, a part of the U.S. Department of Health and Human Services, is the primary federal agency for conducting and supporting medical research.

  http://www.nih.gov/

- **National Institute for Occupational Safety and Health (NIOSH):** NIOSH is the federal agency responsible for conducting research and making recommendations for the prevention of work-related injury and illness. NIOSH is part of the Centers for Disease Control and Prevention in the Department of Health and Human Services.

  http://www.cdc.gov/niosh/homepage.html

- **National Report on Human Exposure to Environmental Chemicals:** The Second Report, released in January 2003, presents biomonitoring exposure data for 116 environmental chemicals for U.S. population over the 2-year period 1999–2000.

  http://www.cdc.gov/exposurereport/

- **National Toxicology Program:** An interagency program to coordinate toxicological testing, strengthen the science base in toxicology, develop and validate improved testing methods, and provide information about potentially toxic chemicals to health regulatory and research agencies, the scientific and medical communities, and the public.

  http://ntp-server.niehs.nih.gov/

- **Occupational Safety and Health Administration (OSHA):** OSHA's mission is to ensure the safety and health of America's workers by setting and enforcing standards; providing training, outreach, and education; establishing partnerships; and encouraging continual improvement in workplace safety and health.

  http://www.osha.gov/

- **Poisonous Plants Informational Database:** Includes plant images, botany, chemistry, toxicology, diagnosis, and prevention of poisoning of animals.

  http://www.ansci.cornell.edu/plants/

- **Recognition and Management of Pesticide Poisonings:** Presented by The National Pesticide Telecommunications Network, 5th edition (1999).

  http://npic.orst.edu/rmpp.htm

- **Right to Know Hazardous Substance Fact Sheets:** New Jersey Department of Health & Senior Services, Division of Epidemiology, Environmental and Occupational Health. Available in English and Spanish.

  http://www.state.nj.us/health/eoh/rtkweb/rtkhsfs.htm

- **Toxicon Multimedia Project:** Medical Toxicology Consortium Including Cook County Hospital, The University of Illinois Hospital, and RUSH Medical Center, Chicago, Illinois. Includes Virtual Toxicology Cases and Virtual Toxicology Lectures.

  http://www.uic.edu/com/er/toxikon/

- **TOXLINE:** Biochemical, pharmacological, physiological, and toxicological effects of drugs and other chemicals: References from toxicology literature.

  http://toxnet.nlm.nih.gov/cgi-bin/sis/htmlgen?TOXLINE

- **Toxics Release Inventory (TRI):** Annual environmental releases of over 600 toxic chemicals by U.S. facilities.

  http://toxnet.nlm.nih.gov/cgi-bin/sis/htmlgen?TRI

- **U.S. Department of Agriculture (USDA):** The USDA's mission is to enhance the quality of life for the American people by supporting the production of agriculture.

  http://www.usda.gov/

- **World Health Organization (WHO):** WHO's objective, as set out in its Constitution, is the attainment by all peoples of the highest possible level of health. Health is defined in WHO's Constitution as a state of complete physical, mental, and social well-being and not merely the absence of disease or infirmity.

  http://www.who.int

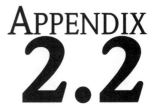

# APPENDIX
# 2.2

## Regulatory Agencies That Maintain Lists for Hazardous Chemicals

Some regulatory agencies maintain lists of environmental and industrial chemicals that are deemed to be hazardous. In addition, technical reports are available from many of these agencies. The following table is compilation of a number of agencies that maintain such lists with contact information, and websites current at the time of this writing.

| Controlling Regulatory Entity | List Name | List Producer and Contact Information | Reference | List Description |
|---|---|---|---|---|
| Canada | Domestic Substances List of Canada | nsn-infoline@ec.gc.ca Notification and Client Services Division New Substances Branch Risk Assessment Directorate Environment Canada Place Vincent Massey, 14th Floor Gatineau QC K1A 0H3 Telephone: (800) 567-1999 (Toll Free in Canada) (819) 953-7156 (Outside of Canada) Facsimile: (819) 953-7155 | http://www.ec.gc.ca/substances/nsb/download/DSL.PDF The final list was developed in several stages: a Core List, a Provisional List, and a Final List in 1994. | Mandated by the Canadian Environmental Protection Act (CEPA), this list covers substances manufactured or imported into Canada for industrial use. |
| | Workplace Hazardous Materials Information System (WHMIS): Ingredient Disclosure List, Canada | Canadian Product Safety Branch, Consumer and Corporate Affairs 50 Victoria St. Hull Quebec OC9, Canada. (819) 953-4763 | Canadian Workplace Hazardous Material Information System. Canada Gazette Part II, 122(2) (1 Jan 1988). http://www.hc-sc.gc.ca/hecs-sesc/whmis/application.htm | A list of chemicals that must be identified on Canadian Material Safety Data Sheets if they are included in products that fall within the Workplace Hazardous Material Information System (WHMIS) hazard criteria specified in the Controlled Products Regulations of Canada. |

*(continues)*

| Controlling Regulatory Entity | List Name | List Producer and Contact Information | Reference | List Description |
|---|---|---|---|---|
| European Union | European Inventory of Existing Commercial Chemical Substances | The European Commission http://europa.eu.int/<br><br>Office for Official Publications of the European Communities, 2 rue Mercier, L-2985 Luxembourg; Telephone: 011-352-49928 425 66 or 011-352-488-573<br><br>North America: European Union Delegation of the European Commission, Attn: Public Affairs, 2300 M Street N.W., Washington, D.C. 20036 1-202-862-9539 1-202-429-1766 (fax) | Official Journal of the European Communities, June 1990. http://stneasy.cas. org/dbss/chemlist/ einecs.html | EINECS is the European counterpart of TSCAINV. It lists chemical substances that were reported by the Member States to the European Commission as existing on the European Community Market between January 1, 1971 and September 18, 1991. |
| | European Inventory of Existing Commercial Chemical Substances Supplement (Elincs) | The European Commission. http://europa.eu.int/<br><br>Office for Official Publications of the European Communities, 2 rue Mercier, L-2985 Luxembourg; Telephone: 011-352-49928 425 66 or 011-352-488-573<br><br>North America: European Union Delegation of the European Commission, Attn: Public Affairs, 2300 M Street NW, Washington, D.C. 20036 1-202-862-9539 1-202-429-1766 (fax) | Official Journal of the European Communities, Dec 17, 1994. http://europa.eu. int/eur-lex/en/ com/cnc/2003/ com2003_ 0642en01.pdf | Elincs supplements EINECS and these two include all substances placed on the community market before August 15, 1993. |
| World Health Organization | International Agency for Research on Cancer List | International Agency for Research on Cancer, World Health Organization, Lyon, France | IARC Monographs http://www.IARC.fr/ | Substances that have been evaluated by the International Agency for Research on Cancer (IARC) for carcinogenic risk to humans and animals. |

| Controlling Regulatory Entity | List Name | List Producer and Contact Information | Reference | List Description |
|---|---|---|---|---|
| World Health Organization (continued) | | For publications, call (518) 436-9686, or write to WHO Publication, Centre USA, 49 Sheriden Avenue, Albany, NY 12210 | | These evaluations are recognized as authoritative sources of information on the carcinogenicity of chemicals. |
| International Maritime Association | Marine Pollutants List | International Maritime Organization, 4 Albert Embankment, London SE1 7SR, United Kingdom Tel +44 (0)20 7735 7611 Fax +44 (0)20 7587 3210 National Response Center, RM 2611, 2100 Second Street SW, Washington, DC 20593 | CFR 49,172.101, App. B, 1995; http://www.myregs.com/dotrspa/ | A list of substances, materials, and articles identified as marine pollutants or severe marine pollutants in the International Maritime Dangerous Goods (IMDG) code and of the not otherwise specified (n.o.s.) and generic entries to be used to offer marine pollutants for shipment. |
| U.S. Environmental Protection Agency | Hazardous Air Pollutants | EPA: (202) 272-0167 200 Pennsylvania Ave NW, Washington, DC 20640 Clean Air Docket, EPA Library, Research Triangle Park, 109 T.W. Alexander Drive, Durham, NC 27711 (919) 541-2777 | Section 112 (b)(1) Hazardous Air Pollutants Section (b)(1) of the Clean Air Act (CAA) http://www.epa.gov/ttn/atw/188polls.html | The Clean Air Act Amendment of 990, Title 3 established this initial list of 189 hazardous pollutants. |
| | Ozone Depletion Chemicals List | Stratospheric Protection Information Hotline at 1-800-296-1996. (202-343-9210 from outside the U.S.) U.S. EPA Mail Code 6205J, 1200 Pennsylvania Avenue NW, Washington, DC 20460-0001 (202) 343-9410 | CRF 40,82, Subpt A. App A and B, 1996. http://www.epa.gov/ozone/ods.html | A list of controlled substances in Sections 602–607 and 616 of the Clear Air Act imposing limits on the production and consumption of certain ozone-depleting substances. |

*(continues)*

| Controlling Regulatory Entity | List Name | List Producer and Contact Information | Reference | List Description |
|---|---|---|---|---|
| | EPA Pesticide List | U.S. EPA Chemical Support Group, Office of Pesticide Programs, Ariel Rios Building, 1200 Pennsylvania Avenue NW, Washington, DC 20460 (703) 305-7090 | 1) Federal Register 54(204), 4388, 1989 (Oct 24). 2) Federal Register 54(34), 7740, 1989 (Feb 22). 3) Federal Register 54(100), 22706, 1989 (May 25). 4) Federal Register 54(140), 30848, 1989 (Jul 24). 5) Federal Register 55(147), 31164, 1990 (Jul 31). http://www4.law. cornell.edu/uscode/ html/uscode07/usc_ sup_01_7_10_6.html | The list contains those chemical substances (active ingredients) for which pesticide Registration Standards have been issued and those subject to reregistration under the Federal Insecticide, Fungicide, and Rodenticide Act (FIFRA). |
| | EPA High Production Volume Chemical List | U.S. Environmental Protection Agency, P.O. Box 1473, Merrifield, VA 22116 Attention: Chemical Right-to-Know Program (202) 564-4770 | http://www.epa.gov/ opptintr/chemrtk/ hpvcolst.htm | Non-Confidential Information Submitted by Companies on Chemicals Under the 1990, 1994, and 1998 Inventory Update Rule (IUR). |
| | List of Pesticide Product Inert Ingredients | Office of Prevention, Pesticide and Toxic Substances U.S. EPA, 401 M Street SW, Washington, DC 20460. Public Response and Program Resources Branch at (703) 305-5805 | List of Pesticide Product Inert Ingredients (May, 1995). http://www.epa.gov/ opprd001/inerts/ inerts_list4.pdf | Pesticide product inert ingredients |
| | Master Testing List (MTL) | Office of Pollution Prevention and Toxic Substances, U.S. Environmental Protection Agency, Washington, DC 20460. TSCA Hotline at (202) 554-1404 TSCA-Hotline @epamail.epa.gov EPA website: http:www.epa.gov/opptintr /main/ctibhome.htm | Publication of the EPA office of Pollution Prevention and Toxics, and Office of Prevention, Pesticides, and Toxic Substances, Washington, DC, December 1, 1996. http://www.epa.gov/ opptintr/chemtest/ mtl.htm | A listing from the EPA Office of Pollution Prevention and Toxics' (OPPT) existing chemical testing priorities, as well as those of other EPA program offices, other federal agencies, the TSCA Inter- agency Testing com- mittee, and interna- tional organizations. |

| Controlling Regulatory Entity | List Name | List Producer and Contact Information | Reference | List Description |
|---|---|---|---|---|
| | CERCLA Hazardous Substances Table 302.4 | U.S. Environmental Protection Agency, 401 M Street SW, Washington, DC 20460 (703) 412-9810 | CFR 40,302.4,1996. http://www.epa.gov/ NCEI/plainlanguage/ documents/epcra.pdf | The Comprehensive Environmental Response, Compensation, and Liability Act (CERCLA) hazardous substances as defined by the Clean Water Act Sections 311 and 307(a); RCRA Section 3001; Clean Air Act, Section 112; and TSCA Section 7. |
| | Superfund Amendments and Reauthorization Act (SARA) of 1986, Section 110, ATSDR/EPA Priority List | The Agency for Toxic Substances and Disease Registry (ATSDR) in conjunction with EPA ATSDR Division of Toxicology, 1600 Clifton Road NE, Mailstop F-32, Atlanta, GA 30333 Phone: 1-888-42-ATSDR (1-888-422-8737) FAX: (770)-488-4178 Email: ATSDRIC@cdc.gov | http://www. atsdr.cdc.gov/ clist.html | The ATSDR Profile Priority List (APPL) ranks the 275 substances of the highest concern at National Priority List (NPL) waste sites from a public health perspective, as per SARA Section 110 and CERCLA Section 104(i)(2)(A), as amended, and likelihood of human exposure, with lowest rank (1) highest priority. Comprehensive reviews of health effect information, available from ATSDR and NTIS. |
| | Superfund Amendments and Reauthorization Act (SARA) of 1986, Section 302, Extremely Hazardous Substances List | Chemical Emergency Preparedness and Prevention RCRA, Superfund, and EPCRA Call Center (800) 424-9346 Toll Free (703) 412-9810 - Metropolitan DC area and international calls | CFR 40,355 App. A, 1996 http://yosemite. epa.gov/oswer/ ceppoehs.nsf/ Alphabetical_ Results?openview d | The list of extremely hazardous substances subject to reporting requirements under Title III of SARA, when stored in amount in excess of a Threshold Planning Quantity (TPQ). |

*(continues)*

| Controlling Regulatory Entity | List Name | List Producer and Contact Information | Reference | List Description |
|---|---|---|---|---|
| | Toxic Chemical Release Inventory | U.S. Environmental Protection Agency Emergency Planning and Community Right To Know Information Hotline, (1-800) 535-0202 | http://www.epa.gov/tri/ | A list of toxic chemicals whose emissions or releases are subject to annual reporting under Title III of SARA. |
| | Toxic Substances Control Act Chemical Substances Inventory | U.S. Environmental Protection Agency, Office of Toxic Substances, Washington, DC 20460 (202) 554-1404 | Toxic Substances Chemical Substance Inventory. http://www.epa.gov/opptintr/newchems/invntory.htm | Existing commercial chemical substances in the U.S. From a regulatory perspective, substances that are not found in the Inventory are considered "new" by EPA and therefore are subject to the Premanufacture Notification requirements of TSCA. The Inventory is not intended to cover all commercial chemical substances. Certain substances such as drugs and pesticides that are regulated by other laws are explicitly excluded. |
| U.S. Department of Transportation (DOT) | DOT Coast Guard Bulk Hazardous Materials | Coast Guard, U.S. DOT Coast Guard Headquarters, Hazardous Materials Branch, 2100 Second Street SW Washington, DC 20593-0001 (202) 267-1577 | CFR 46,150, Table I,1995; CFR 46,30.25, 1995. http://www.access.gpo.gov/nara/cfr/waisidx_01/46cfr30_01.html | Flammable and combustible bulk liquid materials regulated by the Coast Guard. |
| | DOT Coast Guard Noxious Liquid Substances | Coast Guard, U.S. Department of Transportation Coast Guard Headquarters, Hazardous Materials Branch, 2100 Second Street, Washington, DC 20593-0001 (202) 267-1577 | CFR 46,153, Table I, 1995. CHAPTER I— COAST GUARD, DEPARTMENT OF TRANSPORTATION PART 153—SHIPS CARRYING BULK LIQUID, LIQUEFIED GAS, OR COMPRESSED GAS HAZARDOUS MATERIALS | Noxious liquid substances regulated by the Coast Guard. |

| Controlling Regulatory Entity | List Name | List Producer and Contact Information | Reference | List Description |
|---|---|---|---|---|
| | DOT Hazardous Materials Table | U.S. Department of Transportation DOT Docket Office at (202) 366-5046 | FR 59(249),67395, 1994 (Dec 29). http://hazmat.dot. gov/enforce/forms/ ohmforms.htm#101 Title 49 CFR 172.101 Table (List of Hazardous Materials) | Hazardous materials regulated by the U.S. DOT. |
| U.S. Drug Enforcement Administration (DEA) | DEA Controlled Substances | Drug and Chemical Evaluation Section, Office of Diversion Control, Drug Enforcement Administration 600 Army Navy Dr., Arlington, VA 22202 (202) 305-8500 | 1) List of Controlled Substances, Scheduling Actions 2) CFR 21, 1308.11-15,1996. http://www. deadiversion.usdoj. gov/schedules/ | Controlled substances regulated by the DEA, Department of Justice. |
| USDA/FDA | Direct Food Substances Generally Recognized as Safe | U.S. FDA Center for Food Safety and Applied Nutrition, Office of Premarket Approval Division of Petition Control, Direct Additive Branch. (202) 418-3066  Food and Drug Administration 5600 Fishers Lane, Rockville, MD 20857 1-888-463-6332 | CFR 21,184,1996. http://www.access. gpo.gov/nara/cfr/ waisidx_99/ 21cfrv3_99.html | Direct food additives generally recognized by the FDA as safe so long as used as prescribed. |
| | List of Substances Added to Food in the U.S. | U.S. FDA, Center for Food Safety and Applied Nutrition CFSAN Toll free hotline is 1-888-SAFEFOOD CFSAN, 5100 Paint Branch Parkway, College Park, MD 20740-3835 | Priority-Based Assessment of Food Additives (PAFA) File, 1996. http://www.cfsan .fda.gov/~dms/ opa-indt.html | An official FDA listing maintained by the Center for Food Safety and Applied Nutrition (CFSAN) of all substances known to be added to the U.S. food supply, including Generally Recognized As Safe (GRAS) compounds. |
| NTP/HHS | NTP Carcinogens List | National Toxicology Program, Public Health Service, U.S. Department of Health and Human Services NTP, P.O. Box 12233, MD EC-14, Research Triangle Park, NC 27709 Telephone: (919) 541-4096 | Ninth Annual Report on Carcinogens, 2001, U.S. DHHS, PHS, NTP. http://ntp.niehs. nih.gov/index.cfm? objectid=72016262- BDB7-CEBA- FA60E922B18C2540 | A list of substances that are either known to be carcinogens or that may reasonably be anticipated to be carcinogenic to which a significant number of persons residing in the U.S. are exposed. |

*(continues)*

| Controlling Regulatory Entity | List Name | List Producer and Contact Information | Reference | List Description |
|---|---|---|---|---|
| NTP/HHS (continued) | | | | The publication of this list by the National Toxicology Program (NTP) of the Department of Health and Human Services (DHHS) is mandated for information purposes only by Public Law 95-622. |
| | NTP Technical Reports List | National Toxicology Program, Division of Toxicology Research and Testing, U.S. Department of Health and Human Services.<br><br>Central Data Management, Mail Drop A0-01, NIEHS, P.O. Box 12233, Research Triangle Park, NC 27709 (919) 541-3419 | The NTP Technical Report Series. http://ntp.niehs. nih.gov/ntpweb/ index.cfm? objectid=78CC7E4C -F1F6-975E- 72940974DE301C3F | A list of chemicals for which NTP technical reports are available. The reports describe the results of experiments to determine carcinogenicity. |
| NIOSH/ OSHA | OSHA Toxic and Hazardous Substances | Occupational Safety and Health Administration, DO. Technical Service Center at (202) 219-7894 | CFR 29,1910.1000, 1996. http://www.access. gpo.gov/nara/cfr/ waisidx_ 01/29cfr1910a_ 01.html | The U.S. Labor Department List of Regulated Toxic and Hazardous Substances for which occupational exposure limits are defined. |
| | 1989 OSHA Toxic and Hazardous Substances List | Produced by OSHA in 1989, and vacated by Court order in 1992. | OSHA Publication number 3112, 1989 | Although this OSHA list was vacated by court order in 1992, it is still enforced in some states including Utah, Alaska, Michigan, New Mexico, and Vermont. |
| | NIOSH Recommended Exposure Limits List | National Institute for Occupational Safety and Health 1-800-35-NIOSH (1-800-356-4674) Outside the U.S. 513-533-8328 | DHHS (NIOSH) Publication No. 92-100. http://www.cdc.gov/ niosh/92-100.html | The NIOSH list of substances with recommended exposure limits. |

| Controlling Regulatory Entity | List Name | List Producer and Contact Information | Reference | List Description |
|---|---|---|---|---|
| American Conference of Govern-mental Industrial Hygienists (ACGIH) | ACGIH Threshold Limit Value List | ACGIH, 6500 Glenway Avenue, Building D-7, Cincinnati, OH 45211-4438 (513) 742-2020 | Threshold Limit Values and Biological Exposure Indices for 2001 | A list of substances for which the ACGIH recommended Threshold Limit Values (TLV), where TLV is defined as an airborne concentra-tion to which most workers can be exposed without adverse effects. |
| State of California EPA | California List of Chemicals Known to Cause Cancer or Reproduc-tive Effects | CA EPA Office of Environmental Health Hazard Assessment at (916) 445-6900. 1001 Eye Street, Sacramento, CA 95814 | The Safe Drinking Water and Toxic Enforcement Act of 1986 http://www.oehha. org/prop65/prop65_ list/newlist.html | Chemicals (regulated by California) believed to cause cancer or reproductive toxicity. |
| State of Massachu-setts DOH | Massachusetts Substance List | MA Department of Health, Boston, MA 02133 (617) 727-2660 | Massachusetts Substance List for "Right-to-Know" Law (4/11/1994) M.G.L. c. 111F, General Law, Chapter 30A, 28 June 1984, Appendix A of 105 CMR 670.000 Code of MA Regulation. http://www.michigan. gov/deq/0,1607, 7-135-3307_3667_ 4136-12130–, 00.html | Toxic and hazardous substances applicable to the provisions of MA General Law C.111F. |
| State of Michigan DNR | Michigan Critical Materials Register (CMR) | Michigan Department of Natural Resources Great Lakes Environmental Assessment Section Surface Water Quality Division (517)-373-2190 http://www.michigan.gov/ deq | Michigan Department of Natural Resources, Critical Materials Register, January 1, 1994 | Critical materials for which reporting is required under Michigan Act 293, P.A. 1972. This Act requires all businesses discharging waste-water to lagoons, deep wells, the surface of the ground, surface waters, septic tanks, or municipal sewer systems to file a report with Michigan Department of Natural Resources. |

*(continues)*

| Controlling Regulatory Entity | List Name | List Producer and Contact Information | Reference | List Description |
|---|---|---|---|---|
| State of New Jersey DEP | New Jersey Hazardous Substance List | Bureau of Hazardous Substances Division of Environmental Quality, New Jersey Department of Environmental Protection, 401 East State Street, Trenton, NJ 609-984-2202 | New Jersey Worker and Community Right to Know Act, Department of Environmental Protection List of Hazardous Substances, 1995. http://www.state.nj. us/health/eoh/rtkweb/ factsheetlist.pdf | The New Jersey Right to Know Environmental Hazardous Substance List. |
| | New Jersey Extraordinarily Hazardous Substance List | New Jersey Department of Environmental Protection and Energy Division of Environmental Safety, Health and Analytical Programs, Bureau of Release Prevention, CN424 Trenton, NJ 08625 (609) 633-7289 | New Jersey Administration Code 7:31-2.3 (19 Jul 1993). http://www.nj.gov/ dep/enforcement/ relprev/tcpa/ ehslist.htm | Hazardous substances regulated by New Jersey Bureau of Release and Prevention under NJ Administration Code 7:31-2.3. |
| State of Pennsylvania DOLI | Pennsylvania Right to Know List | Department of Labor and Industry, Bureau of PENNSAFE, Labor and Industry Building, P.O. Box 68571, Harrisburg, PA 17120 Voice: (717) 783-2071 FAX: (717) 783-5099 | RTK Publication Number 691 Rev. 11-95 (Pennsylvania Right to Know Compliance Materials for Employers 1995). http://www.dli. state.pa.us/landi/ CWP/view.asp? a=185&Q=167513 | Chemicals regulated under Pennsylvania Worker and Community Right to Know Act. |

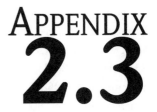

# APPENDIX
# 2.3

## Regional Poison Control Centers

Regional poison control centers represent important local resources for information on the toxic properties of chemicals, both clinical and nonclinical. They provide information to the public on the management of suspected poisonings by animal and plants, household products, over-the-counter and prescription drugs, pesticides, or virtually any substance available. They maintain huge databases of material safety data sheets and provide programs such as "Poisindex" whereby any published information on a chemical can be found rapidly. Regional poison control centers and contact numbers are organized by state.

ALABAMA
*Alabama Poison Center*
2503 Phoenix Drive
Tuscaloosa, AL 35405
Emergency Phone: (800) 222-1222

*Regional Poison Control Center*
Children's Hospital
1600 7th Avenue South
Birmingham, AL 35233
Emergency Phone: (800) 222-1222

ALASKA
*Oregon Poison Center*
Oregon Health Sciences University
3181 SW Sam Jackson Park Road, CB550
Portland, OR 97201
Emergency Phone: (800) 222-1222

ARIZONA
*Arizona Poison & Drug Info Center*
Arizona Health Sciences Center, Room 1156
1501 North Campbell Avenue
Tucson, AZ 85724
Emergency Phone: (800) 222-1222

*Banner Poison Control Center*
901 East Willetta Street
Room 2701
Phoenix, AZ 85006
Emergency Phone: (800) 222-1222

ARKANSAS
*Arkansas Poison & Drug Info Center*
College of Pharmacy
University of Arkansas for Medical Sciences
4301 W. Markham, Mail Slot 522-2
Little Rock, AR 72205
Emergency Phone: (800) 222-1222

CALIFORNIA
California Poison Control System
*California Poison Control System—*
*Fresno/Madera Division*
Children's Hospital Central California
9300 Valley Children's Place, MB 15
Madera, CA 93638-8762
Emergency Phone: (800) 222-1222

*California Poison Control System—*
*Sacramento Division*
UC Davis Medical Center
2315 Stockton Boulevard
Sacramento, CA 95817
Emergency Phone: (800) 222-1222

*California Poison Control System—*
*San Diego Division*
University of California, San Diego,
Medical Center
200 West Arbor Drive
San Diego, CA 92103-8925
Emergency Phone: (800) 222-1222

*California Poison Control System—*
*San Francisco Division*
UCSF Box 1369
San Francisco, CA 94143-1369
Emergency Phone: (800) 222-1222

COLORADO
*Rocky Mountain Poison & Drug Center*
777 Bannock Street
Mail Code 0180
Denver, CO 80204-4028
Emergency Phone: (800) 222-1222

CONNECTICUT
*Connecticut Poison Control Center*
University of Connecticut Health Center
263 Farmington Avenue
Farmington, CT 06030-5365
Emergency Phone: (800) 222-1222

DELAWARE
*The Poison Control Center*
34th & Civic Center Blvd.
Philadelphia, PA 19104-4303
Emergency Phone: (800) 222-1222

DISTRICT OF COLUMBIA
*National Capital Poison Center*
3201 New Mexico Avenue NW
Suite 310
Washington, DC 20016
Emergency Phone: 1-800-222-1222
TTY/TDD: (202) 362-8563 (TTY)

FLORIDA
*Florida Poison Information Center—*
*Jacksonville*
655 West Eighth Street
Jacksonville, FL 32209
Emergency Phone: (800) 222-1222

*Florida Poison Information Center—Miami*
University of Miami, Dept. of Pediatrics
P.O. Box 016960 (R-131)
Miami, FL 33101
Emergency Phone: (800) 222-1222

*Florida Poison Information Center—Tampa*
Tampa General Hospital
P.O. Box 1289
Tampa, FL 33601
Emergency Phone: (800) 222-1222

GEORGIA
*Georgia Poison Center*
CHOA at Hughes Spalding
Grady Health System
80 Jesse Hill Jr. Drive, SE
P.O. Box 26066
Atlanta, GA 30335-3801
Emergency Phone: (800) 222-1222

HAWAII
*Hawaii Poison Center*
1319 Punahou Street
Honolulu, HI 96826
Emergency Phone: (800) 222-1222

Rocky Mountain Poison & Drug Center
777 Bannock Street
Mail Code 0180
Denver, CO 80204-4028
Emergency Phone: (800) 222-1222

IDAHO
*Rocky Mountain Poison & Drug Center*
777 Bannock Street
Mail Code 0180
Denver, CO 80204-4028
Emergency Phone: (800) 222-1222

ILLINOIS
*Illinois Poison Center*
222 S. Riverside Plaza, Suite 1900
Chicago, IL 60606
Emergency Phone: (800) 222-1222

INDIANA
*Indiana Poison Center*
Methodist Hospital, Room AG373
Clarian Health Partners
I-65 at 21st Street
Indianapolis, IN 46206-1367
Emergency Phone: (800) 222-1222

IOWA
*Iowa Statewide Poison Control Center*
Iowa Health System and University of Iowa
Hospitals & Clinics
401 Douglas Street, Suite 402
Sioux City, IA 51101
Emergency Phone: (800) 222-1222

KANSAS
*Mid-America Poison Center*
University of Kansas Medical Center
3901 Rainbow Blvd., Room B-400
Kansas City, KS 66160-7231
Emergency Phone: (800) 222-1222

KENTUCKY
*Kentucky Regional Poison Center*
Medical Towers South, Suite 847
234 East Gray Street
Louisville, KY 40202
Emergency Phone: (800) 222-1222

LOUISIANA
*Louisiana Poison Center*
1521 Wilkinson Street
Shreveport, LA 71103
Emergency Phone: (800) 222-1222

MAINE
*Northern New England Poison Center*
*Serving Maine, New Hampshire, and Vermont*
22 Bramhall Street
Portland, ME 04102
Emergency Phone: (800) 222-1222

MARYLAND
*Maryland Poison Center*
University of MD at Baltimore
School of Pharmacy
20 North Pine Street, PH 772
Baltimore, MD 21201
Emergency Phone: (800) 222-1222

*National Capital Poison Center*
3201 New Mexico Avenue NW
Suite 310
Washington, DC 20016
Emergency Phone: (800) 222-1222

MASSACHUSETTS
*Regional Center for Poison Control and*
*Prevention*
*Serving Massachusetts and Rhode Island*
Children's Hospital Boston
300 Longwood Avenue
Boston, MA 02115
Emergency Phone: (800) 222-1222

MICHIGAN
*Children's Hospital of Michigan*
*Regional Poison Control Center*
4160 John R Harper Professional Office
Building, Suite 616
Detroit, MI 48201
Emergency Phone: (800) 222-1222

*DeVos Children's Hospital*
Regional Poison Center
1300 Michigan NE, Suite 203
Grand Rapids, MI 49503
Emergency Phone: (800) 222-1222

MINNESOTA
*Hennepin Regional Poison Center*
Hennepin County Medical Center
701 Park Avenue
Minneapolis, MN 55415
Emergency Phone: (800) 222-1222

MISSISSIPPI
*Mississippi Regional Poison Control Center*
University of Mississippi Medical Center
2500 N. State Street
Jackson, MS 39216
Emergency Phone: (800) 222-1222

MISSOURI
*Missouri Regional Poison Center*
7980 Clayton Road, Suite 200
St. Louis, MO 63117
Emergency Phone: (800) 222-1222

MONTANA
*Rocky Mountain Poison & Drug Center*
777 Bannock Street
Mail Code 0180
Denver, CO 80204-4028
Emergency Phone: (800) 222-1222

NEBRASKA
*Nebraska Regional Poison Center*
8401 West Dodge Road, Suite 115
Omaha, NE 68114
Emergency Phone: (800) 222-1222

NEVADA
*Oregon Poison Center*
Oregon Health Sciences University
3181 SW Sam Jackson Park Road, CB550
Portland, OR 97201
Emergency Phone: (800) 222-1222

*Rocky Mountain Poison & Drug Center*
777 Bannock Street
Mail Code 0180
Denver, CO 80204-4028
Emergency Phone: (800) 222-1222

NEW HAMPSHIRE
*Northern New England Poison Center*
*Serving Maine, New Hampshire, and Vermont*
22 Bramhall Street
Portland, ME 04102
Emergency Phone: (800) 222-1222

NEW JERSEY
*New Jersey Poison Information and*
*Education System*
University of Medicine and Dentistry at
New Jersey
140 Bergen Street
Newark, NJ 07101
Emergency Phone: (800) 222-1222

NEW MEXICO
*New Mexico Poison & Drug Information*
*Center*
MSC 09 5080
1 University of New Mexico
Albuquerque, NM 87131-0001
Emergency Phone: (800) 222-1222

NEW YORK
*Upstate New York Poison Center*
750 East Adams Street
Syracuse, NY 13210
Emergency Phone: (800) 222-1222

*The Ruth A. Lawrence Poison and Drug*
*Information Center*
*Serving Finger Lakes*
University of Rochester Medical Center
601 Elmwood Avenue, Box 321
Rochester, NY 14642
Emergency Phone: (800) 222-1222

*Long Island Regional Poison and Drug*
*Information Center*
Winthrop University Hospital
259 First Street
Mineola, NY 11501
Emergency Phone: (800) 222-1222

*New York City Poison Control Center*
NYC Bureau of Public Health Labs
455 First Avenue
Room 123, Box 81
New York, NY 10016
Emergency Phone: (800) 222-1222

*Western New York Poison Center*
Children's Hospital of Buffalo
219 Bryant Street
Buffalo, NY 14222
Emergency Phone: (800) 222-1222

NORTH CAROLINA
*Carolinas Poison Center*
P.O. Box 32861
Charlotte, NC 28232
Emergency Phone: (800) 222-1222

NORTH DAKOTA
*Hennepin Regional Poison Center*
Hennepin County Medical Center
701 Park Avenue
Minneapolis, MN 55415
Emergency Phone: (800) 222-1222

OHIO
*Central Ohio Poison Center*
700 Children's Drive, Room E 263
Columbus, OH 43205
Emergency Phone: (800) 222-1222

*Cincinnati Drug & Poison Information Center*
3333 Burnet Avenue
Vernon Place—3rd Floor
Cincinnati, OH 45229
Emergency Phone: (800) 222-1222

*Greater Cleveland Poison Center*
11100 Euclid Avenue/MP 6007
Cleveland, OH 44106-6007

OKLAHOMA
*Oklahoma Poison Control Center*
Children's Hospital at OU Medical Center
940 N.E. 13th Street, Room 3510
Oklahoma City, OK 73104
Emergency Phone: (800) 222-1222

OREGON
*Oregon Poison Center*
Oregon Health & Science University
3181 SW Sam Jackson Park Road, CB550
Portland, OR 97239
Emergency Phone: (800) 222-1222

PENNSYLVANIA
*Pittsburgh Poison Center*
Children's Hospital of Pittsburgh
3705 Fifth Avenue
Pittsburgh, PA 15213
Emergency Phone: (800) 222-1222

*The Poison Control Center at The Children's*
*Hospital of Philadelphia*
34th & Civic Center Blvd.
CHOP North, Suite 985
Philadelphia, PA 19104-4303
Emergency Phone: (800) 222-1222

PUERTO RICO
*Puerto Rico Poison Center*
P.O. Box 367212
San Juan, P.R.
Emergency Phone: (800) 222-1222

RHODE ISLAND
*Regional Center for Poison Control and*
*Prevention*
*Serving Massachusetts and Rhode Island*
300 Longwood Avenue
Boston, MA 02115
Emergency Phone: (800) 222-1222

SOUTH CAROLINA
*Palmetto Poison Center*
College of Pharmacy
University of South Carolina
Columbia, SC 29208
Emergency Phone: (800) 222-1222

SOUTH DAKOTA
*Hennepin Regional Poison Center*
Hennepin County Medical Center
701 Park Avenue
Minneapolis, MN 55415
Emergency Phone: (800) 222-1222

TENNESSEE
*Tennessee Poison Center*
501 Oxford House
1161 21st Avenue South
Nashville, TN 37232-4632
Emergency Phone: (800) 222-1222

TEXAS
*Central Texas Poison Center*
Scott and White Memorial Hospital
2401 South 31st Street
Temple, TX 76508
Emergency Phone: (800) 222-1222

*North Texas Poison Center*
*at Parkland Memorial Hospital*
5201 Harry Hines Blvd.
Dallas, TX 75235
Emergency Phone: (800) 222-1222

*South Texas Poison Center*
The University of Texas Health Science
Center—San Antonio
Department of Surgery
Mail Code 7849, 7703 Floyd Curl Drive
San Antonio, TX 78229-3900
Emergency Phone: (800) 222-1222

*Southeast Texas Poison Center*
The University of Texas Medical Branch
3.112 Trauma Center
901 Harborside Drive
Galveston, TX 77555-1175
Emergency Phone: (800) 222-1222

*Texas Panhandle Poison Center*
1501 S. Coulter
Amarillo, TX 79106
Emergency Phone: (800) 222-1222

*West Texas Regional Poison Center*
Thomason Hospital
4815 Alameda Avenue
El Paso, TX 79905
Emergency Phone: (800) 222-1222

UTAH
*Utah Poison Control Center*
585 Komas Drive, Suite 200
Salt Lake City, UT 84108-1208
Emergency Phone: (800) 222-1222

VERMONT
*Northern New England Poison Center*
*Serving Maine, New Hampshire, and Vermont*
22 Bramhall Street
Portland, ME 04102
Emergency Phone: (800) 222-1222

VIRGINIA
*Blue Ridge Poison Center*
University of Virginia Health System
P.O. Box 800774
Charlottesville, VA 22908-0774
Emergency Phone: (800) 222-1222

*National Capital Poison Center*
3201 New Mexico Avenue NW, Suite 310
Washington, DC 20016
Emergency Phone: (800) 222-1222

*Virginia Poison Center*
Medical College of Virginia Hospitals
Virginia Commonwealth University
Medical Center
P.O. Box 980522
Richmond, VA 23298-0522
Emergency Phone: (800) 222-1222

WASHINGTON
*Washington Poison Center*
155 NE 100th Street, Suite 400
Seattle, WA 98125-8011
Emergency Phone: (800) 222-1222

WEST VIRGINIA
*West Virginia Poison Center*
3110 MacCorkle Ave SE
Charleston, WV 25304
Emergency Phone: (800) 222-1222

WISCONSIN
*Wisconsin Poison Center*
Children's Hospital of Wisconsin
P.O. Box 1997, Mail Station 677A
Milwaukee, WI 53201-1997
Emergency Phone: (800) 222-1222

WYOMING
*Nebraska Regional Poison Center*
8200 Dodge Street
Omaha, NE 68114
Emergency Phone: (800) 222-1222

## Websites

Agency for Toxic Substances and Disease Registry (ATSDR):
http://www.atsdr.cdc.gov/

American Association of Poison Control Centers:
http://www.aapcc.org

American College of Medical Toxicology:
http://www.acmt.net/main/

Carcinogenic Potency Project:
http://potency.berkeley.edu/cpdb.html

Centers for Disease Control and Prevention (CDC):
http://www.cdc.gov/

ChemFinder:
http://chemfinder.cambridgesoft.com/

CCRIS Chemical Carcinogenesis Research Information System:
http://toxnet.nlm.nih.gov/cgi-bin/sis/htmlgen?CCRIS

ClinicalTrials:
http://www.clinicaltrials.gov/

DART/ETIC Developmental & Reproductive Toxicology:
http://toxnet.nlm.nih.gov/cgi-bin/sis/htmlgen?DARTETIC

Environmental Protection Agency (EPA):
http://www.epa.gov/

EXTOXNET:
http://extoxnet.orst.edu/

Extremely Hazardous Substances (EHS):
http://yosemite.epa.gov/oswer/ceppoehs.nsf/EHS_Profile?openform

Food and Drug Administration (FDA):
http://www.fda.gov/

GENE-TOX Genetic Toxicology (Mutagenicity):
http://toxnet.nlm.nih.gov/cgi-bin/sis/htmlgen?GENETOX

Hazardous Materials:
http://www.usfa.fema.gov/subjects/hazmat/

HSDB Hazardous Substances Data Bank:
http://toxnet.nlm.nih.gov/cgi-bin/sis/htmlgen?HSDB

IRIS Integrated Risk Information System:
http://toxnet.nlm.nih.gov/cgi-bin/sis/htmlgen?IRIS

IUPAC:
http://www.iupac.org/dhtml_home.html

Healthy People 2010:
http://www.healthypeople.gov/

ITER International Toxicity Estimates for Risk:
http://toxnet.nlm.nih.gov/cgi-bin/sis/htmlgen?iter

The Library of the Karolinska Institute of Sweden:
http://www.mic.ki.se/Diseases/C21.613.html

Material Safety Data Sheets Online:
http://www.ilpi.com/msds/index.html

MEDLINEplus:
http://medlineplus.gov/

Medwatch Homepage:
http://www.fda.gov/medwatch/report/hcp.htm

National Institute of Environmental Health Sciences (NIEHS):
http://www.niehs.nih.gov/

National Institutes of Health (NIH):
http://www.nih.gov/

National Institute for Occupational Safety and Health (NIOSH):
http://www.cdc.gov/niosh/homepage.html

National Institute of Standards and Technology:
http://webbook.nist.gov/chemistry/

National Report on Human Exposure to Environmental Chemicals:
http://www.cdc.gov/exposurereport/

National Toxicology Program:
http://ntp-server.niehs.nih.gov/

Occupational Safety and Health Administration (OSHA):
http://www.osha.gov/

Poisonous Plants Informational Database:
http://www.ansci.cornell.edu/plants/

Recognition and Management of Pesticide Poisonings:
http://npic.orst.edu/rmpp.htm

Registry of Toxic Effects of Chemical Substances:
http://www.cdc.gov/niosh/97-119.html

Right to Know Hazardous Substance Fact Sheets:
http://www.state.nj.us/health/eoh/rtkweb/rtkhsfs.htm

Toxicon Multimedia Project:
http://www.uic.edu/com/er/toxikon/

TOXLINE:
http://toxnet.nlm.nih.gov/cgi-bin/sis/htmlgen?TOXLINE

TRI Toxics Release Inventory:
http://toxnet.nlm.nih.gov/cgi-bin/sis/htmlgen?TRI

U.S. Department of Agriculture:
http://www.usda.gov/

U.S. National Library of Medicine, National Institutes of Health, Environmental Health and
Toxicology Specialized Information Services (SIS). (2005). *Toxicology tutorial I.* Retrieved from
http://www.sis.nlm.nih.gov/enviro/toxtutor.html

World Health Organization:
http://www.who.int

# Toxicity and the Factors That Modify Toxic Responses

## Cellular Basis of Toxicity

All chemicals have the potential to produce toxicity. As previously indicated, toxicity may be generally defined as any adverse effect of some aspect of normal biology that is causally linked to exposure to a chemical agent. This may occur in many forms ranging from immediate death to subtle changes not realized for months or years. Toxicity can be manifested, for example, as follows:

- Enzyme inhibition (biochemical pathway interruption)
- Cytotoxicity (cell death)
- Inflammation (local or systemic response)
- Covalent binding (e.g., electrophilic metabolites to DNA)
- Receptor interaction (modification of normal effects by interfering with receptor function)
- Necrosis (tissue death)
- Lethal synthesis (toxicant incorporation into a biochemical pathway)
- Lipid peroxidation (free radical oxidation of fatty acids leading to cellular injury or death)
- Immune-mediated hypersensitivity reactions (e.g., allergens producing sensitization)
- Immunosuppression (increased susceptibility to biological and chemical agents)
- Neoplasia (formation of tumors)
- Mutagenic (DNA alterations)

## Spectrum of Adverse Effects

Adverse effects may involve different levels in the body (e.g., macromolecules such as DNA or specific cells, tissues, and organs). For example, cyanide is relatively nonspecific and interrupts electron transport in the mitochondria of all cells, potentially leading to cytotoxicity and death, whereas tetrodotoxin is a specific blocker of sodium channels, especially affecting excitable cells such as nerve and muscle.

The level of toxicity depends on the concentration of the toxicant at the site of action and is influenced by such factors as the rate of absorption, access to the target cell, the degree of biotransformation or bioactivation, and the rate of elimination. Toxicity is essentially the result of a chemical or its metabolite interacting with a molecular target and interfering with critical cellular function. Should the body's efforts at detoxification fail or be impaired by something such as more toxicant present than can be metabolized by available enzymes, dysfunction or injury may occur. Direct injury describes adverse intracellular activities, whereas indirect injury is produced through alteration of extracellular regulatory mechanisms.

Chemicals can interact with molecular targets specifically or nonspecifically, through reactions that are either reversible or irreversible. The binding of botulinum toxin to a nerve terminal to block the release of a neurotransmitter is an example of a specific interaction. Specific effects usually describe interactions with lipids, proteins, and receptors. Nonspecific effects describe those interactions that alter a protein–lipid or lipid–lipid relationship, as detergents do when they alter the conformation or permeability of the membrane by interfering with ionic bonding. Whether the adverse effects produced are reversible or not depends on many factors, including the level of sensitivity of the specific cell(s) affected.

Chemicals can affect the structure of the cellular DNA by binding to it. Some carcinogens and anticancer drugs form covalent adducts in precisely this fashion. Chemicals can interfere with energy production and the synthesis or function of proteins. Extracellular interactions are referred to as indirect injuries. These are injuries that arise from the disruption of the overall processes of the organism like energy production and growth, electrolyte and acid–base regulation, waste product removal, and cellular and tissue interactions governed by the endocrine and nervous systems. Chemicals can modify the extracellular environment, which in turn affects metabolic needs and cell activity regulation. Carbon monoxide is an excellent example; it binds preferentially to the hemoglobin molecule in red blood cells, and toxicity results in all cells of the body as a consequence of the lowered oxygen-carrying capacity of the blood.

Regulatory mechanisms in the nervous, endocrine, and immune systems are targeted by chemicals. In the nervous system acute ethanol exposure can effect physiological changes in enough central nervous system cells to produce reversible behavioral and performance changes and decrements, methylmercury can irreversibly damage neuron cell bodies, and inorganic lead can produce a loss of myelin. Toxicants can interfere with normal hormonal mechanisms, as is the case with environmental "hormone disruptors" such as dioxins. Dioxin in laboratory tests with rodents is relatively specific in nature and can mimic estrogen hormone, thus disrupting the fetus early on in the pregnancy. Interactions with the immune system can be localized, as in the case of a rash, or systemic, as with anaphylaxis.

There are a number of outcomes to chemical injury:

- Cells and tissues repair sufficiently to resume normal function.
- Incomplete repair is only sufficient to resume some function.
- Complete death of an organ or the organism occurs.
- Neoplastic growth occurs, which may result in the death of the organism.

Cellular swelling, a sign of early injury, is due to disruption of energy-producing mechanisms and is accompanied by disruption of the sodium–potassium pump in the cellular membrane. The resultant intracellular change allows the influx of sodium and water. Cellular swelling can be considered reversible if it disappears when the toxicant is removed. Fatty changes are a more serious form of reversible cellular injury. Small vacuoles of lipids build up within the cell; this can occur in several organs but is most commonly observed in the liver, the main site of lipid synthesis and metabolism. It is possible to reverse fatty changes, but it takes far longer to effect a recovery. When the damage to the cell is so severe that it cannot survive, cell death occurs by apoptosis or necrosis.

Necrosis is the end-stage response to cellular injury that culminates with irreversible deterioration and death. It describes a progressive failure of essential functions. Necrosis normally affects contiguous tissues, and the rapid degeneration of cells triggers an inflammatory response. It begins as a reduced production of cellular proteins, a change in the cell's electrolytic gradient, and compromised membrane integrity. Some cytoplasmic organelles swell (mitochondria and endoplasmic reticulum), whereas others shrink (ribosomes in particular). The early phase leads to fluid accumulation that can be seen microscopically as "pale staining." Some cells lose the ability to metabolize fatty acids, and this leads to an accumulation of lipid vacuoles. In the final stages of necrosis, the cell and nucleus shrink and disintegrate. Apoptosis, programmed cell death, is a normal part of the life cycle of a cell. It is an orderly process that destroys an individual cell and recycles its contents. Apoptosis occurs in a single cell within the damaged tissue or in several noncontiguous cells.

After toxic damage, cells and tissues attempt to restore homeostasis and prevent further injury to important structural and functional components by removing or replacing damaged molecules or cells. Repair at the tissue and organ levels is complex. There are two basic cell types in an organ—parenchymal and stromal. Stromal components are supportive, for example, blood vessels and connective tissue to provide a structural framework. Parenchymal components, like hepatocytes of the liver and pneumocytes (alveolar cells) of the lungs, are the functional cells that we associate with normal function. Repair can be accomplished by regeneration of parenchymal cells or repair or replacement of stromal cells. The ultimate aim of repair is to restore the functionality of the organ or, failing that, to regain structural integrity. The ability of a parenchymal cell to regenerate depends on its type. Regenerating cells can be classified as permanent, labile, or stabile. Permanent cells such as neurons and skeletal and cardiac muscle cells do not replace themselves. Labile cells, like epithelial cells or fibroblasts, can replicate easily. Stabile cells such as hepatocytes and kidney tubular cells are capable of regeneration to a lesser extent but are dependent on stromal cells for structural support. If the stromal framework is damaged, the cells can end up scattered in the surrounding tissue. This leads to diminished organ function.

After necrosis the body frequently attempts to replace the dead tissue. If the injury is minimal, function may never be compromised. If the damage is extensive, the body may not be able to provide enough cells of the appropriate type to resume normal function. Using the liver as an example, when complete functional repair cannot be accomplished by replacement of hepatocytes, structural repair ensues. Cirrhosis, with its extensive loss of hepatocytes, is characterized by fibrosis (deposition of collagen) due to structural repair by fiber-producing cells (fibrocytes). The result is scarring and diminished function (Figure 3.1).

Humans cannot avoid contact with toxic compounds; however, it takes more than contact alone to produce adverse effects in an organism. Toxicity is determined by the chemical and physical properties of the compound, the absorbed dose, the method and duration of exposure, the overall health of the organism exposed, and the ability of the organism to dispose of the toxicant. Toxicity and adverse effects are manifested only after the organism has exhausted its protective mechanisms (Figure 3.2).

## Factors That Modify Toxicity

### Age

As we age, from fetus to senior citizen, the body undergoes developmental and metabolic changes. Fetuses are especially vulnerable to toxic insult because their cells are rapidly differentiating, dividing, and migrating during organogenesis. The rapidity of fetal tissue differentiation and division provides increased opportunities for mistakes to occur during DNA replication, for example, or disruption of the differentiation and migration processes of cells, leading to dramatic effects on the fetus. One needs only to think about the effects of thalidomide, which was prescribed to pregnant women as a sleep aid and for relief of nausea, and the resulting fetal abnormalities produced in over 12,000 children.

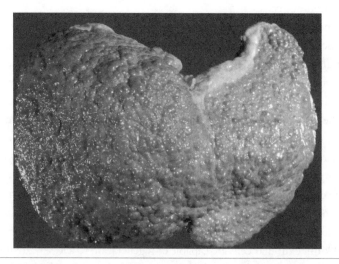

**FIGURE 3.1** Cirrhosis of the liver. *Source:* Courtesy of Leonard V. Crowley, M.D., Century College.

**Toxic Damage to Cells**

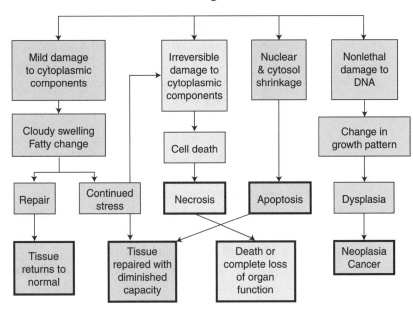

**FIGURE 3.2**    Toxic damage to cells. *Source:* Accessed from: http://sis.nlm.nih.gov/ enviro/toxtutor/Tox3/fig13.gif.

Infants and children, rapidly undergoing behavioral and physical development, are more likely to be adversely affected by toxicants than adults. Lead in children is a well-documented example of a great public health concern. Lead produces changes in calcium metabolism in the developing brain and may disrupt interneuronal programming and levels of neurotransmitters. Altered calcium levels interfere with normal signal transduction pathways, leading to disruption of critical processes involved in brain development such as cell–cell communication, organization, and development of the blood–brain barrier.

In the elderly decreased organ function places them at greater risk from exposure to neuro, hepatic, and renal toxicants, for example. Decreased ability to regulate body temperature, lowered immunological function, reduced cardiac efficiency, and numerous other concerns about their health status are important contributing factors of concern. Decreased biotransforming ability in the elderly can affect elimination rates that may result in prolonged retention times for some toxicants and drugs, thus leading to amplified effects at similar exposures in the younger adult.

## Gender

Gender differences in metabolism, body fat composition, body water, and hormones may all contribute to susceptibility. In males certain chemicals have been demonstrated to adversely affect sperm production and fertility. In women some toxicants impact conception or produce gestational problems. Many toxicants are structurally similar to hormones. They have been shown experimentally to disrupt the endocrine systems as well. These agents include phthalates, alkyl phenolic compounds, polychlorinated biphenyls (PCBs), and polychlorinated dibenzodioxins. An important example of an estrogen agonist is diethylstilbestrol (DES). During the mid-20th century women who were prone to miscarry were prescribed DES as a pregnancy stabilizer. Unfortunately, it produced severe effects in their children, such as reproductive (uterine, vaginal) effects in female offspring and abnormalities in the prostate gland in male offspring.

A difference in something as simple as total body water can result in altered concentrations of a toxicant at the same dose. Consider alcohol consumption, for example. In the United States, presumptive intoxication is defined as a blood alcohol concentration (BAC) of 80 mg (or higher) of ethanol per 100 ml of blood (0.08% BAC). Blood alcohol tables have been developed that generally correlate well with actual measured levels and are routinely used by the courts to assess legal (presumptive) intoxication and driving impairment (Figure 3.3).

The table is different for females due to a greater percentage of body fat composition. This means women will have a higher concentration of blood alcohol on average for the same number of drinks consumed. This is, of course, an oversimplification; however, a gender difference in overall body water is a contributing factor. So whereas three drinks in a 140-pound male will result in a 0.08 BAC, the corresponding value is 0.11 in a female under the same conditions of consumption, time, and measurement.

## Disease

The overall health of an individual can also have a dramatic effect on the response to toxicants. People with impaired liver and kidney function have increased risks of toxic damage because of the decreases in biotransformation and excretion capability. Individuals with suppressed immune function, such as individuals with human immunodeficiency virus (HIV)/acquired immune deficiency syndrome, are possibly more susceptible to carcinogenic agents. Some studies have suggested that exposure to opioids like methadone may in fact induce rapid progression toward HIV-associated dementia.

## Lifestyle and Diet

Lifestyle considerations factor in how well the body can handle toxicants. In humans the number of alveolar macrophages is increased from three- to fivefold in smokers compared with nonsmokers. One of the causative agents for emphysema is cigarette smoke. Nearly all fish and shellfish contain traces of mercury, which may be harmful to the developing fetus. Where one resides may increase exposures to certain pollutants that may contribute to or exacerbate disease. Living in an area where there are industrial discharges of air or water contaminants may place susceptible individuals at greater risk.

## Genetics

Much of the interest in studying genetics and toxicology (toxicogenomics) has come from the field of pharmacogenetics, which deals with studying human variation in relation to drug efficacyand toxic response to drugs. It has long been known that there are variable responses to drugs,

| Men | | | | | | | | | |
|---|---|---|---|---|---|---|---|---|---|
| **Approximate Blood Alcohol Percentage** | | | | | | | | | |
| Drinks | **Body Weight in Pounds** | | | | | | | | **Sample Behavioral Effects** |
| | 100 | 120 | 140 | 160 | 180 | 200 | 220 | 240 | |
| 0 | .00 | .00 | .00 | .00 | .00 | .00 | .00 | .00 | Only Completely Safe Limit |
| 1 | .04 | .03 | .03 | .02 | .02 | .02 | .02 | .02 | Impairment Begins |
| 2 | .08 | .06 | .05 | .05 | .04 | .04 | .03 | .03 | Driving Skills Significantly Affected: Information Processing Altered |
| 3 | .11 | .09 | .08 | .07 | .06 | .06 | .05 | .05 | |
| 4 | .15 | .12 | .11 | .09 | .08 | .08 | .07 | .06 | |
| 5 | .19 | .16 | .13 | .12 | .11 | .09 | .09 | .08 | |
| 6 | .23 | .19 | .16 | .14 | .13 | .11 | .10 | .09 | Legally Intoxicated Criminal Penalties; Reaction of Time Slowed; Loss of Balance; Impaired Movement; Slurred Speech |
| 7 | .26 | .22 | .19 | .16 | .15 | .13 | .12 | .11 | |
| 8 | .30 | .25 | .21 | .19 | .17 | .15 | .14 | .13 | |
| 9 | .34 | .28 | .24 | .21 | .19 | .17 | .15 | .14 | |
| 10 | .38 | .31 | .27 | .23 | .21 | .19 | .17 | .16 | |
| One drink is 1.5 oz. shot of hard liquor, 12 oz. of beer, or 5 oz. of table wine. | | | | | | | | | |

**FIGURE 3.3** Blood alcohol tables. *Source:* Adapted from BAC Charts produced by the National Clearinghouse for Alcohol and Drug Information.

ranging from individuals who exhibit no therapeutic effect to those who exhibit toxic response at the same doses. Differences in the genetic expression of important detoxification enzymes can result in altered rates of biotransformation. Polymorphism has been shown to result in human variation of observed toxicity. For example, a variant in a xenobiotic metabolizing enzyme may result in a toxic response if the variant has a lower level of activity when compared with other variants. An important example of the evolving knowledge regarding variation in toxic response and genetics involves exposure to aromatic amines, bladder cancer, and smoking and variations of the *N*-acetylation polymorphism (*NAT2*). Studies suggest that bladder cancer incidence in smokers, for example, exposed to aromatic amines differed depending on which *NAT2* phenotype the subject exhibited. Depending on the *NAT2* variant, some of the subjects were considered "slow acetylators," whereas others were "normal acetylators." The former may be at a moderately increased risk of developing bladder cancer as opposed to "fast" or "normal acetylator" variants of *NAT2*. A number of other genes have been implicated in other toxicities (Table 3.1).

## Toxicogenomics and Its Importance in Public Health

It is important that we understand the role that genetic polymorphism plays in the response of populations to chemical exposures. Toxicogenomics is a relatively new discipline that has as its goal the elucidation of gene expression in response to toxicants. This is important in further developing public health risk assessments. In 2001 guidance from the International Programme on Chemical Safety (IPCS) called for the replacement of default uncertainty factors with chemical specific adjustment factors (CSAFs). The magnitude of the CSAFs could be calculated based on human variability depending on age, sex, and genetic polymorphisms. Currently, a default uncertainty factor of 10 is applied to encompass the range of variability in human response to toxicants; however, if more specific values could be developed from genetic variation studies, the risk assessment process could become more accurate and reliable in protecting the public's health. Using CSAFs in place of default uncertainty factors enhances the risk assessment process by allowing assessors to make more data-informed biologically based decisions about the risks associated with a toxic exposure.

In addition to enhancing the risk assessment process for public health, toxicogenomics could also be useful in the occupational public health setting. An increasing number of businesses, particularly industrial businesses, are using genetic screening to test potential employees for polymorphisms related to increased risk of toxic response with exposure to certain chemicals. The problem is that many of these tests have yet to be validated for their value in predicting toxic response and are mostly being used on an experimental voluntary basis. If a potential employee or current employee screens positive for a polymorphism related to increased risk of toxic response, the employee can choose to be relocated to a different position that does not involve the exposure. However, this leaves many opportunities for discrimination in the workplace because many people believe that being "susceptible" to a disease or toxic response is viewed as an undesirable status. There is great concern that the genetic data on employees could be used in an unethical and illegal manner, causing more problems than if the ability to obtain these data never existed. Thus companies and public health agencies are proceeding with caution in using genetic screening.

All in all, the field of toxicogenomics is evolving rapidly as more information on the human genome is released. One thing to keep in mind about the data and evidence presented on genetic variation and toxic response is that these studies are mostly preliminary studies done on small samples of populations. The degree to which these polymorphisms increase variability in toxic response is still not well established, and the findings presented thus far only *suggest* that genetic variation is the major cause of toxic response variation. It also must not be overlooked that biotransformation of a xenobiotic toxicant can involve a number of different enzymes and chemical pathways; thus a single polymorphism may have no major effect on response at all. Toxicogenomics is an exciting and important field to public health and will hopefully help us to develop more accurate and reliable ways to protect the public's health.

## Bibliography

Aldridge, J. E., Flaherty, M., Gibbons, J., Kreider, M., Levin, E., & Romano, J. (2003). Heterogeneity of toxicant response: Sources of human variability. *Toxicological Sciences, 76,* 3–20.

Burke, W., Khoury, M. J., & Thomson, E. (2000). *Genetics and public health in the 21st century: Using genetic information to improve health and prevent disease.* New York: Oxford University Press.

Carroquino, M., Pastino, G., & Yap, W. (2000). Human variability and susceptibility to trichloroethylene. *Environmental Health Perspectives Supplements, 108*(S2), 201–214.

Clewell, H., Gentry, P. R., Hack, C. E., Haber, L., & Maier, A. (2002). An approach for the quantitative consideration of genetic polymorphism data in chemical risk assessment. *Toxicological Sciences, 70,* 120–139.

Commission on Geosciences, Environment and Resources. (1997). *Building a foundation for sound environmental decisions.* Washington, D.C.: National Academy Press.

Eaton, D., Kelada, S., Khoury, M., Rothman, N., & Wang, S. (2003). Applications of human genome epidemiology to environmental health. In M. J. Khoury, J. Little, W. Burke (Eds.), *Human genome epidemiology: A scientific foundation for using genetic information to improve health and prevent disease.* New York: Oxford University Press.

Klaassen, C. D. (2001). *Casarett & Doull's toxicology. The basic science of poisons.* New York: McGraw-Hill.

Klaassen, C. D., & Watkins, J. B. (2003). *Casarett & Doull's essentials of toxicology.* New York: McGraw-Hill.

Macgregor, J. T. (2003). The future of toxicology: impact of the biotechnology revolution. *Toxicological Sciences, 75,* 236–248.

Mohrenweiser, H. W. (2004). Genetic variation and exposure related risk estimation: Will toxicology enter a new era? *Toxicologic Pathology, 32*(Suppl. 1), 136–145.

National Institutes of Health. (Undated). *Toxicology tutor I: Dose response.* Retrieved June 2005 from http://sis.nlm.nih.gov/enviro/toxtutor/Tox1/a22.htm.

Nebert, D. W., & McKinnon, R. A. (Undated). *Genetic determinants of toxic response.* Retrieved from http://www.ilo.org/encyclopedia/?doc&nd=857400325&nh=0.

U.S. National Library of Medicine, National Institutes of Health, Environmental Health, and Toxicology Specialized Information Services (SIS). (2005). *Toxicology tutorial II.* Retrieved June 2005 from http://www.sis.nlm.nih.gov/enviro/toxtutor.html.

# Biological Poisons: Plant and Animal Toxins

Earth is home to an impressive array of toxic and venomous organisms that are capable of inflicting injury or death to humans. When it comes to producing poisons, nature in general produces chemicals far more toxic than anything a human can concoct. Many have been used for research purposes to study physiological mechanisms, a number are used clinically, and others have served as prototypes to develop synthetic chemicals of medical importance. Toxins are poisonous substances produced by living things, usually for the purpose of defense or predation. They are effective in very small amounts (Table 4.1).

The term *toxin* is reserved for any toxicant of biological origin. Toxins fall into several broad categories based on the organism that produces them:

- Bacteria
- Fungi: mycotoxins
- Algae: phycotoxins
- Plants: phytotoxins
- Animals: zootoxins

Venom is an animal toxin that is produced in a poison gland or group of cells and is delivered to another animal through a bite or sting. This is referred to as envenomation.

**Table 4.1**   LD$_{50}$ Values of Some Common Animal Toxins

| Species | Route of Administration | Family | LD$_{50}$ (mg/kg) Mouse | Locality |
|---------|------------------------|--------|------------------------|----------|
| **Scorpions** | | | | |
| *Androctonus mauretanicus* | sc | Buthidae | 0.31 | N. Africa |
| *Centruroides exilicauda*, bark scorpion | sc | Buthidae | 1.12–1.46 | Arizona, USA |
| **Spiders** | | | | |
| *Latrodectus mactans tredecimgluttatus* (black widow spider ssp.) | sc | Latrodectus | 0.90 | Europe, N. America |
| **Insects** | | | | |
| Common bee sting | iv | Apidae | 6.00 | Wide distribution |
| Wasp | iv | Vesperidae | 2.5 (purified toxin) | Wide distribution |
| **Centipedes** | | | | |
| *Scolopendra viridicornis* | im | | 12.5 | |
| | iv | Scolopendra | 1.5 | Tropics |
| *Scolopendra subspinipes* | im | | 60 | |
| | iv | Scolopendra | 2.35 | Tropics |
| **Fish** | | | | |
| *Pterois* spp. (Lionfish) | iv | Scorpaenidae | 1.1 | Tropics |
| *Synanceja* spp. (stonefish) | iv | Scorpaenidae | 0.2 | Tropics |
| Puffer fish | oral | Tetraodontidae | 0.008 | Wide distribution |
| **Snakes** | | | | |
| *Agkistrodon contortrix*, copperhead | iv | Crotalidae | 10.5 | N. America |
| *Crotalus scutulatus*, Mojave rattler | iv | Crotalidae | 0.23 | N. America |
| *Crotalus atrox*, W. diamondback | iv | Crotalidae | 4.2 | N. America |
| *Crotalus adamanterus*, E. diamondback | iv | Crotalidae | 1.89 | N. America |
| *Naja naja* ssp., cobra | iv | | 0.13 | |
| | sc | Elapidae | 0.29 | Asia |
| *Ophiophagus hannah*, King cobra | iv | Elapidae | 0.35 | Asia |

im, intramuscular; iv, intravenous; sc, subcutaneous.

# Bacterial Toxins

## Botulinum Toxin

Botulinum toxin refers to a collection of neurotoxic proteins that are produced under anaerobic conditions by the bacterium *Clostridium botulinum.* There are seven serologically distinct toxin types, designated A through G, with similar toxicities as determined experimentally in laboratory rodents. The amount of toxin to produce a lethal effect is approximately 0.0002 µg/kg body weight. It is likely the most acutely toxic substance known, with a lethal dose of about 200–300 pg/kg, meaning that about 100 grams could kill most of the humans on earth. To place its toxicity in perspective, sodium cyanide has an $LD_{50}$ of 10,000 µg/kg (Table 4.2).

*Clostridium* spores are ubiquitously found in soil globally. The foodborne illness results from ingestion of food that has become contaminated with spores that germinate and grow, especially in an anaerobic environment. The germinating spores vegetate, produce, and release the toxin that causes botulism. A form of botulism results from infection of wounds with spores that subsequently germinate, resulting in production of toxin and symptoms of botulism. The toxin is composed of two polypeptide chains that are connected by a disulfide bond: a 50-kDa light chain and a 100-kDa heavy chain.

The light chain of the toxin

- Is a protease enzyme that attacks one of the fusion proteins at the neuromuscular junction, preventing neurotransmitter vesicles from anchoring to the membrane (a requirement to release acetylcholine).
- Inhibits acetylcholine release, and then the toxin interferes with nerve impulses.
- Produces paralysis of muscles.

The heavy chain of the toxin

- Is important for targeting the toxin to specific types of axon terminals.
- Attaches the toxin to proteins on the surface of axon terminals so that it can be taken into neurons by endocytosis.

Botulism is characterized by general muscular weakness that first affects ocular and throat muscles and then extends to all the muscles. In severe intoxications generalized flaccid paralysis is accompanied by impairment of respiration and of autonomic functions, resulting in death. Experimentally, the time to the onset of paralysis in animals injected with the neurotoxins depends on dose, species, and route of injection, with a latent period of hours to days between injection and symptoms. After entering the general circulation, the toxin binds to the presynaptic membranes of motor neuron nerve terminals, enters the neuronal cytosol, and blocks the release of acetylcholine, thus causing a flaccid paralysis. The toxin is used in very small amounts both as a cosmetic treatment and to treat painful muscle spasms (e.g., the esophagus) and is sold under the brand names, respectively, Botox and Dysport.

**Table 4.2** Comparison of the Toxicity of Botulinum Toxin with Several Other Chemical Substances

| Toxin | $LD_{50}$ (µg/kg) | Molecular Weight |
|---|---|---|
| Botulinum toxin | 0.00025 | 150,000 |
| Batrachotoxin (amphibian dart poison) | 2 | 538 |
| Tetrodotoxin (puffer fish poison) | 9 | 319 |
| Sodium cyanide | 10,000 | 65 |

In humans the latency period may be greater than a week, and symptoms initially are difficulty speaking and swallowing, which may progress to generalized paralysis and even death. The symptoms of botulism can be prevented by antitoxin antibodies; the general public is not vaccinated against botulism because it is very rare in developed countries.

## Tetanus Toxin

Tetanus, from the Greek *tetanos* meaning stretched, rigid, was described by Hippocrates 25 centuries ago. Tetanus toxin produces a hypercontracted state of the skeletal muscle that is often fatal. Death results from respiratory and heart failure. The bacterium *Clostridium tetani* is the causal agent. It is an anaerobic bacterium whose spores germinate under very low oxygen levels and is introduced into the body generally through skin wounds such as lacerations, abrasions, and occasionally from body piercing or tattooing. Tetanus toxin is an extremely potent neuromuscular toxin that is responsible for all the symptoms produced in humans and other mammals.

The toxin is referred to as tetanospasmin or spasmogenic toxin. Once introduced into the body, the spores of the bacteria vegetate and release toxin into the capillary and lymphatic vessels to peripheral nerves and by retrograde transport travels to the spinal cord and accumulate in the ventral horn of the gray matter.

Like botulinum toxin, the tetanus toxin is a peptide that contains two chains: a heavy 100-kDa chain connected by a disulfide bond to a 50-kDa light chain. The heavy chain binds onto the cell membrane of the neuron, whereas the light chain, which is a zinc-containing endopeptidase, interferes with the protein vesicles that contain the neurotransmitters (Figure 4.1). The action effectively blocks the release of important central nervous system inhibitory neurotransmitters such as glycine and gamma-aminobutyric acid (GABA), thus inhibiting the inhibitory neurons. Their inhibition leaves the stimulatory components for neuromuscular effects largely unregulated, and

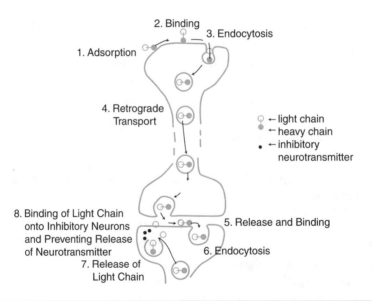

FIGURE 4.1    Tetanus toxin movement from peripheral to central nervous system.

this produces a central nervous system tetanic spasm of the skeletal muscles of the body. The muscular spasms associated with severe toxicity are so strong that fractures of the long bones can occur.

Clinically, the muscles of the face and jaw are first affected, thus giving rise to the common term "lockjaw." A tetanus shot is most often given for any significant skin wound to supplement the immunization conferred in childhood through the diphtheria/tetanus/pertussis vaccination series.

Tetanus toxin has a similar mechanism of action to botulinum toxin, but the two have different sites of action: The former affects neurotransmitter release in the central nervous system, and the latter affects neurotransmitter release in the peripheral nervous system at the neuromuscular junction. They are both exotoxins (liberated from the living bacteria) with the heavy chains involved in targeting and binding to the appropriate cell membranes and the lighter chains interfering with neurotransmitter release.

### Endotoxins

Bacterial endotoxins are known to cause an inflammatory response in the human respiratory tract. Endotoxin is not secreted in soluble form by live bacteria as are exotoxins but rather is a chemical component in the cell wall of the bacteria that is released when the bacteria lyses. The main endotoxin is the lipopolysaccharide (LPS) complex associated with the outer bacterial wall in most gram-negative bacteria. LPS is often used synonymously with endotoxin and consists of a polysaccharide chain and a lipid, often referred to as lipid A, the latter of which produces the toxic effects of the bacteria. Endotoxins are associated with fever, inflammation, and lowering of blood pressure. LPS binds to serum protein and through a complex series of transfers to the cells of the immune system triggers a signal for the secretion of chemical mediators of inflammation. If significant endotoxin is present, the individual can go into "septic shock" characterized by life-threatening symptoms, including the deregulation of blood pressure and electrolyte–water balance.

Bacterial endotoxins have been associated with the exacerbation of respiratory conditions both directly (e.g., exacerbation of existing asthma) and indirectly (e.g., increased incidence of colds, which in turn can exacerbate existing asthma). The response is mediated by a number of proinflammatory cytokines (e.g., interleukin-1, -6, and -8 and tumor necrosis factor-alpha) and clinically gives rise to such general symptoms as headache, fever, tightness of the chest, nonproductive cough, decreased lung function, and general malaise.

## Fungal Toxins

### Poison Mushrooms

A common name that is recognized for poisonous mushrooms is "toadstool" or "death's stool," which comes from the German *Todesstuhl*. These toxins are produced by fungi and cannot be made nontoxic by cooking, freezing, or other forms of food processing. Unless one is a true expert in the identification of mushrooms, it is best to avoid consuming any that have been collected in the wild or obtained from a questionable source. Unfortunately, poisonings occur in the United States and elsewhere from the consumption of misidentified species or through the intentional consumption of species that have psychotropic properties by individuals who desire this effect.

Mushroom poisonings result in a wide variety of clinical effects. The prognosis depends on the species and the amount of consumption. The general types of illness produced fall within four categories based on the primary toxicity associated with the mushroom:

1. Gastrointestinal: producing transient nausea, vomiting, abdominal cramping, and diarrhea
2. Disulfiram-like effects: no symptoms occur unless alcohol is consumed within 2–3 days after ingestion of the mushrooms, resulting in the typical unpleasant effects associated with the use of "antabuse"
3. Neurotoxic: producing coma, convulsions, hallucinations, excitement, and depression
4. Cytotoxic: resulting in generalized destruction of cells, especially the liver and kidneys, followed by organ failure

## Mushroom Toxins

Mushroom poisoning can result from the consumption of a number of species of mushrooms that contain the following toxins:

- Amanitin
- Coprine
- Gyromitrin
- Ibotenic acid
- Muscarine
- Muscimol
- Orellanine
- Psilocybin

## Gastrointestinal Effects

Numerous mushrooms contain toxins that can cause gastrointestinal distress, including but not limited to nausea, vomiting, diarrhea, and abdominal cramps. Some examples of these mushrooms are as follows:

- Jack O'Lantern (*Omphalotus illudens*)
- Tigertop (*Tricholoma pardinum*)
- Early False Morel (*Verpa bohemica*)
- Green Gill (*Chlorophyllum molybdites*)
- Horse mushroom (*Agaricus arvensis*)
- Gray Pinkgill (*Entoloma lividum*)
- Pepper bolete (*Boletus piperatus*)

Consumption of these mushrooms produces symptoms similar to mushrooms that produce cytotoxicity and sometimes death. Diagnostically, the primary difference between the two types of poisonings is that the gastrointestinal toxins have a rapid onset, whereas the latter (although gastrointestinal disturbances occur) have a 12- to 48-hour latency period before symptom onset.

Fatalities from the gastrointestinal toxins are extremely rare and related to poor or unsuccessful supportive measures to maintain hydration and electrolyte balance, especially for very old or young patients. Little is known about the chemical properties of these toxins other than they are a collection of peptides, resins, and compounds that produce irritation.

### Disulfiram-Like Effects

A few species of mushrooms produce an unusual amino acid, coprine, which is metabolized in humans to cyclopropanone, a compound that interferes with the metabolism of ethanol. Consumption of alcoholic beverages within approximately 3 days of consumption of these mushrooms produces nausea, headache, flushing, vomiting, and other unpleasant effects over the course of several hours, similar to those produced in individuals taking "antabuse" in combination with alcohol. The Inky Cap Mushroom (*Coprinus atramentarius*) is the mushroom most commonly responsible for this poisoning. Apart from alcohol-induced toxicity, this mushroom is generally considered to be edible, with no apparent adverse effects.

### Neurotoxic Effects

A neurotoxic poisoning can result from ingestion of a number of mushroom species containing the toxin muscarine (e.g., *Clitocybe dealbata, Inocybe geophylla*). These mushrooms typically have muscarine concentrations of several percent. Within minutes of consumption and over the course of several hours, increased salivation, lacrimation, sweating, nausea, abdominal pain, diarrhea, blurred vision, and difficulty breathing (in severe cases) result.

Ibotenic acid and muscimol poisonings occur from consumption of mushrooms such as the Fly Agaric (*Amanita muscaria*) and Panthercap (*Amanita pantherina*). Both toxins are present; however, muscimol is several times more potent than ibotenic acid. Within 1 to 2 hours after consumption, dizziness and drowsiness may occur, with the individual sometimes falling asleep as well. This is followed by excitability, illusions, and delirium that alternate with periods of drowsiness over the course of a few hours. Severe intoxications may result in convulsions and coma.

A number of mushrooms when ingested produce hallucinations and effects similar to alcohol intoxication. Several of these mushrooms (e.g., *Psilocybe cubensis, P. mexicana, Conocybe cyanopus*) are eaten for their psychotropic effects. Most of the psychotropic mushrooms are small, brown, and leathery in appearance ("Little Brown Mushrooms"), not easily confused with the edible nontoxic species of mushrooms. The toxic effects are caused by psilocybin, a psychedelic alkaloid of the tryptamine family. These mushrooms have been commonly called "magic mushrooms" or "shrooms," and their effects are similar to lysergic acid diethylamide (LSD). The onset of effects is generally rapid and subsides within several hours, except for severe cases, usually seen in children, where hallucinations, fever, coma, and death have been reported.

### Cytotoxic Effects

The cyclic peptides collectively referred to as the amanitins are produced by a number of different species of poison mushrooms, including Death Cap or Destroying Angel (*Amanita phalloides and Amanita virosa*), Autumn Skullcap (*Galerina autumnalis*), and Fool's Mushroom

(*Amanita verna*). Consumption of these mushrooms generally does not result in immediate ill-ness, but rather its course is divided into two phases. In the first phase symptoms begin to appear within 12–48 hours and are extremely intense. Symptoms include diarrhea, excessive urination, thirst, abdominal pain, and seizures. During this phase the patient appears to have recovered for a period of several hours to days; however, this gives way to a second phase of rapid downhill deterioration due to organ system failure, jaundice, cyanosis, and coma, which results in a 50–90% death rate over the course of about a week (less depending on the amount of con-sumption). If the patient survives there is permanent liver injury.

A cytotoxic mushroom poisoning that resembles *Amanita* poisoning but is less intense comes from the consumption of the False Morels (e.g., *Gyromitra esculenta, G. gigas*), which contain the hydrazine derivative gyromitrin, which is hepatotoxic and affects the nervous system as well. The mortality rate is approximately 2%. There is again a latent period lasting approximately 10 hours after consumption in which the individual is apparently symptom free. This is followed by a rapid onset of abdominal bloating, headache, diarrhea, and vomiting.

Another cytotoxic mushroom poisoning that is characterized by an extremely long latent period of several days to several weeks is from consumption of the Sorrel Webcap mushroom (*Cortinarius orellanus*) and some of its relatives. The toxin orellanine results in intense thirst, uri-nation, nausea, muscle aches, and, in severe cases, kidney tubular necrosis, liver degeneration, and renal failure. The course of the illness can last for several weeks and is accompanied by a death rate of approximately 15%.

## Mycotoxins

### Aflatoxins

The mycotoxins, which are collectively referred to as aflatoxins, are produced by molds that infest peanuts, corn, wheat, rice, tree nuts, dairy products, and other agricultural plants consumed by both humans and animals. They are produced primarily by members of the genus *Aspergillus*. These molds grow especially well in tropical and subtropical areas where temperature and humidity are high. Exposure to the toxin can occur from the consumption of contaminated food and its han-dling. Respiratory exposure to airborne spores can be of special concern to grain handlers. Aflatoxicosis, an acute illness of exposure, although relatively rare in humans, is more likely to occur in underdeveloped countries. Acutely, the consumption of food with large amounts of aflatoxin can result in liver damage, which may be fatal. In India in the early 1970s, approximately 400 people developed aflatoxicosis and 108 people died from eating very heavily contaminated grains.

Chronic exposure to aflatoxin has been associated with a specific form of liver cancer. Epidemiological studies have shown that humans who were positive for hepatitis B had a 30-fold increase in the carcinogenic potential of aflatoxin when compared with those who were negative, thus suggesting a synergistic-like effect.

Humans are not the only animals affected by aflatoxins; they have been shown to injure or kill chickens, turkeys, pheasants, cattle, sheep, pigs, and dogs. In 1960 aflatoxin killed about 100,000 turkeys that were eating moldy peanuts. That same year aflatoxins were shown to pro-duce liver cancer in laboratory animals. Today we know that aflatoxins are known human mutagens and hepatocarcinogens. Aflatoxin B1 is the most potent hepatocarcinogen known; however, it must first be metabolized to the carcinogenic form. Mammals such as cows that are fed contaminated feed metabolize aflatoxin, and therefore it may be found in milk and other dairy products; thus regulatory limits have been set for human food sources (e.g., 15 ppb for peanut butter) and also for the feed given to agricultural animals.

## Trichothecenes

The trichothecenes are represented by several toxins (e.g., T-2 toxin, diacetoxyscirpenol, deoxynivalenol) and are produced by species of *Fusarium,* a mold that grows under cool to cold conditions on grains, alfalfa, tomatoes, fruits, and other substrates. The trichothecenes are a group of sesquiterpenes produced by various *Fusarium* species, such as *F. graminearum, F. sporotrichioides, F. poae,* and *F. equiseti.*

The most important structural features causing the biological activities of trichothecenes are the 12,13-epoxy ring, the presence of hydroxyl or acetyl groups at appropriate positions on the trichothecene nucleus, and the structure and position of the side chain. The toxins have been called radiomimetic toxins (referring to radiation effects) because they affect the following rapidly reproducing cells:

- Bone marrow
- Lymphocytes in lymph nodes
- Seminiferous tubules of testicle
- Fetus and placenta
- Cells with high metabolic rates
- Immunosuppression

These toxins have been observed to produce effects in both laboratory animals and agriculturally important species. Exposure of certain farm animals has been associated with increased abortions, abdominal pain, diarrhea, and testicular damage. In humans the main toxins produced by *Fusarium* are the fumonisins, which have been related (very limited evidence) to esophageal cancer.

Members of the genus *Stachybotrys* are filamentous molds generally growing on cellulose-rich substrates. These molds have been associated with "sick building syndrome," especially in buildings where there has been evidence of water intrusion. Complaints include

- Eye, nose, or throat irritation
- Headache
- Dry cough
- Dry or itchy skin
- Difficulty in concentrating
- Dizziness and nausea
- Fatigue
- Sensitivity to odors

The nature of this "syndrome" with respect to causality continues to be a topic of controversy.

### Ergolines

Contamination of rye by *Claviceps purpurea* (ergot fungus) produces several powerful ergoline derivatives (e.g., methylergometrine, ergotamine). The symptoms, from either high doses or when moderate doses interact with potentiators such as certain antibiotics (e.g., azithromycin), include

- Convulsive symptoms (e.g., painful seizures and spasms, diarrhea, paresthesias, itching, headaches, nausea, and vomiting)
- Central nervous system symptoms (e.g., hallucinations, hysteria, mania, or psychosis)
- Gangrenous symptoms (e.g., dry gangrene due to vasoconstriction of distal structures, such as the fingers and toes; weak peripheral pulse; loss of peripheral sensation; edema; and ultimately the death and loss of affected tissues)

Ergot has an interesting history and was first mentioned in the early Middle Ages as the cause of outbreaks of mass poisonings affecting thousands of individuals. The illness appeared in two characteristic forms: convulsive (ergotismus convulsivus) and gangrenous (ergotismus gangraenosus). The gangrenous form has been referred to as "St. Anthony's Fire" because ergotism victims in the Middle Ages, numbering in the thousands, were treated by the monks of the Order of St. Anthony. Other outbreaks of ergot poisoning approaching epidemic proportions were recorded in more recent times in European countries and in certain areas of Russia. In 1951, 150 people were hospitalized in Pont-Saint-Esprit, France; 5 died and a number of others became psychotic, believing they were pursued by snakes and demons. In 2001 there was an outbreak in Ethiopia from consumption of contaminated barley.

The chemicals in ergot have been used to synthesize chemicals that may be of medicinal importance. One attempt resulted in the production of LSD by Dr. Albert Hoffman of Switzerland. He wrote the following:

> Last Friday, April 16, 1943, I was forced to stop my work in the laboratory in the middle of the afternoon and to go home, as I was seized by a peculiar restlessness associated with a sensation of mild dizziness. On arriving home, I lay down and sank into a kind of drunkenness which was not unpleasant and which was characterized by extreme activity of imagination. As I lay in a dazed condition with my eyes closed (I experienced daylight as disagreeably bright) there surged upon me an uninterrupted stream of fantastic images of extraordinary plasticity and vividness and accompanied by an intense, kaleidoscope-like play of colors. This condition gradually passed off after about two hours.

His "experience" was the direct result of his consumption of the chemicals that he produced synthetically.

## Algal Toxins

The Cyanobacteria of the plant kingdom Monera are known by the common name blue-green algae. They are primitive photosynthetic organisms, with about a dozen toxic species found on land, in freshwater, and in the oceans. Some marine blue-green algae are responsible for a form of contact dermatitis known as "swimmers itch," characterized by skin and mucous membrane inflammation. Other species of blue-green algae have been responsible for the deaths of large populations of wild and domestic animals, including migrating ducks and geese and cattle and sheep that have consumed contaminated water. Their toxins are released when their cells die or if entire intact cells are consumed. Humans drinking from these contaminated water sources are also at risk for potentially severe toxicity as well. The species *Microcystis* produces cyclopeptide hepatotoxins (nodularin and microcystin). These toxins inhibit enzymes in the liver that are important in maintaining its structural support (e.g., protein phosphatases) and have been used as a research tool as well. The toxins have also been linked to liver cancer in parts of the world where frequent algae blooms occur.

*Anabaena* produces the neurotoxin saxitoxin and an extremely neurotoxic alkaloid, anatoxin, also referred to as the "very fast death factor." The anatoxins affect the nervous system, often causing death due to paralysis of the respiratory muscles due to its irreversible binding to the nicotinic acetylcholine receptor; that is, it functions like acetylcholine but is not broken down. This results in a condition whereby the sodium channels in the muscle are locked in the open position and the muscles become overstimulated and eventually paralyzed. This can affect the diaphragm, resulting in respiratory failure and death within minutes if a sufficient amount of the toxin is consumed.

Saxitoxins are also neurotoxins; however, they function in a fashion similar to tetrodotoxin in that they block sodium channels in neurons, thus inhibiting the transmembrane movement of sodium ions and effectively blocking neural action potentials. This can result in an understimulation of muscles at the neuromuscular junction, and respiratory paralysis will result if the dose is sufficiently high. Small doses obtained from oral consumption of any mollusk or fish that may concentrate this toxin is a tingling and numbness of the mouth, tongue, and face, similar to that of tetrodotoxin.

In the plant kingdom a number of different true algae are present, most of which are of little toxicological concern. They fall within a number of divisions:

- Division Chrysophyta: Diatoms are abundant and important economically due to the presence of silica in their cellular wall and represent an important source of food in both freshwater and marine environments.
- Division Euglenophyta: Euglenoids are flagellated unicellular plants that make up part of the diet of aquatic invertebrates.
- Division Chlorophyta: The green algae are represented by numerous species abundant in freshwater and represent an important part of the aquatic food chain.
- Division Rhodophyta: The red algae include seaweeds, which represent an important food source for many herbivores and are also consumed by humans. It is a source of carbohydrates such as carrageen and agar, which are widely used.
- Division Phaeophyta: The brown algae or seaweed that occurs in coastal waters, often referred to as kelp, is an important food source for marine organisms and humans as well.
- Division Pyrrophyta: The dinoflagellates are unicellular algae that are important sources of food in freshwater and marine environments. These algae are of toxicological importance because they are associated with massive fish kills and contamination of shellfish

and fish, especially during times of the year when blooms occur. They have also been shown to be respiratory irritants in humans.

## Dinoflagellates and Red Tides

The red tide refers to the reddish orange-brown color of coastal water during outbreaks of certain species of dinoflagellates, in the Gulf of Mexico, Caribbean, and other coastal areas around the world. Red tide blooms, especially in the late summer and autumn months, occur almost every year off the west coast of Florida and are associated with massive fish and bird kills. Several species, especially *Karenia brevis,* produce toxins that can cause these massive fish kills in coastal fish that swim through the bloom. The toxins are released into the water when dinoflagellate is fragmented, largely from the action of the waves. The toxins that are released damage the gills and cardiovascular systems of these fish, resulting in death. Many thousands of them are washed onto the beaches, where they lie until consumed by birds and other animals or until they are collected and incinerated. Clams, oysters, and mussels may continue to filter feed during these outbreaks, thereby accumulating toxins in their tissues.

The toxins are of several types of lipid-soluble chemicals that are neurotoxic to mammals. These toxins have been collectively referred to as brevetoxins. They are depolarizing toxins in that they open voltage-gated sodium ion channels in neural cell membranes, thus leading to unregulated sodium influx into the cell. It is believed that the respiratory problems associated with the inhalation of aerosolized Florida red tide toxins are due in part to the opening of sodium channels by the brevetoxins, causing the release of neurotransmitters from autonomic nerve endings in the airways. In particular, the release of acetylcholine from peripheral nerve endings leads to airway smooth muscle depolarization and contraction.

During a red tide, the aerosol of contaminated salt spray, which contains toxins and fragmented organisms, can be carried inland depending on wind and other environmental conditions. The brevetoxins can be highly concentrated in the aerosol of sea spray generated by waves hitting the shore during a red tide. This has been associated with respiratory irritation in nonasthmatic individuals and may be particularly offending to individuals that are asthmatic. Aerosolized red tide toxin-induced effects include conjunctival irritation, copious catarrhal exudates, rhinorrhea, nonproductive cough, and bronchoconstriction.

Red tide was associated with the deaths of a large number of manatees during a 1996 bloom. Necropsy showed severe catarrhal rhinitis, pulmonary hemorrhage and edema, and evidence of neurotoxicity in the dead manatees.

# Higher Plant Toxins

Many higher plants produce harmful substances that if ingested can produce injury and sometimes death. Young children are especially at risk for toxicity from plants due to their curious nature and attraction to brightly colored leaves and berries. Some plants contain chemicals that are potent sensitizing agents and can invoke an immunologically mediated dermatitis. Ingestion of toxic plants affects primarily the gastrointestinal, cardiovascular, and central nervous systems.

Plant toxins can be classified based on their general chemical structure. Examples of the types of toxins contained in plants are as follows:

- Alkaloids (e.g., Yew, Poison Hemlock, Nightshade, Jimsonweed)
- Proteins and amino acids (e.g., Castor bean)
- Glycosides (e.g., Lily of the Valley, Foxglove, Oleander)
- Oxalates (e.g., Philodendron, Dieffenbachia, Rhubarb)
- Phenols, resins, and volatile oils (e.g., Poison Ivy, Poison Oak, Poison Sumac, Rhododendrons)
- Phototoxins (e.g., St. John's wort)

Plant toxins can be present even in fruit and vegetable plants. The pits and leaves of cherries, peaches, and apricots contain cyanogenic (cyanide-containing) glycosides. Harmful alkaloids are present in the foliage of common tomato plants, and the green parts of potatoes contain solanine, a glycoalkaloid.

Garden, outdoor ornamental, and wild plants also contain toxins, some of which are extremely dangerous if consumed. Examples of these types of plants are as follows:

- Oleander (*Nerium oleander*): contains saponins, oleandroside, nerioside, and other cardio-glycosides, especially the woody stems and leaves
- Lilies: most are poisonous, especially to domestic animals
- Foxglove (*Digitalis purpurea*): contains cardioglycosides, which can be fatal if ingested
- Privet (*Ligustrum* sp.): produces berries that contain syringin and ligustrin, which can be fatal to humans
- Castor Oil Plant (*Ricinus communis*): oil used as a purgative; however, the water-soluble fraction contains the highly toxic protein ricin
- Yew (*Taxus baccata*, the "English yew"): all parts of the plant, except for the fleshy red bit of the fruit, contain poisons
- Nightshade (*Atropa belladonna*): contains the parasympathetic blocking agent, atropine
- Mayapple (*Podophyllum peltatum*): the green portions of the fruit and rhizomes contain podophyllotoxin
- Poison Hemlock (*Conium maculatum*): contains the alkaloid coniine
- Wolfsbane or Monkshood (*Aconitum napellus*): seed pods and roots concentrate the poison aconitum
- Poison Ivy (*Toxicodendron radicans*), Poison Oak (*T. diversilobum*), and Poison Sumac (*T. vernix*): contain a highly irritating and sensitizing oil, urushiol

Plants containing oxalates include *Brassaia* and *Schefflera* spp. (Umbrella Tree) and *Dieffenbachia* spp. (Dumbcane); both are popular indoor plants. The oxalates are capable of producing contact dermatitis and can produce significant local irritation such as severe swelling and stinging of the mouth and tongue (*Dieffenbachia* spp. is also referred to as "Mother-in-Law's Tongue.")

Chili pepper (*Capsicum annum*), also commonly referred to as cayenne pepper or red pepper, is used as a spice, ornamental plant, and as a repellent for common pests. It produces local effects, the intensity of which depends on the area of the skin contacted, the length of exposure, and the sensitivity of the individual. Cutaneous contact produces pain and a burning/stinging sensation, and contact with sensitive areas such as the eye can result in intense pain, tearing, blepharospasm, and conjunctivitis. For this reason it is commonly used for personal self-defense in the form of pepper spray. It is also used as a topical anesthetic to relieve pain due to its ability to interfere with substance P (a neurogenic mediator of inflammation) in sensory nerve endings.

Holly (*Ilex* spp.) produces small red or black berries during winter months to which children are particularly attracted. Consumption results in severe gastrointestinal symptoms such as vomiting, abdominal cramping, and diarrhea. Contained within the berries are a mixture of phenols, alkaloids, saponins, and triterpenes that are very irritating to the mucosa of the gastrointestinal tract. Medical treatment is usually unnecessary except in severe cases, which may require the use of fluid replacement, activated charcoal, and general supportive care.

Philodendron (*Philodendron* spp.), also referred to as Parlor Ivy or Panda Plant, can produce mucosal irritation of the mouth and gastrointestinal tract and mild dermatitis. The plant contains resorcinol and small amounts of calcium oxalate.

Pokeweed (*Phytolacca americana*) is often processed to be used as a salad or tea. Pokeweed contains phytolaccatoxin and phytolaccigenin, which can be severely irritating to the gastrointestinal tract. Traditionally, pokeweed leaves are processed by boiling them two times and discarding the water. Pokeweed salad has been a common staple of Southern cuisine in the United States for decades despite its well-publicized toxicity, even after boiling. Symptoms begin several hours after digestion and include gastrointestinal disturbances such as cramping, vomiting, and diarrhea, which can be severe; these symptoms usually resolve within 24 hours.

Poison ivy, oak, and sumac (*Toxicondendron* spp.) are the cause of most cases of allergic contact dermatitis in the United States. These plants contain a mixture of volatile oily chemicals that are potent sensitizing agents, including the antigen urushiol, to which most individuals become sensitized upon dermal exposure to the plant(s). Within 36 hours after a sensitized individual is exposed to these plants, a blistery itching rash develops. The oil upon contact with skin binds to skin proteins; however, if the area is thoroughly washed with soap and water within 10 to 15 minutes after contact, a reaction may be prevented. After the antigen is fixed, however, it cannot be washed off or transferred to other areas. Scratching or oozing blisters cannot spread the antigen to other areas of the body or to other persons. New lesions that appear a few days after the primary lesions represent less sensitive areas where lesser amounts of antigen were deposited. The dermatitis can be treated with antihistamines and corticosteroids.

*Euphorbia pulcherrima* (Poinsettia) is included here because of the common misconception that the plant is toxic if consumed. This misconception centers on a legend in 1919 of a 2-year-old child dying after eating the leaves of the plant. Any toxicity associated with this plant pertains to those individuals who are allergic to latex; they may suffer an allergic response upon contact with the diterpene esters of the plant.

The Aconitum family (e.g., *Aconitium napellus*), commonly referred to as Monkshood, Wolfsbane, Friars Cap, and Aconitine, contain alkaloids that can produce severe cardiovascular effects that have a rapid onset, severe gastrointestinal disturbances, numbness, and paresthesia.

Severe poisoning can result in ventricular tachycardia, conduction blocks, premature ventricular contractions, ventricular fibrillation, and respiratory muscle paralysis, with death as a real outcome unless very aggressive supportive care is obtained quickly.

# Animal Toxins

## Spider Venoms

If asked to name a spider, more likely than not the black widow spider comes to mind, even though most people will never see one in their lifetime despite a range covering most of the United States and many localities in other countries as well. This infamous arachnid is one of several species of widow spiders (*Lactrodectus* spp.) similar in body shape and size. They have similar life cycles as well; the female lays approximately 250 eggs that hatch within several weeks. Most black widow spider bites are from females. The adult black widow, both male and female, has a jet black and rounded abdomen with two red or orange-yellowish triangular emaculations (markings) on the underside that form the characteristic hourglass shape. The Southern black widow spider is the most widespread in Florida. It is glossy black with the characteristic red hourglass on the underside of its abdomen. The other variants differ in coloration and the appearance of the hourglass. The spider is approximately 1.5 inches wide with spread legs. It builds webs outdoors in garages and sheds, outhouses, and woodpiles but sometimes indoors as well. *Lactrodectus* spiders are not aggressive.

Widow spider venom is neurotoxic, and envenomations result in a syndrome that develops within 1–2 hours after being bitten. Referred to as latrodectism, this syndrome is characterized by

- Pain first localized at the lymph nodes
- Nausea
- Abdominal muscle rigidity
- Generalized muscle contractions and cramps
- Hypertension
- Transient tachycardia
- Bradycardia
- Profuse sweating
- Oliguria

The bite of black widow spiders is minimally painful and may even go unnoticed until symptoms occur. Severe envenomations are frequently treated with antivenin, without which respiratory distress and even death may result. On a worldwide basis more deaths have been attributed to black widow spider bites than to any other species of spider. When one considers that a mature female black widow spider injects venom into the skin at a depth of about 0.1 mm and that the amount injected is about 0.02 mg, which is distributed in the human body, this makes the animal one of the most venomous creatures on the planet. For comparison, the Brazilian Wandering Spider injects approximately 1 to 2 mg of venom (Table 4.3).

**Table 4.3    Comparison of the Toxicity of Three Species of Spiders**

| Genus | Species | Common Name | LD$_{50}$ |
|---|---|---|---|
| Latrodectus | mactans | Black widow | 0.002 mg/kg |
| Loxosceles | reclusa | Brown recluse | 0.48 mg/kg |
| Phoneutria | bahiensis | Brazilian wandering spider | 0.00061–0.00157 mg/kg |

The black widow spider has been responsible for approximately 100 deaths reported in the United States from 1950 to 1990. Before the development of widow antivenin, approximately 5% of bites resulted in fatalities, which are rare today if medical treatment is promptly sought.

There are approximately a dozen species of recluse spiders of which the brown recluse, *Loxosceles reclusa,* is the most commonly encountered in the United States. The range of the *L. reclusa* in the United States is approximately the lower two-thirds of the country by the eastern three-fourths of the country. Bites of *Loxosceles* spiders found in South America are more serious in their consequences than their North American relatives.

The brown recluse ranges in color from tan to dark brown and is approximately an inch in length with long (~1.5") thin legs. The most distinguishing characteristic of the spider is a violin-shaped emaculation behind the three pairs of semicircularly arranged eyes. The neck of the violin points toward the abdomen. The spider has also been popularly referred to as the "violin" or "fiddleback spider." They are essentially nonaggressive and slow moving; however, if disturbed they may bite. Typically, the spiders are found both inside and outside of buildings in dark, quiet, undisturbed places, especially where things are stored, such as in the attic.

The venom of the recluse spider can produce significant and sometimes life-threatening tissue destruction, beginning at the site of envenomation and extending outward and downward into deeper tissues. The bite is slightly painful, but over the course of several hours severe pain at the site of an envenomation occurs, radiating outward to surrounding tissue. For such a relatively small creature, the extent of tissue necrosis is astounding. The medical condition that results is referred to as *loxoscelism*, which describes the local and systemic effects of this type of envenomation. Recluse spider venom is cytotoxic and hemolytic. About a dozen components make up this complex mixture, including the protein sphingomyelinase D, which is largely responsible for the extensive tissue damage. Over the course of 24 hours, a central vesicle appears at the center of the bite with hemorrhagic tissue radiating outward, giving a "bull's-eye" appearance to the lesion. Medical treatment includes tissue debridement and supportive measures for infection and pain. Deep tissue involvement of connective tissue and muscles can result from envenomation, which may require the attention of a wound care specialist and tissue grafting.

## Scorpions

Scorpion venom is generally neurotoxic and interferes with neurotransmission. Although most species are relatively harmless to humans in that their stings produce local pain and perhaps swelling or numbness, several species in the Buthidae family can be dangerous to humans. The "death stalker," *Leiurus quinquestriatus,* has potent venom that has resulted in fatalities. Other species, such as *Androctonus, Parabuthus,* and *Tityus,* also have potent venoms. Scorpion envenomations usually do not deliver enough venom to kill a healthy adult, and most reported fatalities have occurred in the young, elderly, or individuals with illnesses such as cardiac conduction abnormalities.

## Hymenopterans

These stinging insects can produce envenomations that can be painful and produce local tissue injury; however, the amount of venom from single stings is essentially insufficient to produce systemic toxicity. This, of course, is not the case for individuals who are allergic to certain insect venom. In this case even a single sting from a bee, for example, may result in a life-threatening anaphylactic response.

There have been very unfortunate instances where individuals have received multiple envenomations from members of a colony of insects (e.g., bees, yellow jackets) that have resulted in severe nonimmunologically mediated toxicity and sometimes death. The toxicities of venoms from a number of species are provided in Table 4.4.

## Cnidarians

The Phylum Cnidaria comprises jellyfish, hydroids, corals, and anemones. They are structurally simple radially symmetrical animals. They are referred to as polyps if they are attached to a substrate and medusas if in the free-swimming state. Their venom apparatus is the nematocyst that contains a coiled thread-like structure with a skin-piercing barb on the end. Even when dead they are capable of discharge upon chemical or mechanical stimulation.

The Box Jellyfish, *Chironex Fleckeri,* may have upward of 60 tentacles, each with 5,000 nematocysts. The tentacles can detach onto the skin and the nematocysts discharge. The venom requires immediate treatment with an antivenin or the encounter may be fatal. The stings of a Box Jellyfish are considered so excruciating that victims are in danger of going into shock and drowning before they can reach medical attention. The stings of jellyfish in this family should be treated immediately by dousing the affected area with vinegar and applying ice packs. The vinegar has no analgesic properties; it reduces further nematocyst discharges.

The Portuguese Man-of-War (*Physalia*), or Bluebottle, is a colony of four distinct types of polyps, each with a specialized function. Stings from this animal require slightly different first

**Table 4.4**    Examples of Hymenopterans and Toxicity of Their Venoms

| Family | Common Name | Species | $LD_{50}$ (mg/kg) |
|---|---|---|---|
| Apidae | Honey bee | *Apis mellifera* | 2.8 |
| Mutillidae | Velvet ant | *Dasymutilla klugii* | 71 |
| Vespidae | Paper wasp | *Polistes canadensis* | 2.4 |
| Vespidae | Yellow jacket | *Vespula squamosa* | 3.5 |
| Formicidae | Harvester ants (fire ants) | *Pogonomyrmex* spp. | 0.66 |

aid than that of the Box Jellyfish. In the case of a Man-of-War, the tentacles should be gently tweezed out of the victim to prevent further firing of nematocysts. Neither vinegar nor ice is recommended for Man-of-War injuries. The remaining members of Cnidaria include sponges, corals, and anemones. Anemone stings may resemble those of *Physalia*, and treatment should begin with nematocyst removal followed by palliative measures.

## Mollusks

There are two species of blue-ringed octopus, *Hapalochlaena lunulata* and *Hapalochlaena maculosa*, differing in size and distribution. They share the ability to painlessly kill a human within 5 minutes. They inject paralytic neuromuscular venom that contains both maculotoxin and tetrodotoxin. Both block nerve conduction by interfering with sodium channels. There is no known antidote. The octopi are capable of delivering one of two venoms that differ markedly in strength. They possess two poison glands, each as large as their brain. One gland contains mild toxin reserved for prey, whereas the other contains a vastly more potent toxin used for defense.

The bivalve mollusks are associated with toxicities related to their consumption. Shellfish poisonings are usually classified as

- Amnesic shellfish poisoning
- Diarrheic shellfish poisoning
- Neurotoxic shellfish poisoning
- Paralytic shellfish poisoning

Amnesic shellfish poisoning is caused by the unusual amino acid, domoic acid, as the contaminant of shellfish from its filter feeding of dinoflagellates and other algae. Both gastrointestinal and neurological symptoms occur within 2 days after the consumption of contaminated organisms. Symptoms include nausea, vomiting, diarrhea, confusion, seizure, and short-term memory loss (hence the designation amnesic shellfish poisoning). Outbreaks have resulted in several deaths, such as the one in 1987 on Prince Edward Island in Canada where 156 cases occurred from eating contaminated mussels (3 deaths and 12 cases of permanent short-term memory loss).

Diarrheic shellfish poisoning results from the consumption of mollusks feeding on algae, such as *Dinophysis* and *Prorocentrum* spp. These algae produce the toxin okadaic acid and its derivatives. The onset of symptoms occurs within minutes to several hours after consumption of contaminated shellfish. Symptoms include nausea, abdominal pains, headache, fever, and diarrhea. The poisoning lasts approximately 2–3 days without any apparent lasting effects.

Neurotoxic shellfish poisoning occurs when bivalves accumulate brevetoxins from the dinoflagellate *Karenia brevis*. The toxins produce gastrointestinal and neurological symptoms in humans that are not life-threatening within minutes to hours. Symptoms include vomiting; diarrhea; muscle aches; dizziness, numbness and tingling about the lips, tongue, and throat; and a reversal of the sensations of hot and cold. These symptoms may last for several days.

Paralytic shellfish poisoning results from the consumption of shellfish that feed on species of algae such as *Alexandrium, Pyrodinium,* and *Gymnodinium*. The onset of symptoms occurs 1–2 hours after consumption of contaminated shellfish and includes symptoms such as numbness, tingling, difficulty speaking, and difficulty breathing that may require clinical respiratory support over the course of 12 to 24 hours. The potent neurotoxin, saxitoxin, is primarily responsible for the illness.

Some species of cone snails are responsible for the recorded deaths of several dozen humans. When curious individuals pick them up, the snails fire a harpoon-like tongue that pierces the skin. A species, *Conus geographus,* is known colloquially as the "cigarette snail" in the belief that the victim often has only a short time to live after envenomation. Symptoms of a cone snail sting can start immediately or can be delayed in onset for days. Symptoms include intense pain, numbness and tingling, swelling, and muscle paralysis that can lead to death if appropriate supportive measures are not taken. Life support in cases of severe envenomation remains the only option until such time as the venom is metabolized and eliminated by the individual. There is no antivenin.

A number of peptides that have been isolated from cone snails may show promise as potent pain-killing drugs. The first painkiller, Ziconotide, derived from cone snail toxins was approved by the U.S. Food and Drug Administration in December 2004.

## Amphibians

More than 100 toxins have been identified in the skin secretions of poison dart frogs, especially *Dendrobates* and *Phyllobates*. These brightly colored and commonly found frogs are also known as "poison dart" or "poison arrow" frogs; however, only members of the genus *Phyllobates* produce the extremely potent neurotoxin, batrachotoxin, and its derivatives. *Phyllobates terribilis* contains the highly toxic steroidal alkaloid, batrachotoxin, which has been used by native South American tribes for hunting purposes. Tribe members treat their blowgun darts by dipping the tips in the secretions of the skin of the frog. When these darts pierce the skin of prey, they quickly become paralyzed and can be captured.

The toxin may be derived from the metabolism of chemicals obtained through the frog's diet of primarily insects because when these wild frogs are brought into captivity and fed nonindigenous insects, they lose their toxicity. The toxin is sufficiently potent that if a human was to lick the skin on the back of the frog, a lethal dose of toxin could be absorbed. It has been estimated that a lethal dose for an average adult male can be lower than 50 µg.

The mechanism of action of batrachotoxin is similar to that of tetrodotoxin; however, it is 10 times as potent. Tetrodotoxin is also produced from some amphibian species, for example, the California newt, *Taricha torosa*.

Some toads produce biogenic amines like epinephrine and norepinephrine that can have effects on the cardiovascular system. Some toads of the family Bufonidae produce a toxin known as bufotoxin that has effects similar to those of digitalis. Other species in this family produce indolalkamines like bufotenin, a potent hallucinogen. The practice of "frog licking" to get high has resulted in some individuals being hospitalized due to severe hallucinations.

## Reptiles

Snakes have historically enjoyed a fearsome mythology; however, most snakes shun human contact and reserve attack for predation and defense. There are close to 3,500 species of snakes worldwide, approximately 400 of which can be considered dangerous to humans. Venomous snakes fall into six families:

- Elapidae (cobras, kraits, mambas, and coral snakes)
- Hydrophiidae (sea snakes)
- Laticaudidae (sea kraits)
- Viperidae (Old World vipers and adders)
- Colubridae (boomslang and keelback)
- Crotalidae (rattlesnakes, water moccasins, copperheads, and bushmasters)

The United States is home to more than 20 species of venomous snakes; all but three states (Alaska, Hawaii, and Maine) have at least one indigenous species. Venomous snakes native to the United States belong to either the New World Crotalidae or Elapidae families. The majority are crotalids, primarily rattlesnakes, water moccasins, and copperheads. The largest and most dangerous of American snakes is the Diamondback Rattlesnake. It can be recognized by the distinctive pattern of yellow-bordered diamond-shaped markings on the back. The tail is a rattling mechanism of brittle, button-shaped, horny growth. The arrow-shaped head is much wider than the neck. They may commonly be found in flatlands, pine woods, abandoned fields, and brushy, treed, or grassy areas. The Pigmy Rattlesnake, or "ground rattler," normally measures less than 18 inches in length. The body is grayish in color, with several rows of rounded dusky spots, often with a bit of reddish color along the midline of the back, near the head. This species is found in areas of pine and wiregrass but may be found in almost any locality where there are lakes, ponds, or marshes.

The Cottonmouth (water moccasin) is always found near water such as stream banks, river swamps, and lake margins. The color pattern of the body is variable and may be olive, brownish, or blackish. The body is stout for the length, the tail abruptly tapers, the broad head is much wider than the neck, and the mouth has a whitish interior lining—hence the name "cottonmouth."

The coral snake belongs to the *Elapidae* family. The coral snake normally measures less than 24 inches and is brightly colored with red, black, and yellow bands. It has a black nose, and there are no red rings on the tail portion of the body. The band of color in the coral snake is always in sequence of black, yellow, and red. The coral snake is a small slender-bodied species that prefers damp areas, living around rotting logs, old lumber piles, leaf mold, and piles of decaying vegetation.

Snake venom is a form of modified saliva whose potency and effect vary between both species and individuals. Venoms can be broadly classified as hemotoxic, cytotoxic, or neurotoxic depending on the damage elicited by envenomation. Hemotoxic venoms affect the heart and cardiovascular system, cytotoxic venoms produce local damage, and neurotoxic venoms damage the brain and nervous system. Most venom triggers more than one type of damage. The venom of proteroglyphous snakes such as the Elapidae is neurotoxic, and death results from respiratory suppression. The venom of Viperidae is hemotoxic and cytotoxic so it elicits both local and systemic damage. The neurotoxic venom of the Laticaudidae and Hydrophiidae families is extremely dangerous. Most of the snakes in the Colubridae family are not venomous. The Boomslang is an exception; its hemotoxic venom is quite potent.

Snake venom is an incredibly complex mixture of proteins, peptides, inorganic cations, and small amounts of metals. Venoms may also contain lipids, carbohydrates, biogenic amines, and amino acids. The polypeptides found in snake venoms are low-molecular-weight proteins without enzymatic activity; like venom, they can be classified as hemotoxic, cytotoxic, and neurotoxic. The typical snake venom consists of at least 25 different enzymes. Arginine ester hydrolase; collagenase; phospholipases A, B, and C; phosphomonoesterase; phosphodiesterase; and hyaluronidase are among the most important proteolytic enzymes commonly found in snake venom. 5'-Nucleotidase, L-amino oxidase, and phosphodiesterase are among the few enzymes found in the venom of all poisonous snakes. The effects of some common enzymes are seen in Table 4.5.

Most damaging effects are the result of proteolytic enzyme activity. They catalyze the breakdown of proteins integral to membrane and tissue integrity. There can be more than one proteolytic enzyme in a snake's venom; they include peptide hydrolases, proteases, peptidases, and proteinases. Phospholipase A hydrolyzes phospholipids, the primary components of biological membranes. The resultant membrane breakdown releases membrane-bound compounds such as amino acid oxidase, lactate dehydrogenase, phosphatase, phosphodiesterase, acetylcholinesterase, and NAD nucleotidase. The presence of RNase and DNase 5'-nucleotidase leads to RNA and DNA degradation.

Crotalid venom is rich in proteolytic enzyme activity. Viperids have significantly less and elapids have almost none. This correlates with the levels of tissue destruction associated with envenomation by snakes from each family. Thrombin-like enzymes are distributed in the same fashion as proteolytic enzymes, with the most found in crotalids and the least in elapids. *In vitro,* these enzymes convert fibrinogen to fibrin and promote clot formation. Hypotension and shock are the primary cause for mortality in crotalid bites. There is a paradoxic effect observed *in vivo* with thrombin-like enzymes acting as defibrinating agents.

**Table 4.5**   Common Snake Venom Enzymes and Their Effects

| Enzyme | Effect |
| --- | --- |
| Phosphodiesterase | Acts as exonucleotidase, decreases blood pressure, interferes with cardiac function |
| Collagenase | Digests collagen (principal protein of the skin, tendons, cartilage, bone, and connective tissue) |
| Hyaluronidase (also referred to as "the spreading factor") | Hydrolyzes mucopolysaccharides, such as hyaluronic acid, increasing viscosity of connective tissues by increasing tissue permeability, thought to be related to edema |
| Phospholipase | Hydrolyzes phospholipids, membrane breakdown |
| Arginine ester hydrolase | Hydrolyzes peptide or ester linkages, may be responsible for bradykinin release |
| Thrombin-like enzymes (crotalase, ancrod, batroxobin) | Prevents thrombin formation |
| Acetylcholinesterase | Causes paralysis |

The first antivenin was described more than 100 years ago. Antivenins are physiological antidotes that counter the effects without changing the properties of the venom. Horses or sheep are exposed to graduated doses of venom until they become hyperimmunized. The animal's blood is then drawn, the serum is removed, and the blood is reinfused. The serum obtained is refined for release into humans; the finished product contains immunoglobulins digested by pepsin to isolate the antigen capable of neutralizing the venom. The fact that the antivenins are animal derived increases the potential for hypersensitivity reactions and anaphylaxis. There are several types of hypersensitivity reactions; type I is an immediate response caused by antigen-IgE cross-linking on mast cells and basophils, whereas type III is a delayed onset serum sickness that is largely limited to diffuse inflammatory responses.

The complexity of snake venom hinders the development of an effective polyvalent antivenin. A "cocktail" of antivenins can be used against a broad range of venoms; however, the addition of each antivenin decreases the overall efficacy of the sera. Although antivenins exist for the majority of snake venom, it is not always the treatment of choice. For example, compression bandages are favored for neurotoxic venoms such as that of the coral snake and other elapids. There is some disagreement among physicians regarding viper bites. The venom is cytotoxic so the local damage may be magnified by compression bandages, but this can be seen as preferable to systemic damage. Hypotension and shock are the primary causes for mortality in crotalid bites; swift administration of intravenous fluids can prevent death if given in sufficient quantity.

## Bibliography

Ascenzi, P., Polticelli, F., & Visca, P. (2003). *Bacterial, plant & animal toxins.* Kerala, India: Scientific Research Flash.

*A small dose of toxin.* Retrieved July 2005 from www.asmalldoseof.org/toxicology/an_pl_toxin.php.

Atheris Laboratories. Retrieved July 2005 from http://www.atheris.ch/ven_data1.htm.

Baden, D. G. (1983). Marine food-borne dinoflagellate toxins. *International Review of Cytology, 82,* 99–150.

Baden, D. G., & Mende, T. J. (1982). Toxicity of two toxins from the Florida red tide marine dinoflagellate, *Gymnodinium breve. Toxicon, 20,* 457–461.

Blum, M. S. (1981). *Chemical defenses in arthropods.* New York: Academic Press.

Bryson, P. D. (Ed.). (1996). Mushrooms. In *Comprehensive review in toxicology for emergency clinicians* (3rd ed., pp. 685–693). New York: Taylor & Francis.

Cohen, S. G., & Bianchine, P. J. (1995). Hymenoptera, hypersensitivity, and history: A prologue to current day concepts and practices in the diagnosis, treatment, and prevention of insect sting allergy. *Annals of Allergy, Asthma, & Immunology, 74,* 198–217.

*Dangers on the reef.* Retrieved July 2005 from http://www.barrierreefaustralia.com/the-great-barrier-reef/blueringedoctopus.htm.

*Desert USA.* Retrieved July 2005 from http://www.desertusa.com/oct96/du_scorpion.html.

Diaz, J. H. (2004). The global epidemiology, syndromic classification, management, and prevention of spider bites. *American Journal of Tropical Medicine and Hygiene, 71*(2), 239–250.

*For goodness snakes! Treating and preventing venomous bites.* Retrieved July 2005 from http://www.fda.gov/FDAC/features/995_snakes.html.

Franz, D. R., & LeClaire, R. D. (1989). Respiratory effects of brevetoxin and saxitoxin in awake guinea pigs. *Toxicon I, 27,* 647–654.

Gill, D. M. (1982). Bacterial toxins: A table of lethal amounts. *Microbiological Reviews, 46,* 86–94.

Keeler, R. F., & Tu, A. T. (Eds.) (1991). *Toxicology of plant and fungal compounds.* New York: Marcel Dekkar.

Klaassen, C. D. (2001). *Casarett & Doull's toxicology. The basic science of poisons.* New York: McGraw-Hill.

Klaassen, C. D., & Watkins, J. B. (2003). *Casarett & Doull's essentials of toxicology.* New York: McGraw-Hill.

Lampe, K. F., & McCann, M. A. (1985). *AMA handbook of poisonous and injurious plants.* Chicago: American Medical Association.

Lindstrom, M., & Korkeala, H. (2006). Laboratory diagnostics of botulism. *Clinical Microbiology Reviews, 19*(2), 298–314.

Pappas, G., Panagopoulou, P., Christou, L., & Akritidis, N. (2006). Category B potential bioterrorism agents: Bacteria, viruses, toxins, and foodborne and waterborne pathogens. *Infectious Disease Clinics of North America, 20*(2), 395–421.

Pierce, R. H., Henry, M. S., Proffitt, L. S., & Hasbrouck, P. A. (1990). Red tide toxin (brevetoxin) enrichment in marine aerosol. In E. Graneli, S. Sundstron, L. Elder, & D. M. Anderson, Eds.), Toxic marine phytoplankton: Proceedings of the Fourth International Conference on Toxic Marine Phytoplankton. New York: Elsevier.

*Poisonous animals.* Retrieved July 2005 from http://www.vency.com/poisonousanimals.html.

Rochat, H., & Martin-Eauclaire, M. F. (Eds.) (2000). *Animal toxins: Facts and protocols.* New York: Birkhauser Verlag.

Schmidt, J. O. (1982). Biochemistry of insect venoms. *Annual Review of Entomology, 27,* 339–368.

Schmidt, J. O. (1990). Hymenopteran venoms: Striving towards the ultimate defense against vertebrates. In D. L. Evans and J. O. Schmidt (Eds.), *Insect defenses: adaptive mechanisms and strategies of prey and predators* (pp. 387–419). Albany, NY: SUNY Press.

Steidinger, K. A., & Baden, D. G. (1984). Toxic marine dinoflagellates. In D. L. Spector (Ed.), *Dinoflagellates* (pp. 201–261). New York: Academy Press.

Stocklin, G. (2006). *Handbook of animal toxins.* Hoboken, NJ: John Wiley & Sons.

Stocklin, R. (2004). *A handbook of animal toxins: Peptides and proteins.* Hoboken, NJ: John Wiley & Sons.

*U.S. FDA CFSAN bad bug book.* Retrieved July 2005 from http://www.cfsan.fda.gov/~mow/saxitoxn.html.

U.S. National Library of Medicine, National Institutes of Health, Environmental Health, and Toxicology Specialized Information Services (SIS). (2005). *Toxicology Tutorial III.* Retrieved July 2005 from http://www.sis.nlm.nih.gov/enviro/toxtutor.html.

# CHAPTER 5

# Environmental Pollutants and Their Fate

The environment in which we live contains a vast multitude of chemical agents that affect not only our species, but many others as well. We are a part of the ecology; although we like to view ourselves as being insulated from it, we must recognize that all the components of the environment are necessary for our continued survival as a species on this delicately balanced rock called planet Earth. A relatively new discipline of toxicology, ecotoxicology, can be viewed as a study of the harmful effects of chemicals on ecosystems. It deals with the delivery, transport, transformation, and effects of pollutants on the physical environment and on the species that live here. Pollutants enter into ecosystems through discharges into the atmosphere, contamination of land, and entry into water.

Central to this discipline is the recognition that a multidisciplinary approach to the problems of solving environmental issues is fundamental. Clearly, human activities (including the discharge of environmental pollutants) have had a negative effect on plant and animal species globally. Thousands of species are currently recognized as being endangered or threatened (Table 5.1), and their loss would be a tragic occurrence, especially when human activities are a significant contributing factor. Chemical pollution has been linked to

- Loss of parental attention in birds
- Decreased fertility in invertebrates, fish, reptiles, birds, and mammals
- Decreased hatching success in fish, turtles, and birds

- Abnormal thyroid function in birds and mammals
- Feminization in males and masculinization in females in birds, fish, and invertebrates
- Altered immune function in birds and mammals

Environmental engineers, epidemiologists, chemists, toxicologists, and others must work with government officials and the public to determine and develop the best rational management approaches and their implementation in dealing with environmental issues. The goal, of course, is to develop methods and approaches to better preserve the natural structure and function of our delicately balanced biosphere.

**Table 5.1    Examples of Threatened (T) or Endangered (E) Animal Species**

| Common Name | Scientific Name | Species Group | Range | Listing Status |
|---|---|---|---|---|
| Abalone, white | *Haliotis sorenseni* | Snails | North America | E |
| Acornshell, southern | *Epioblasma othcaloogensis* | Clams | U.S.A. (AL, GA, TN) | E |
| Addax | *Addax nasomaculatus* | Mammals | North Africa | E |
| Akepa, Hawaii (honeycreeper) | *Loxops coccineus coccineus* | Birds | U.S.A. (HI) | E |
| Akepa, Maui (honeycreeper) | *Loxops coccineus ochraceus* | Birds | U.S.A. (HI) | E |
| Akialoa, Kauai (honeycreeper) | *Hemignathus procerus* | Birds | U.S.A. (HI) | E |
| Akiapola`au (honeycreeper) | *Hemignathus munroi* | Birds | U.S.A. (HI) | E |
| Ala balik (trout) | *Salmo platycephalus* | Fishes | Turkey | E |
| Albatross, Amsterdam | *Diomedia amsterdamensis* | Birds | Indian Ocean, Amsterdam Island | E |
| Albatross, short-tailed | *Phoebastria (=Diomedea) albatrus* | Birds | North Pacific Ocean and Bering Sea, Canada, China, Japan, Mexico, Russia, Taiwan, U.S.A. (AK, CA, HI, OR, WA) | E |
| Alethe, Thyolo | *Alethe choloensis* | Birds | Malawi, Mozambique | E |

**Table 5.1    Examples of Threatened (T) or Endangered (E) Animal Species (continued)**

| Common Name | Scientific Name | Species Group | Range | Listing Status |
|---|---|---|---|---|
| Alligator, American | *Alligator mississippiensis* | Reptiles | Southeastern U.S.A. | T |
| Alligator, Chinese | *Alligator sinensis* | Reptiles | China | E |
| Ambersnail, Kanab | *Oxyloma haydeni kanabensis* | Snails | U.S.A. (AZ, UT) | E |
| Amphipod, Hay's Spring | *Stygobromus hayi* | Crustaceans | U.S.A. (DC) | E |
| Amphipod, Illinois cave | *Gammarus acherondytes* | Crustaceans | U.S.A. (IL) | E |
| Amphipod, Kauai cave | *Spelaeorchestia koloana* | Crustaceans | U.S.A. (HI) | E |
| Amphipod, Noel's | *Gammarus desperatus* | Crustaceans | U.S.A. (NM) | E |
| Amphipod, Peck's cave | *Stygobromus (=Stygonectes) pecki* | Crustaceans | U.S.A. (TX) | E |
| Anoa, lowland | *Bubalus depressicornis* | Mammals | Indonesia | E |
| Anoa, mountain | *Bubalus quarlesi* | Mammals | Indonesia | E |
| Anole, Culebra Island giant | *Anolis roosevelti* | Reptiles | U.S.A. (PR, Culebra Island) | |
| Antelope, Tibetan | *Pantholops hodgsonii* | Mammals | China, India, Nepal | E |
| Antelope, giant sable | *Hippotragus niger variani* | Mammals | Angola | E |
| Argali | *Ovis ammon* | Mammals | Afghanistan, China, India, Kazakhstan, Kyrgyzstan, Mongolia, Nepal, Pakistan, Russia, Tajikistan, Uzbekistan | E, T |
| Armadillo, giant | *Priodontes maximus* | Mammals | Venezuela and Guyana to Argentina | E |
| Armadillo, pink fairy | *Chlamyphorus truncatus* | Mammals | Argentina | E |
| Ass, African wild | *Equus asinus* | Mammals | Somalia, Sudan, Ethiopia | E |
| Ass, Asian wild | *Equus hemionus* | Mammals | Southwestern and Central Asia | E |
| Avahi | *Avahi laniger* (entire genus) | Mammals | Malagasy Republic (=Madagascar) | E |
| Aye-aye | *Daubentonia madagascariensis* | Mammals | Malagasy Republic (=Madagascar) | E |
| Ayumodoki (loach) | *Hymenophysa curta* | Fishes | Japan | E |
| Babirusa | *Babyrousa babyrussa* | Mammals | Indonesia | E |
| Baboon, gelada | *Theropithecus gelada* | Mammals | Ethiopia | T |
| Bandicoot, barred | *Perameles bougainville* | Mammals | Australia | E |

*(continues)*

**Table 5.1**    Examples of Threatened (T) or Endangered (E) Animal Species (continued)

| Common Name | Scientific Name | Species Group | Range | Listing Status |
|---|---|---|---|---|
| Bandicoot, desert | *Perameles eremiana* | Mammals | Australia | E |
| Bandicoot, lesser rabbit | *Macrotis leucura* | Mammals | Australia | E |
| Bandicoot, pig-footed | *Chaeropus ecaudatus* | Mammals | Australia | E |
| Bandicoot, rabbit | *Macrotis lagotis* | Mammals | Australia | E |
| Bankclimber, purple (mussel) | *Elliptoideus sloatianus* | Clams | U.S.A. (AL, GA, FL) | T |
| Banteng | *Bos javanicus* | Mammals | Southeast Asia | E |
| Bat, Bulmer's fruit (=flying fox) | *Aproteles bulmerae* | Mammals | Papua New Guinea | E |
| Bat, bumblebee | *Craseonycteris thonglongyai* | Mammals | Thailand | E |
| Bat, gray | *Myotis grisescens* | Mammals | Central and Southeastern U.S.A. | E |
| Bat, Hawaiian hoary | *Lasiurus cinereus semotus* | Mammals | U.S.A. (HI) | E |
| Bat, Indiana | *Myotis sodalis* | Mammals | Eastern and Midwestern U.S.A | E |
| Bat, lesser long-nosed | *Leptonycteris curasoae yerbabuenae* | Mammals | U.S.A. (AZ, NM), Mexico, Central America | E |
| Bat, little Mariana fruit | *Pteropus tokudae* | Mammals | Western Pacific Ocean, U.S.A. (Guam) | E |
| Bat, Mariana fruit (=Mariana flying fox) | *Pteropus mariannus mariannus* | Mammals | Western Pacific Ocean, U.S.A. (GU, MP) | T |
| Bat, Mexican long-nosed | *Leptonycteris nivalis* | Mammals | U.S.A. (NM, TX), Mexico, Central America | E |
| Bat, Ozark big-eared | *Corynorhinus (=Plecotus) townsendii ingens* | Mammals | U.S.A. (MO, OK, AR) | E |
| Bat, Rodrigues fruit (=flying fox) | *Pteropus rodricensis* | Mammals | Indian Ocean, Rodrigues Island | E |
| Bat, Singapore roundleaf horseshoe | *Hipposideros ridleyi* | Mammals | Malaysia | E |
| Bat, Virginia big-eared | *Corynorhinus (=Plecotus) townsendii virginianus* | Mammals | U.S.A. (KY, NC, WV, VA) | E |
| Bean, Cumberland (pearlymussel) | *Villosa trabalis* | Clams | U.S.A. (AL, KY, TN, VA) | E |
| Bean, purple | *Villosa perpurpurea* | Clams | U.S.A. (TN, VA) | E |
| Bear, American black | *Ursus americanus* | Mammals | North America | T |

**Table 5.1**    Examples of Threatened (T) or Endangered (E) Animal Species (continued)

| Common Name | Scientific Name | Species Group | Range | Listing Status |
|---|---|---|---|---|
| Bear, Baluchistan | *Ursus thibetanus gedrosianus* | Mammals | Iran, Pakistan | E |
| Bear, brown | *Ursus arctos arctos* | Mammals | Palearctic | E |
| Bear, brown | *Ursus arctos pruinosus* | Mammals | China (Tibet) | E |
| Bear, grizzly | *Ursus arctos horribilis* | Mammals | Holarctic | T |
| Bear, Louisiana black | *Ursus americanus luteolus* | Mammals | U.S.A. (LA, all counties; MS, all counties south of or touching a line from Greenville, Washington County, to Meridian, Lauderdale County; TX, all counties east of or touching a line from Linden, Cass County, SW to Bryan, Brazos County, thence SSW to Rockport, Aransas County) | T |
| Bear, Mexican grizzly | *Ursus arctos* | Mammals | Holarctic | E |
| Beaver (Mongolian) | *Castor fiber* ssp. *birulai* | Mammals | Mongolia | E |
| Beetle, American burying | *Nicrophorus americanus* | Insects | U.S.A. (eastern states south to FL, west to SD and TX), eastern Canada | E |
| Beetle, Coffin Cave mold | *Batrisodes texanus* | Insects | U.S.A. (TX) | E |
| Beetle, Comal Springs dryopid | *Stygoparnus comalensis* | Insects | U.S.A. (TX) | E |
| Beetle, Comal Springs riffle | *Heterelmis comalensis* | Insects | U.S.A. (TX) | E |
| Beetle, delta green ground | *Elaphrus viridis* | Insects | U.S.A. (CA) | T |
| Beetle, Helotes mold | *Batrisodes venyivi* | Insects | U.S.A. (TX) | E |
| Beetle, Hungerford's crawling water | *Brychius hungerfordi* | Insects | U.S.A. (MI, Canada) | E |
| Beetle, Kretschmarr Cave mold | *Texamaurops reddelli* | Insects | U.S.A. (TX) | E |
| Beetle, Mount Hermon June | *Polyphylla barbata* | Insects | U.S.A. (CA) | E |

*(continues)*

**Table 5.1**     Examples of Threatened (T) or Endangered (E) Animal Species (continued)

| Common Name | Scientific Name | Species Group | Range | Listing Status |
|---|---|---|---|---|
| Beetle, Tooth Cave ground | *Rhadine persephone* | Insects | U.S.A. (TX) | E |
| Beetle, valley elderberry longhorn | *Desmocerus californicus dimorphus* | Insects | U.S.A. (CA) | T |
| Bison, wood | *Bison bison athabascae* | Mammals | Canada, northwestern U.S.A | E |
| Blackbird, yellow-shouldered | *Agelaius xanthomus* | Birds | U.S.A. (PR) | E |
| Blindcat, Mexican (catfish) | *Prietella phreatophila* | Fishes | Mexico | E |
| Blossom, green (pearlymussel) | *Epioblasma torulosa gubernaculum* | Clams | U.S.A. (TN, VA) | E |
| Blossom, tubercled (pearlymussel) | *Epioblasma torulosa torulosa* | Clams | U.S.A. (AL, IL, IN, KY, TN, WV) | E, T |
| Blossom, turgid (pearlymussel) | *Epioblasma turgidula* | Clams | U.S.A. (AL, TN) | E, T |
| Blossom, yellow (pearlymussel) | *Epioblasma florentina florentina* | Clams | U.S.A. (AL, TN) | E, T |
| Boa, Jamaican | *Epicrates subflavus* | Reptiles | Jamaica | E |
| Boa, Mona | *Epicrates monensis monensis* | Reptiles | U.S.A. (PR) | T |
| Boa, Puerto Rican | *Epicrates inornatus* | Reptiles | U.S.A. (PR) | E |
| Boa, Round Island bolyeria | *Bolyeria multocarinata* | Reptiles | Indian Ocean, Mauritius | E |
| Boa, Round Island casarea | *Casarea dussumieri* | Reptiles | Indian Ocean, Mauritius | E |
| Boa, Virgin Islands tree | *Epicrates monensis granti* | Reptiles | U.S.A. (PR), British Virgin Islands | E |
| Bobcat, Mexican | *Lynx (=Felis) rufus escuinapae* | Mammals | Central Mexico | E |
| Bobwhite, masked (quail) | *Colinus virginianus ridgwayi* | Birds | U.S.A. (AZ), Mexico (Sonora) | E |
| Bontebok | *Damaliscus pygarus (=dorcas) dorcas* | Mammals | South Africa | E |
| Bonytongue, Asian | *Scleropages formosus* | Fishes | Thailand, Indonesia, Malaysia | E |
| Booby, Abbott's | *Papasula (=Sula) abbotti* | Birds | Indian Ocean, Christmas Island | E |
| Bristlebird, western | *Dasyornis longirostris (=brachypterus l.)* | Birds | Australia | E |

**Table 5.1**     Examples of Threatened (T) or Endangered (E) Animal Species (continued)

| Common Name | Scientific Name | Species Group | Range | Listing Status |
|---|---|---|---|---|
| Bristlebird, western rufous | *Dasyornis broadbenti littoralis* | Birds | Australia | E |
| Bulbul, Mauritius olivaceous | *Hypsipetes borbonicus olivaceus* | Birds | Indian Ocean, Mauritius | E |
| Bullfinch, Sao Miguel (finch) | *Pyrrhula pyrrhula murina* | Birds | Eastern Atlantic Ocean, Azores | E |
| Bush-shrike, Ulugura | *Malaconotus alius* | Birds | Tanzania | T |
| Bushwren, New Zealand | *Xenicus longipes* | Birds | New Zealand | E |
| Bustard, great Indian | *Ardeotis (=Choriotis) nigriceps* | Birds | India, Pakistan | E |
| Butterfly, bay checkerspot | *Euphydryas editha bayensis* | Insects | U.S.A. (CA) | T |
| Butterfly, Behren's silverspot | *Speyeria zerene behrensii* | Insects | U.S.A. (CA) | E |
| Butterfly, callippe silverspot | *Speyeria callippe callippe* | Insects | U.S.A. (CA) | E |
| Butterfly, Corsican swallowtail | *Papilio hospiton* | Insects | Corsica, Sardinia | E |
| Butterfly, El Segundo blue | *Euphilotes battoides allyni* | Insects | U.S.A. (CA) | E |
| Butterfly, Fender's blue | *Icaricia icarioides fenderi* | Insects | U.S.A. (OR) | E |
| Butterfly, Homerus swallowtail | *Papilio homerus* | Insects | Jamaica | E |
| Butterfly, Karner blue | *Lycaeides melissa samuelis* | Insects | U.S.A. (IL, IN, MA, MI, MN, NH, NY, OH, PA, WI), Canada (Ont.) | E |
| Butterfly, Lange's metalmark | *Apodemia mormo langei* | Insects | U.S.A. (CA) | E |
| Butterfly, lotis blue | *Lycaeides argyrognomon lotis* | Insects | U.S.A. (CA) | E |
| Butterfly, Luzon peacock swallowtail | *Papilio chikae* | Insects | Philippines | E |
| Butterfly, mission blue | *Icaricia icarioides missionensis* | Insects | U.S.A. (CA) | E |
| Butterfly, Mitchell's satyr | *Neonympha mitchellii mitchellii* | Insects | U.S.A. (IN, MI, NJ, OH) | E |

*(continues)*

**Table 5.1** Examples of Threatened (T) or Endangered (E) Animal Species (continued)

| Common Name | Scientific Name | Species Group | Range | Listing Status |
|---|---|---|---|---|
| Butterfly, Myrtle's silverspot | *Speyeria zerene myrtleae* | Insects | U.S.A. (CA) | E |
| Butterfly, Oregon silverspot | *Speyeria zerene hippolyta* | Insects | U.S.A. (CA, OR, WA) | T |
| Butterfly, Palos Verdes blue | *Glaucopsyche lygdamus palosverdesensis* | Insects | U.S.A. (CA) | E |
| Butterfly, Queen Alexandra's birdwing | *Troides alexandrae* | Insects | Papua New Guinea | E |
| Butterfly, Quino checkerspot | *Euphydryas editha quino (=E. e. wrighti)* | Insects | U.S.A. (CA), Mexico | E |
| Butterfly, Saint Francis' satyr | *Neonympha mitchellii francisci* | Insects | U.S.A. (NC) | E |
| Butterfly, San Bruno elfin | *Callophrys mossii bayensis* | Insects | U.S.A. (CA) | E |
| Butterfly, Schaus swallowtail | *Heraclides aristodemus ponceanus* | Insects | U.S.A. (FL) | E |
| Butterfly, Smith's blue | *Euphilotes enoptes smithi* | Insects | U.S.A. (CA) | E |
| Butterfly, Uncompahgre fritillary | *Boloria acrocnema* | Insects | U.S.A. (CO) | E |
| Cahow | *Pterodroma cahow* | Birds | North Atlantic Ocean, Bermuda | E |
| Caiman, Apaporis River | *Caiman crocodilus apaporiensis* | Reptiles | Colombia | E |
| Caiman, black | *Melanosuchus niger* | Reptiles | Amazon basin | E |
| Caiman, broad-snouted | *Caiman latirostris* | Reptiles | Brazil, Argentina, Paraguay, Uruguay | E |
| Caiman, brown | *Caiman crocodilus fuscus (includes Caiman crocodilus chiapasius)* | Reptiles | Mexico, Central America, Colombia, Ecuador, Venezuela, Peru | T |
| Caiman, common | *Caiman crocodilus crocodilus* | Reptiles | Brazil, Colombia, Ecuador, French Guiana, Guyana, Suriname, Venezuela, Bolivia, Peru | T |
| Caiman, Yacare | *Caiman yacare* | Reptiles | Bolivia, Argentina, Peru, Brazil | T |

**Table 5.1** Examples of Threatened (T) or Endangered (E) Animal Species (continued)

| Common Name | Scientific Name | Species Group | Range | Listing Status |
|---|---|---|---|---|
| Camel, Bactrian | *Camelus bactrianus* | Mammals | Mongolia, China | E |
| Campeloma, slender | *Campeloma decampi* | Snails | U.S.A. (AL) | E |
| Caracara, Audubon's crested | *Polyborus plancus audubonii* | Birds | U.S.A. (AZ, FL, LA, NM, TX) south to Panama; Cuba | T |
| Caribou, woodland | *Rangifer tarandus caribou* | Mammals | U.S.A. (AK, ID, ME, MI, MN, MT, NH, VT, WA, WI), Canada | E |
| Cat, Andean | *Felis jacobita* | Mammals | Chile, Peru, Bolivia, Argentina | E |
| Cat, Asian golden (=Temmnick's) | *Catopuma (=Felis) temminckii* | Mammals | Nepal, China, Southeast Asia, Indonesia (Sumatra) | E |
| Cat, black-footed | *Felis nigripes* | Mammals | Southern Africa | E |
| Cat, flat-headed | *Prionailurus (=Felis) planiceps* | Mammals | Malaysia, Indonesia | E |
| Cat, Iriomote | *Prionailurus (=Felis) bengalensis iriomotensis* | Mammals | Japan (Iriomote Island, Ryukyu Islands) | E |
| Cat, leopard | *Prionailurus (=Felis) bengalensis bengalensis* | Mammals | India, Southeast Asia | E |
| Cat, marbled | *Pardofelis (=Felis) marmorata* | Mammals | Nepal, Southeast Asia, Indonesia | E |
| Cat, Pakistan sand | *Felis margarita scheffeli* | Mammals | Pakistan | E |
| Cat, tiger | *Leopardus (=Felis) tigrinus* | Mammals | Costa Rica to northern Argentina | E |
| Catfish | *Pangasius sanitwongsei* | Fishes | Thailand | E |
| Catfish, Thailand giantE | *Pangasianodon gigas* | Fishes | Thailand | |
| Catfish, Yaqui | *Ictalurus pricei* | Fishes | U.S.A. (AZ), Mexico | T |
| Catspaw (=purple cat's paw pearlymussel) | *Epioblasma obliquata obliquata* | Clams | U.S.A. (AL, IL, IN, KY, OH, TN) | E, T |
| Catspaw, white (pearlymussel) | *Epioblasma obliquata perobliqua* | Clams | U.S.A. (IN, MI, OH) | E |
| Cavefish, Alabama | *Speoplatyrhinus poulsoni* | Fishes | U.S.A. (AL) | E |
| Cavefish, Ozark | *Amblyopsis rosae* | Fishes | U.S.A. (AR, MO, OK) | T |
| Cavesnail, Tumbling Creek | *Antrobia culveri* | Snails | U.S.A. (MO) | E |
| Chamois, Apennine | *Rupicapra rupicapra ornata* | Mammals | Italy | E |

*(continues)*

**Table 5.1    Examples of Threatened (T) or Endangered (E) Animal Species (continued)**

| Common Name | Scientific Name | Species Group | Range | Listing Status |
|---|---|---|---|---|
| Cheetah | *Acinonyx jubatus* | Mammals | Africa to India | E |
| Chimpanzee | *Pan troglodytes* | Mammals | Africa; see 17.40(c)(3) | E |
| Chimpanzee, pygmy | *Pan paniscus* | Mammals | Zaire | E, T |
| Chinchilla | *Chinchilla brevicaudata boliviana* | Mammals | Bolivia | E |
| Chub, bonytail | *Gila elegans* | Fishes | U.S.A. (AZ, CA, CO, NV, UT, WY) | E |
| Chub, Borax Lake | *Gila boraxobius* | Fishes | U.S.A. (OR) | E |
| Chub, Chihuahua | *Gila nigrescens* | Fishes | U.S.A. (NM), Mexico (Chihuahua) | T |
| Chub, Gila | *Gila intermedia* | Fishes | U.S.A. (AZ, NM), Mexico | E |
| Chub, humpback | *Gila cypha* | Fishes | U.S.A. (AZ, CO, UT, WY) | E |
| Chub, Hutton tui | *Gila bicolor* ssp. | Fishes | U.S.A. (OR) | T |
| Chub, Mohave tui | *Gila bicolor mohavensis* | Fishes | U.S.A. (CA) | E |
| Chub, Oregon | *Oregonichthys crameri* | Fishes | U.S.A. (OR) | E |
| Chub, Owens tui | *Gila bicolor snyderi* | Fishes | U.S.A. (CA) | E |
| Chub, Pahranagat roundtail | *Gila robusta jordani* | Fishes | U.S.A. (NV) | E |
| Chub, slender | *Erimystax cahni* | Fishes | U.S.A. (TN, VA) | T |
| Chub, Sonora | *Gila ditaenia* | Fishes | U.S.A. (AZ), Mexico | T |
| Chub, spotfin | *Erimonax monachus* | Fishes | U.S.A. (AL, GA, NC, TN, VA) | T |
| Chub, Virgin River | *Gila seminuda (=robusta)* | Fishes | U.S.A. (AZ, NV, UT) | E |
| Chub, Yaqui | *Gila purpurea* | Fishes | U.S.A. (AZ), Mexico | E |
| Chuckwalla, San Esteban Island | *Sauromalus varius* | Reptiles | Mexico | E |
| Cicek (minnow) | *Acanthorutilus handlirschi* | Fishes | Turkey | E |
| Civet, Malabar large-spotted | *Viverra civettina (=megaspila c.)* | Mammals | India | E |
| Clubshell | *Pleurobema clava* | Clams | U.S.A. (AL, IL, IN, KY, MI, OH, PA, TN, WV) | E, T |
| Clubshell, black | *Pleurobema curtum* | Clams | U.S.A. (AL, MS) | E |
| Clubshell, ovate | *Pleurobema perovatum* | Clams | U.S.A. (AL, GA, MS, TN) | E |

**Table 5.1**    Examples of Threatened (T) or Endangered (E) Animal Species (continued)

| Common Name | Scientific Name | Species Group | Range | Listing Status |
|---|---|---|---|---|
| Clubshell, southern | Pleurobema decisum | Clams | U.S.A. (AL, GA, MS, TN) | E |
| Cochito | Phocoena sinus | Mammals | Mexico (Gulf of California) | E |
| Combshell, Cumberlandian | Epioblasma brevidens | Clams | U.S.A. (AL, KY, MS, TN, VA) | E, T |
| Combshell, southern | Epioblasma penita | Clams | U.S.A. (AL, MS) | E |
| Combshell, upland | Epioblasma metastriata | Clams | U.S.A. (AL, GA, TN) | E |
| Condor, Andean | Vultur gryphus | Birds | Colombia to Chile and Argentina | E |
| Condor, California | Gymnogyps californianus | Birds | U.S.A. (AZ, CA, OR), Mexico (Baja California) | E, T |
| Coot, Hawaiian | Fulica americana alai | Birds | U.S.A. (HI) | E |
| Coqui, golden | Eleutherodactylus jasperi | Amphibians | U.S.A. (PR) | T |
| Cotinga, banded | Cotinga maculata | Birds | Brazil | E |
| Cotinga, white-winged | Xipholena atropurpurea | Birds | Brazil | E |
| Crane, black-necked | Grus nigricollis | Birds | China (Tibet) | E |
| Crane, Cuba sandhill | Grus canadensis nesiotes | Birds | West Indies, Cuba | E |
| Crane, hooded | Grus monacha | Birds | Japan, Russia | E |
| Crane, Japanese | Grus japonensis | Birds | China, Japan, Korea, Russia | E |
| Crane, Mississippi sandhill | Grus canadensis pulla | Birds | U.S.A. (MS) | E |
| Crane, Siberian white | Grus leucogeranus | Birds | C.I.S. (Siberia) to India, including Iran and China | E |
| Crane, white-naped | Grus vipio | Birds | Mongolia | E |
| Crane, whooping | Grus americana | Birds | Canada, U.S.A. (Rocky Mountains east to Carolinas), Mexico | E, T |
| Crayfish, cave | Cambarus aculabrum | Crustaceans | U.S.A. (AR) | E |
| Crayfish, cave | Cambarus zophonastes | Crustaceans | U.S.A. (AR) | E |
| Crayfish, Nashville | Orconectes shoupi | Crustaceans | U.S.A. (TN) | E |
| Crayfish, Shasta | Pacifastacus fortis | Crustaceans | U.S.A. (CA) | E |
| Creeper, Hawaii | Oreomystis mana | Birds | U.S.A. (HI) | E |

*(continues)*

**Table 5.1**    Examples of Threatened (T) or Endangered (E) Animal Species (continued)

| Common Name | Scientific Name | Species Group | Range | Listing Status |
|---|---|---|---|---|
| Creeper, Molokai | *Paroreomyza flammea* | Birds | U.S.A. (HI) | E |
| Creeper, Oahu | *Paroreomyza maculata* | Birds | U.S.A. (HI) | E |
| Crocodile, African dwarf | *Osteolaemus tetraspis tetraspis* | Reptiles | West Africa | E |
| Crocodile, African slender-snouted | *Crocodylus cataphractus* | Reptiles | Western and Central Africa | E |
| Crocodile, American | *Crocodylus acutus* | Reptiles | U.S.A. (FL), Mexico, Caribbean, Central and South America | T |
| Crocodile, Ceylon mugger | *Crocodylus palustris kimbula* | Reptiles | Sri Lanka | E |
| Crocodile, Congo dwarf | *Osteolaemus tetraspis osborni* | Reptiles | Congo River drainage | E |
| Crocodile, Cuban | *Crocodylus rhombifer* | Reptiles | Cuba | E |
| Crocodile, Morelet's | *Crocodylus moreletii* | Reptiles | Mexico, Belize, Guatemala | E |
| Crocodile, mugger | *Crocodylus palustris palustris* | Reptiles | India, Pakistan, Iran, Bangladesh | E |
| Crocodile, Nile | *Crocodylus niloticus* | Reptiles | Africa, Middle East | T |
| Crocodile, Orinoco | *Crocodylus intermedius* | Reptiles | South America, Orinoco River basin | E |
| Crocodile, Philippine | *Crocodylus novaeguineae mindorensis* | Reptiles | Philippine Islands | E |
| Crocodile, saltwater | *Crocodylus porosus* | Reptiles | Southeast Asia, Australia, Papua New Guinea, Islands of the West Pacific Ocean | E, T |
| Crocodile, Siamese | *Crocodylus siamensis* | Reptiles | Southeast Asia, Malay Peninsula | E |
| Crow, Hawaiian (='alala) | *Corvus hawaiiensis* | Birds | U.S.A. (HI) | E |
| Crow, Mariana (=aga) | *Corvus kubaryi* | Birds | Western Pacific Ocean, U.S.A. (Guam, Rota) | E |
| Crow, white-necked | *Corvus leucognaphalus* | Birds | U.S.A. (PR), Dominican Republic, Haiti | E |
| Cuckoo-shrike, Mauritius | *Coquus typicus* | Birds | Indian Ocean, Mauritius | E |

**Table 5.1    Examples of Threatened (T) or Endangered (E) Animal Species (continued)**

| Common Name | Scientific Name | Species Group | Range | Listing Status |
|---|---|---|---|---|
| Cuckoo-shrike, Reunion | *Coquus newtoni* | Birds | Indian Ocean, Reunion | E |
| Cui-ui | *Chasmistes cujus* | Fishes | U.S.A. (NV) | E |
| Curassow, razor-billed | *Mitu mitu mitu* | Birds | Brazil (Eastern) | E |
| Curassow, red-billed | *Crax blumenbachii* | Birds | Brazil | E |
| Curassow, Trinidad white-headed | *Pipile pipile pipile* | Birds | West Indies, Trinidad | E |
| Curlew, Eskimo | *Numenius borealis* | Birds | Alaska and northern Canada to Argentina | E |
| Dace, Ash Meadows speckled | *Rhinichthys osculus nevadensis* | Fishes | U.S.A. (NV) | E |
| Dace, blackside | *Phoxinus cumberlandensis* | Fishes | U.S.A. (KY, TN) | T |
| Dace, Clover Valley speckled | *Rhinichthys osculus oligoporus* | Fishes | U.S.A. (NV) | E |
| Dace, desert | *Eremichthys acros* | Fishes | U.S.A. (NV) | T |
| Dace, Foskett speckled | *Rhinichthys osculus ssp.* | Fishes | U.S.A. (OR) | T |
| Dace, Independence Valley speckled | *Rhinichthys osculus lethoporus* | Fishes | U.S.A. (NV) | E |
| Dace, Kendall Warm Springs | *Rhinichthys osculus thermalis* | Fishes | U.S.A. (WY) | E |
| Dace, Moapa | *Moapa coriacea* | Fishes | U.S.A. (NV) | E |
| Darter, amber | *Percina antesella* | Fishes | U.S.A. (AL, GA, TN) | E |
| Darter, bayou | *Etheostoma rubrum* | Fishes | U.S.A. (MS) | T |
| Darter, bluemask (=jewel) | *Etheostoma* | Fishes | U.S.A. (TN) | E |
| Darter, boulder | *Etheostoma wapiti* | Fishes | U.S.A. (AL, TN) | E |
| Darter, boulder | *Etheostoma wapiti* | Fishes | U.S.A. (AL, TN) | E |
| Darter, Cherokee | *Etheostoma scotti* | Fishes | U.S.A. (GA) | T |
| Darter, duskytail | *Etheostoma percnurum* | Fishes | U.S.A. (TN, VA) | E |
| Darter, Etowah | *Etheostoma etowahae* | Fishes | U.S.A. (GA) | E |
| Darter, fountain | *Etheostoma fonticola* | Fishes | U.S.A. (TX) | E |
| Darter, goldline | *Percina aurolineata* | Fishes | U.S.A. (AL, GA, TN) | T |
| Darter, leopard | *Percina pantherina* | Fishes | U.S.A. (AR, OK) | T |
| Darter, Maryland | *Etheostoma sellare* | Fishes | U.S.A. (MD) | E |
| Darter, Niangua | *Etheostoma nianguae* | Fishes | U.S.A. (MO) | T |
| Darter, Okaloosa | *Etheostoma okaloosae* | Fishes | U.S.A. (FL) | E |

From http://ecos.fws.gov/tess_public/SpeciesReport.do?dsource=animals.

## Unfortunate Lessons Learned

Environmental pollutants can relocate from their original source through interface transport processes. An interface is that theoretical boundary between air and water, air and soil, and soil and water. Unfortunately, plants and animals are located in or on these compartments and form a biological interface as well that can be adversely affected. When we think about lessons learned in environmental toxicology, pesticides such as DDT may come to mind. DDT, or dichlorodiphenyltrichloroethane, is a chlorinated hydrocarbon that was developed in the 1930s by the chemist Paul Muller. DDT was a very effective insecticide and did not easily degrade in the environment. Effectiveness and persistence were deemed to be very favorable aspects for adopting its use on a global scale. Indeed, it became very popular during World War II, was instrumental in the reduction of such disease vectors as typhoid and malaria, and is responsible for saving millions of lives. After World War II, DDT was in wide use agriculturally in the United States and abroad because of its cost-effectiveness. Scientists feared its ubiquity would have long-term detrimental effects on wildlife with possible human ramifications. Rachel Carson eloquently described such a horror in her classic antichemical book, *Silent Spring,* in 1962. She helped launch the modern environmental movement when excerpts of her book, describing the potential long-lasting effects that this chemical may exact on birds, fish, and other wildlife in the environment, were published in *The New Yorker. Silent Spring* fueled public opinion against the continued use of this pesticide and was probably the single most important factor to establish public awareness of serious environmental issues.

Experimental studies suggested that DDT may produce reproductive, teratogenic, neurological, and other effects in laboratory animals. It has been implicated in eggshell thinning in raptors and song birds; however, the validity of some older studies has been questioned for failure to adequately assess contributing influences such as the effect of bird age, seasonal variations, and mineral deficiencies. A 1998 study asserted that eggshell thinning actually began 50 years before DDT was widely used.

Because DDT is very lipophilic, it is persistent in the body as well, being stored in adipose tissue, and has been shown to be present in breast milk as well. In 1972 the pesticide was essentially banned for use in the United States, but because of its persistence, due to a half-life in soil of greater than a decade, its effects on the biota continued. And although the U.S. Environmental Protection Agency (EPA) considers DDT a probable human carcinogen, 40 years of tireless scrutiny have failed to conclusively link DDT to a single cancer in humans.

An unfortunate consequence of DDT's withdrawal from the world market was a spike in global malaria infection rates. Today, malaria infects 300 to 500 million people annually; more than 2.7 million people, primarily children under 5, die from malaria each year. As a result, all but the most ardent anti-DDT activists have stepped back from the global ban to support the WHO in its call for limited reintroduction.

The infamous outbreak of mercury poisoning in 1956 among the residents of the Minamata Bay region on the island of Kyushu, Japan, resulted from exposure to high levels of methylmercury from fish and shellfish consumption. It was linked to a local plastics factory that was dumping mercury into the bay. The mercury was then biotransformed by microorganisms into its organic form, methylmercury. Many hundreds of people were affected so severely that they exhibited serious neurological problems such as difficulty walking, swallowing, speaking, and hearing. Examination of the brains from individuals who died revealed that many had a marked loss of brain weight and volume (brain atrophy). Children born to exposed mothers had a high rate of birth defects, including severe brain damage, mental impairment, and delayed development. The link to mercury was not immediately recognized, and exposures to manganese and selenium were first suspected until epidemiological experts were called on to investigate this tragedy. The link to mercury contamination then became clear. It resulted from the bioaccumulation of organic mercury in the marine food chain that was transferred to humans as the final consumers.

Many other unfortunate incidents have occurred from chemicals polluting our environment, and whether the risk to the environment is real or perceived to be real, one needs only to think about public perception when we hear "Love Canal" or "Times Beach" as examples. Public outcry can initiate great change. Hundreds of families were moved from Love Canal, and the Comprehensive Environmental Response, Compensation and Liability Act (CERCLA), commonly recognized as Superfund, was passed by Congress. This Act mandated the EPA to develop the National Priority List for toxic waste site cleanup and/or its remediation.

## Pollution versus Contamination

The commonly used terms *pollution/pollutants* and *contamination/contaminants* are chemical levels that are judged to be above those that would "normally" occur (pristine levels) in any particular component of the environment. The term *pollutant* is commonly taken to refer to any chemical as producing or having the potential to produce actual environmental harm, whereas the term *contaminant* has no implication of harmful. The EPA has categorized pollutants; however, the classification is redundant and allows one to place any specific chemical pollutant into more than one category:

- Agricultural Chemicals
- Air Pollutants
- Biological Contaminants
- Carcinogens
- Chemicals
- Extremely Hazardous Substances
- Microorganisms
- Radiation
- Soil Contaminants
- Toxic Substances (Persistent Bioaccumulative Toxic Pollutants, Persistent Organic Pollutants)
- Water Pollutants

*The Third National Report on Human Exposure to Environmental Chemicals* is part of a long-range biomonitoring project conducted by the Centers for Disease Control and Prevention at the National Center of Environmental Health (NCEH). The project attempts to identify and quantify exposure to 148 common environmental chemicals to which humans have been exposed. For the purpose of the study the NCEH defines an environmental chemical as "a compound or chemical element present in air, water, food, soil, dust, or other environmental media." Exposure was assessed by measuring the level of the chemical or its metabolite in serum and urine specimens collected from participants in the National Health and Nutrition Examination Survey. Simple detection of the chemical or its metabolite in the specimen was not causally linked to an adverse effect or disease.

The chemicals chosen for study had to meet several criteria; the cost and performance of the available analytical methods were a major consideration. Included in the biomonitoring were metals, polycyclic aromatic hydrocarbons (PAH), polychlorinated dibenzo-p-dioxins, polychlorinated dibenzofurans, polychlorinated biphenyls (PCBs), phthalates, organochlorine pesticides, organophosphate pesticides, herbicides, and carbamate insecticides. The Centers for Disease Control and Prevention solicited suggestions for new candidate chemicals for study in October 2002; they added 38 chemicals, including pyrethroids, additional phthalate metabolites, polycyclic aromatic hydrocarbons, dioxins, furans, and PCBs. In subsequent studies it will be possible to determine whether individuals are experiencing exposures to chemicals and their metabolites outside the baseline reference ranges established in the current study. Because this marks the first effort to develop a national exposure profile for some of these chemicals, there are no other numbers available. The report is not yet capable of analyzing the statistical significance of trends; that will be possible in the future with additional data.

The findings for each of the 148 chemicals in the report are summarized individually. The results are reported in both raw numbers and corrected for creatinine (for urine specimens) and total lipids (for serum specimens assaying lipophilic chemicals). Creatinine corrects for dilution in urine specimens, and lipid-corrected values for serum reflect the amount of chemical stored in body fat. The summaries contain general information about the properties of the substance, its method of action, known toxicity, common sources of exposure, reference ranges if known, exposure routes, and target organs. Additional discussion about demographic differences is provided when applicable. Almost without exception, each summary ends with a note advising that simply finding a detectable level of the chemical in question does not mean that the amount is sufficient to cause adverse health effects. We have seen, however, both acute and chronic adverse effects from many of these chemicals in other species in the environment and this, at least in part, is a rationale for continued monitoring of the public.

## The Environment Viewed as Compartments and Ecosystems

An ecosystem comprises populations and communities residing in a defined area. Ecosystems are aquatic (marine and freshwater) or terrestrial. They can be viewed as being composed of a number of compartments:

- An abiotic compartment (nonliving): contains air, water, soils, and sediments
- A biotic compartment (living): composed of animal and plant life

These compartments are complex and not homogeneous in nature. Movement of toxicants from one compartment to another is an important area of concern. One needs only to consider acid rain, which is the result of the movement of acidic chemicals from the atmosphere into rain that in turn finds its way into water and soil, or the movement of pesticides from the soil into bodies of water where it can affect aquatic plant and animal life. A toxicant such as mercury, for example, once released into the environment, can be distributed or partitioned into other compartments based on physical and chemical properties. Within a compartment a toxicant can enter into reactions that may alter its properties. The toxicant and any chemically altered forms of it may produce adverse responses in the organisms that not only reside within that compartment, but also to other organisms that depend on its resources.

## The Atmosphere

The atmosphere is composed of a number of layers that (from the lowest to the highest) are the troposphere, stratosphere, mesosphere, and thermosphere. Our principal concern is the troposphere, which extends from the surface of the earth to an altitude of about 10 km. Contained within the $3 \times 10^{15}$ tons of atmospheric air are also "trace amounts" of chemicals such as carbon monoxide, sulfur dioxide, hydrogen sulfide, nitric acid, ammonia, formaldehyde, lead, oxides of nitrogen, particulates, and many others that we recognize as pollutants. The troposphere contains most of the atmospheric water, and this is where we observe clouds, storms, and other conditions of weather. Contained in this region are the gases necessary to maintain life on this planet, in a mixture that we commonly referred to as air. Air contains about 78% nitrogen at about 21% oxygen by volume and also contains small amounts of hydrogen, helium, carbon dioxide, and methane as well as water, dust, and aerosols. The term *aerosol* is used to refer to particulate matter found in the atmosphere in the form of droplets. Aerosols can adsorb chemicals in the atmosphere such as metals, halogenated organics, and polycyclic aromatic hydrocarbons.

Most airborne pollutants are confined to the first several thousand feet of atmosphere; however, their distribution may not be uniform and may become more concentrated in the immediate zone of air that we breathe, which represents the distance between our feet and nose when vertical. These pollutant chemicals have been linked to contributing to either the development or the exacerbation of diseases including asthma, cardiovascular disease, and cancer.

Circumstances of weather can be especially important in affecting the local concentration of airborne toxicants. For example, during late fall and winter the temperature on land can fall faster than the air above, resulting in a thermal inversion. This reduces the rise of warm air through it, thus trapping pollutants, especially in the absence of wind activity.

### Fate of a Chemical in Air

The Toxics Release Inventory estimates that about half of atmospheric pollutants result directly from their input into the air from industrial discharges. Pollutants reach the atmosphere directly (e.g., emissions from industrial stacks, aerial application of pesticides) or through transport from other compartments. Airborne chemicals can enter into chemical reactions, such as oxidation and photolysis. This ability to enter into chemical reactions results in the production of other pollutants. For example, methane can be oxidized to carbon monoxide via its catalysis by oxides of nitrogen such as $NO_2$ and $NO$, which can then react with oxygen to produce ozone ($O_3$).

The fate of a chemical in the air depends on

- Input (e.g., rate, type of pollutant, source, etc.)
- Dispersion (e.g., mixing from the wind and turbulence)
- Transport (e.g., vertical and horizontal by wind)
- Reactions and formation of secondary pollutants (e.g., chemical reactions such as oxidation hydrolysis and photolysis and physical reactions such as absorption and adsorption)
- Removal (e.g., through precipitation)

An example of an undesirable movement of chemicals in air is pesticide spray drift. The EPA defines pesticide spray drift as the physical movement of a pesticide through air at the time of application or soon thereafter, *to any site other than that intended for application* (referred to as off-target). When pesticide solutions are sprayed by using ground equipment or aerially, droplets are produced, some of which are small enough to stay suspended in the air to be carried by the wind until they fall to the ground or contact another surface. Some examples of these surfaces might include children playing outdoors, farm workers, and wildlife! In estimating risk to populations from such activities, this is taken into consideration; although risk is minimal for most people, some sensitive people in the population may respond poorly. For example, during the Medfly eradication program in Florida in the 1990s, in which the organophosphate pesticide malathion was used in aerial spraying, there were reports of individuals with signs and symptoms consistent with the kinds of cholinergic effects produced by these types of pesticides (e.g., nausea, diarrhea).

## The Hydrosphere

Water covers approximately 70% of the surface of the earth. From the beginning of human civilization, water has provided humans with not only a chemical necessary for survival, but a source of nourishment and a means to travel from one place to another. Unique cultures have developed along oceans, rivers, and lakes. More than 50% of the population of the United States resides in cities surrounding seaports and lakes. The use of vast amounts of water has enabled us to thrive as an agricultural and industrial society.

Along with the activities of society comes the inevitable contamination of waters from manufacturing plant discharges, accidental chemical spills, domestic sewage, agricultural, urban and rural runoff, and atmospheric deposition. Chemical contaminants, once having reached water, can move within that medium because of water turbulence and diffusion. Chemicals in the water can interact, in complex ways, with the sediments and suspended particulates in the water column as well as the plants and animals that reside there.

## Soils

What we commonly refer to as soil is a complex mixture of organic matter, inorganic matter such as silica and clay, water, and air. The composition of soils can vary greatly, in part due to the deliberate changing of its composition to meet specific needs. Thus agricultural soil, for example, may be quite different from a typical urban soil due to the addition of organic matter, fertilizer, and pesticides for optimal plant growth. Chemicals can be put into the soil directly from deliberate or accidental (unintentional) means or indirectly as the result of their translocation from water and air. The direct and deliberate addition of chemicals into the soil would include the addition of agrochemicals such as fertilizer and pesticides, whereas the direct but unintentional addition could be from chemical leaks or spills. Like water and air, chemicals can move about in this medium, undergo chemical reactions, and be transported to plant and animal life. Surface chemicals can move vertically and have the potential to reach groundwater.

## The Biosphere

In the environment chemicals reach plant and animal life, where they may be directly absorbed through the lungs, skin, or gills, for example, or indirectly through the consumption of food. The direct absorption of chemicals from the environmental medium can result in *bioaccumulation* or *bioconcentration*. The *bioavailability* of the chemical refers to that portion present within the medium that is potentially available for direct uptake by the organism. If a chemical is in high concentration in the sediment of a lake, for example, and a fish (which we will refer to as "our fish") spends most of its time residing in the water column, then the bioavailability of this chemical to our fish is low. This of course depends on many factors, including sediment turbulence during certain times of the year or on our fish's dependence for food from sedimentary organisms that enter into the water column. In addition, and depending on the physicochemical properties, a chemical may be concentrated in our fish as well.

A very lipophilic and environmentally persistent chemical such as DDT can be stored and accumulated in its fatty tissue compartments. This is referred to as *bioconcentration,* and in the case of DDT, for example, bioconcentration can result in levels of a thousand orders of magnitude greater than what might be observed as a background level in the water. We can describe what is known as a *bioconcentration factor* (BCF), which is equal to the concentration of the pollutant in our fish divided by its concentration in the water. The BCF is calculated from the ratio of the toxicant concentration in the whole animal (or a particular tissue) at steady state, to its concentration in its environment. If the BCF is greater than 1, it indicates that accumulation is occurring at a level higher in our fish than in the medium in which it resides. It only takes on relevance, however, for substances that remain long enough in the body for quantitative assessment. Chemicals such as DDT and methylmercury are examples of those types of chemicals with biological half-lives long enough to make meaningful quantitative assessments. A short-lived chemical such as ozone would not be amenable to this type of analysis despite its high reactivity and injury-producing potential.

If the concentration of DDT in the water of the lake in which our fish resides is 0.2 ppb and 2 ppm in the fish, then the BCF would be 10,000. The problem here, however, is that the DDT concentration in our fish represents one that has resulted from both direct uptake from water as well as uptake through dietary accumulation. Ecologists like to refer to this as *biomagnification* to designate the accumulation of a pollutant from trophic transfer: from primary producers (plant life) to herbivores to first-level carnivores to second or higher levels and ultimately to the "final" consumer. If our hypothetical fish is one that is a second or higher level carnivore, then it is under-standable why we as consumers may be placed at greater risk for potential toxicity. One needs only to think about the public's concern about mercury from the consumption of tuna fish.

## Toxicity in a Population

Like humans, the toxicity of chemicals on a population depends on many factors. Ecosystems are complex and made up of a multitude of animals and plants. The level of effect(s) of any chemical, on any one particular population of species, may be different from another in that community. Toxicity depends on many factors:

- Species
- Age
- Gender
- Exposure route
- Form and activity of the chemical
- Concentration or dose
- Bioavailability
- Primary route of exposure
- Ability to be absorbed
- Metabolism
- Distribution within the body
- Excretion
- Presence of other chemicals

There can be no doubt that species other than humans develop illnesses in response to environ-mental exposures to pollutants. In the 1980s large numbers of fish from the Great Lakes were observed with a variety of tumors. These tumors were likely produced from their continuous expo-sure to a medium containing polycyclic aromatic hydrocarbons from petroleum. Neoplasms have also been observed in other species as well. Similarly, reproductive and developmental abnormalities have been observed in many different species due to dysfunction of endocrine regulatory mecha-nisms. A great deal of research has been devoted to the study that various pollutants have on the endocrine system. Many have shown that some chemicals can mimic natural hormone and/or block hormone receptors (e.g., some pesticides, dioxins, environmental discharges of hormones). These types of chemicals have been called "endocrine disrupters," and they as well as others may have long-term consequences on population growth, environmental "tolerance," and genetic diversity.

Pollutant-induced mutations can have effects on populations, especially if they are made up of a small number of individuals. The smaller the population's gene pool, the less its genetic variation, and the population will be more prone to a reduction in the number of individuals and possible extinction.

Environmental toxicants can affect the growth and dynamics of the population in a commu-nity (Figure 5.1). Acute toxicity, for example, can result in an increased rate of mortality. Chronic

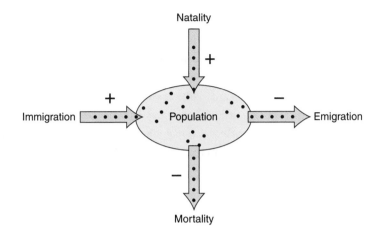

**FIGURE 5.1**   Factors affecting population growth. *Source:* Courtesy of SOFIA/USGS.

effects can result in decreases in birth rate (natality). In a population there may be a wide range of responses to a similar toxic insult (Figure 5.2). Responses to similar insults range from hyposensitivity (no to low response) to hypersensitivity (extreme/life-threatening response).

It is incorrect to believe that the most resistant individuals in a population exposed to a toxicant will also make up for any overall loss to the population due to death or disability of the more sensitive individuals. Although these individuals may be more tolerant to a particular chemical exposure, they may not be the best reproducers within the population.

The increase or decrease in the population of any one species in a community may result in changes in the size of other populations within that community. If, for example, one species in a community serves as an important food source for another, excess mortality due to toxicity in that food source will lead to a decline in the dependent population due to decreased food supply

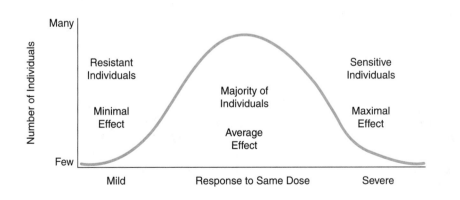

**FIGURE 5.2**   Graphical representation of the majority of responses to toxic insult.

to sustain population growth or current population size. If the species can physically relocate, it may emigrate to find a more suitable environment. Similarly, immigration into the community may occur when conditions are more favorable (see Figure 5.1).

In summary, our environment is an enormously complex system that has no "steady state." It is changing continuously due to both natural events and the activities of society. We as public health officials need to support efforts to rationally deal with environmental issues and recognize that what at the moment may appear "insignificant" may later develop into a public health concern. Recognition of potential problems and rational approaches to problem solving early on is always preferable and more cost-effective than retrofitting our efforts to a situation that has developed into a global monster.

# Bibliography

Bacci, E. (1993). *Ecotoxicology of organic contaminants*. Boca Raton, FL: CRC Press.

Cal/EPA Office of Environmental Health Hazard Assessment. Retrieved September 2005 from www.oehha.ca.gov/ecotox.html.

*Ecological risk analysis*. Retrieved September 2005 from http://www.esd.ornl.gov/programs/ecorisk/ecorisk.html.

*ECOTOX*. Retrieved September 2005 from www.epa.gov/ecotox/.

The Extension Toxicology Network. Retrieved September 2005 from http://ace.orst.edu/info/extoxnet/.

Hinton, D. E., Kullman, S. W., Hardman, R. C., Volz, D. C., Chen, P. J., Carney, M., & Bencic, D. C. (2005). Resolving mechanisms of toxicity while pursuing ecotoxicological relevance? *Pollution Bulletin, 51*(8–12), 635–648.

Johann, F., Moltmann, J. F., & Rawson, D. M. (1995). *Applied ecotoxicology*. Boca Raton, FL: CRC Press.

Klaassen, C. D. (2001). *Casarett & Doull's toxicology. The basic science of poisons*. New York: McGraw-Hill.

Klaassen, C. D., & Watkins, J. B. (2003). *Casarett & Doull's essentials of toxicology*. New York: McGraw-Hill.

Luttik, R., Mineau, P., & Roelofs, W. (2005). A review of interspecies toxicity extrapolation in birds and mammals and a proposal for long-term toxicity data. *Ecotoxicology, 14*(8), 817–832.

Manahan, S. E. (2004). *Environmental chemistry* (8th ed.). Columbia, MO: University of Missouri.

Mineau, P. (2005). A review and analysis of study endpoints relevant to the assessment of "long term" pesticide toxicity in avian and mammalian wildlife. *Ecotoxicology, 14*(8), 775–799.

Newman, M. C., & Jagoe, C. H. (1996). *Ecotoxicology: A hierarchical treatment*. Boca Raton, FL: CRC Press.

Newman, M. C., & Unger, M. A. (2002). *Fundamentals of ecotoxicology* (2nd ed.). Boca Raton, FL: CRC Press.

Sram, R. J., Binkova, B., Dejmek, J., & Bobak, M. (2005). Ambient air pollution and pregnancy outcomes: A review of the literature. *Environmental Health Perspective, 113*(4), 375–382.

*Total Risk Integrated Methodology (TRIM)—TRIM.FaTE*. Retrieved September 2005 from http://www.epa.gov/ttn/fera/trim_fate.html.

U.S. EPA. *Mid-Atlantic threatened and endangered species*. Retrieved September 2005 from http://www.epa.gov/maia/html/te-1.html.

U.S. Fish and Wildlife Species Information. *Threatened and endangered animals and plants.* Retrieved September 2005 from http://www.fws.gov/Endangered/wildlife.html#Species.

U.S. National Library of Medicine, National Institutes of Health, Environmental Health, and Toxicology Specialized Information Services (SIS). (2005). *Toxicology tutorial III.* Retrieved September 2005 from http://www.sis. nlm. nih.gov/enviro/toxtutor.html.

Van Wijngaarden, R. P., Brock, T. C., & Van den Brink, P. J. (2005). Threshold levels for effects of insecticides in freshwater ecosystems: A review. *Ecotoxicology, 14*(3), 355–380.

Vighi, M., Finizio, A., & Villa, S. (2006). The evolution of the Environmental Quality concept: From the US EPA Red Book to the European Water Framework Directive. *Environmental Science and Pollution Research, 13*(1), 9–14.

# Dose and Response

The most fundamental of all principles in toxicology is that of the relationship between the amount of a toxicant that is received by the organism (the *dose*) and the effect(s) that results from that dose (the *response*). The basis for establishing this relationship, for most chemicals, comes primarily from experimental data using laboratory animals, *in vitro* studies, and, to a much lesser extent, information from humans.

The dose–response relationship

- Can establish the lowest dose where an objectively measurable effect first occurs (threshold level)
- Establishes a quantitative relationship between the dose and the response
- Provides the basis for establishing a causal relationship between the dose and the response
- Provides information to assess the relative toxicity of a chemical when compared with others tested under similar conditions of exposure

A true dose–response relationship *that has as its objective* the determination of some aspect of toxicity as an end-point is quantitative and determined experimentally using laboratory animals (*in vivo* studies) or in an appropriate *in vitro* system (e.g., cell cultures). Although dose–response information can be studied experimentally in humans (e.g., clinical trials of new drug candidates), the primary objective is *not* to produce toxicity but rather to establish safe dose ranges for efficacy. Information concerning toxicity in humans therefore most often comes from attempts to reconstruct doses from published accounts of accidental or intentional poisonings, retrospective epidemiological studies, adverse events associated with a chemical intended to produce a beneficial effect on the body's physiology (e.g., a pharmaceutical), or *in vitro* studies using human tissues.

The relationship between dose and response was recognized by Paracelsus in the 16th century as fundamental to understanding how the same chemical can produce benefit or injury to a person. His statement "solely the dose determines that a thing is not a poison" was the recognition that any substance could be a poison and that the right dose differentiates whether that substance will act as a poison or as a remedy. Paracelsus hypothesized that there must be a dose below which no response can occur or can be measured. He also hypothesized that there must be a maximum response in which any further increase in the dose will not result in any corresponding further increase in the effect.

In toxicology the purpose of toxicity testing is to determine the nature and extent of injury produced by exposure to chemicals. Today, we clearly recognize that the dose of a chemical is going to determine the intensity of the effect that it produces in the body, whether the chemical is one that provides some benefit to us or whether it is one that has no benefit to our body at all and may indeed be recognized as a "poison."

Dose can be defined several ways:

- The *administered* or *applied dose* is the amount presented to an absorption barrier and available for absorption (although not necessarily having yet crossed the outer boundary of the organism). This is the dose referred to in toxicity testing unless otherwise specified.
- The *absorbed dose* is the amount crossing a specific absorption barrier (e.g., the exchange boundaries of the skin, lung, and digestive tract) through uptake processes.
- The *internal dose* is a more general term denoting the amount absorbed without respect to specific absorption barriers or exchange boundaries.
- The *delivered dose* is the amount of the chemical available for interaction with any particular organ or cell.

The unit most often used to express dose amount is the gram (Table 6.1).

## Relating Dose to Response

For a dose–response relationship to be scientifically valid in toxicology, a number of conditions must be satisfied:

1. A method is needed to objectively measure an adverse response.
2. The adverse response occurs after the dose is administered.
3. The adverse response is due solely to the dose.
4. The type of adverse response(s) measured is the same or similar for each individual or *in vitro* system that is used for testing.
5. The intensity of the adverse response is proportional to the dose.

The dose–response relationship in toxicology is therefore important in establishing both causality and the lowest dose capable of producing an adverse effect. The lowest dose that produces an adverse effect can be considered a *threshold dose*. At this dose level the first appearance of an adverse effect can be causally linked to the chemical. In other words, the response observed is

**Table 6.1** The Gram

| Unit | Gram Equivalents | Exponential Representation |
| --- | --- | --- |
| Kilogram (kg) | 1000.0 g | $1 \times 10^3$ g |
| Milligram (mg) | 0.001 g | $1 \times 10^{-3}$ g |
| Microgram (μg) | 0.000001 g | $1 \times 10^{-6}$ g |
| Nanogram (ng) | 0.000000001 g | $1 \times 10^{-9}$ g |
| Picogram (pg) | 0.000000000001 g | $1 \times 10^{-12}$ g |

not a random or spontaneous event but rather one that is causally linked to the lowest dose given. Doses above the threshold result in the same type of adverse effect(s) but at correspondingly higher levels of intensity. As the dose is further increased, other types of adverse effects may appear, until a point is reached where the chemical has produced injuries so overwhelming that substantial toxicity or even death may result. Many of us may have personally conducted an acute dose–response study on the effects of increasing doses of ethanol. For those who have, a point may have been reached where significant adverse effects were produced, and although the final toxicological end-point was fortunately not reached, it may have been perhaps wished for!

In humans it may be unclear that any one individual's adverse response is causally linked to a specific chemical exposure even if the exposure preceded the onset of an illness or injury. Other factors may be responsible for this observed illness or injury and must be ruled out before toxicological causation can be established. If this obstacle can be hurdled, it may still be particularly difficult to determine what an actual "dose" was from an exposure to a chemical agent(s) through one or possibly more exposure pathways.

A clear quantitative relationship between the dose and the magnitude of a toxic response may break down when we talk about allergic reactions. In individuals who have been sensitized to some chemical, it is not the chemical that causes the allergic response but rather it is the mediators of inflammation that are produced secondary to the chemical that act as an "allergic trigger."

## Dose–Response Graphs

Experimentally, the dose–response relationship is typically depicted as a two-dimensional graph that plots the intensity of the measured response on the y-axis of the graph (the dependent variable) and the dose on the x-axis (the independent variable). The y-axis is the toxic end-point that is being measured and could represent toxicity observed at the molecular, cellular, tissue, organ, or organism levels (Figure 6.1). The data have been plotted both arithmetically and logarithmically for comparison. You can see that the right curve (log of dose) is more revealing in the sense that it expands the lower doses so that a clearer picture of the response emerges, particularly at the lower dose levels.

The shape of the dose–response curve is generally sigmoidal. The dose at which one can first see a response occurring is generally referred to as the threshold level (Figure 6.2). Theoretically,

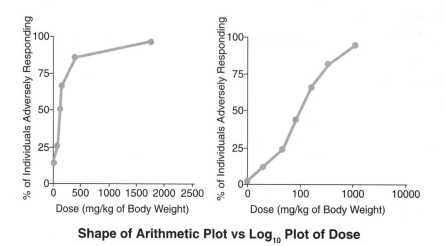

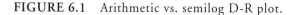

**Shape of Arithmetic Plot vs Log₁₀ Plot of Dose**

**FIGURE 6.1**   Arithmetic vs. semilog D-R plot.

the threshold dose represents a dose that is large enough to show an inability of normal repair mechanisms to keep pace with the level of chemical insult. This of course would need to be referenced to the toxic end-point that we are measuring. If we were using death as an end-point, then the threshold dose for a chemical that first produced liver cell injury (threshold dose for liver cell injury) would not be observable using death as an end-point, because sufficient liver cells would still remain functional to maintain normal body physiology. If on the other hand an *in vitro* end-point was used to measure the threshold for liver cell toxicity (direct cytotoxicity of liver cells in cell culture), then one might observe that the dose (standardized so that *in vivo* and

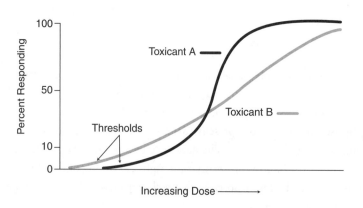

**FIGURE 6.2**   Dose–response curves for two toxicants showing the thresholds for responses.

*in vitro* concentrations of the chemical were similar) that produced no effect in the whole animal produced liver cell death using an *in vitro* toxicity test.

Two terms found in the toxicological literature that represent empirically determined dose levels are the *lowest observed adverse effect level,* or LOAEL, and the *no observed adverse effect level,* or NOAEL. The former represents the lowest data point measured (i.e., the lowest dose at which an observed toxic or adverse effect occurred), whereas the latter represents the highest dose at which there was no measurable toxic or adverse response. Occasionally, one sees the terms *NOEL* and *LOEL* in the scientific literature; by omitting the "A" these terms are applicable to both adverse and beneficial effects.

The slope of a dose–response curve is the most rapidly rising portion and represents the change in the intensity of the response per unit of increase in the dose. Different chemicals may have very different slopes. As depicted in Figure 6.2, chemicals with similar thresholds do not need to have correspondingly similar slopes. Each toxicant has its own characteristic progression of toxicity. Toxicant A rises more sharply to reach its maximum intensity far sooner than the gradually rising toxicant B. The slope of a dose–response curve then reveals something about the potency of the chemical. Potency is a measure of the strength of a chemical relative to that of other chemicals. The sharper the rise in toxicity of one chemical compared with another (or the larger the numerical value of the slope), the more potent the chemical (Figure 6.3).

## How Individuals May Respond in a Population

In a population of individuals, you can observe biological variation in response to the same dose of chemical. Consider a hypothetical group of 100 individuals exposed in exactly the same manner to a chemical in the air that typically produces respiratory irritation (e.g., sulfur dioxide).

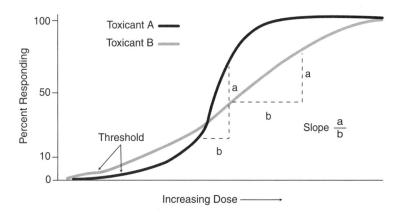

FIGURE 6.3    Slopes of dose–response curves. *Source:* Courtesy of the Toxicology and Environmental Health Information Program of the National Library of Medicine, U.S. Department of Health and Human Services.

Furthermore, consider hypothetically that the concentration of that chemical in the air is the same for each person and that each person receives the same internal dose. We see a bell-shaped distribution curve that theoretically never reaches 0 or 100%.

This bell-shaped curve demonstrates that within this hypothetical population, the majority of responses to the toxicant are similar (some coughing and eye irritation); however, because of biological variability some individuals may be more or less susceptible to the effects of exposure. The individuals toward the left of the curve may have only a barely perceptible sensation of eye irritation, with no tears or coughing. These individuals appear to be less susceptible and we can refer to them as "resistant" or as "hyporesponsive" (Figure 6.4).

Similarly, there are other individuals who are very susceptible to this exposure and respond intensely; they are shown on the right of the curve, and they will likely experience severe coughing, tightness in the chest, and difficulty breathing. We refer to these individuals as being "sensitive" or as "hyperresponsive." The responses have a typically Gaussian distribution and can be expressed as plus or minus one or two standard deviations of that mean. One standard deviation includes 68% of the individuals, and two standard deviations include 95% of the individuals (Figure 6.5).

## The Dose Must Be Referenced to Time

A dose can be a single event or multiple events over a specified period of time. For example, an adult male may take a total dose of 500 mg of amoxicillin three times a day (1,500 mg/day) for 10 consecutive days over the course of a month (total dose, 15,000 mg or 15 g). The antibiotic, if properly taken by this individual, should have therapeutic value. If he were to take the total dose on day 1, then there would be little therapeutic value and indeed there may be adverse effects, including injury to the liver and kidneys. If this individual weighed 70

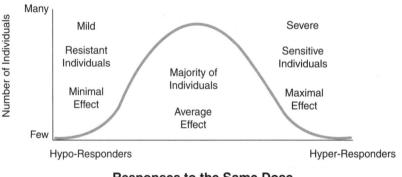

**FIGURE 6.4**    Responses of individuals to the same dose.

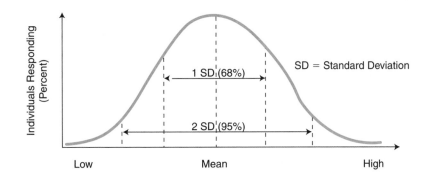

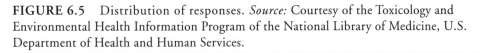

**FIGURE 6.5**   Distribution of responses. *Source:* Courtesy of the Toxicology and Environmental Health Information Program of the National Library of Medicine, U.S. Department of Health and Human Services.

approximately 21.4 mg/kg of body weight (1,500 mg/70 kg). Compare this with all the antibiotic taken as a single total dose of 214 mg/kg of body weight (15,000 mg/70 kg), or a dose 10 times greater than the daily therapeutic level. If we were to reference the doses over an 8-hour period instead of a 24-hour period, then if correctly taken the therapeutic dose becomes 7.14 mg/kg (500 mg/70 kg) compared with 214 mg/kg (15,000 mg/70kg) if all the antibiotic is taken as a single dose. This latter dose is approximately 30 times greater than the therapeutic dose. Clearly then, the way that time is referenced with respect to dose can greatly impact our assessment about toxicity.

## Dose Standardization Based on Body Weight

For both efficacy studies and toxicity studies, doses are standardized based on body weight. For example, if a single daily dose of 0.1 mg/kg of a pharmaceutical has been shown to be efficacious in men, then a 120-kg male should receive a daily dose of 12 mg, whereas a 70-kg male would require only 7 mg. If these same two men were drinking at a pub and each consumed the same amount of the toxicant ethanol, over the same period of time they would have very different blood alcohol concentrations based on weight differences alone, assuming that their blood alcohol levels were similarly determined. For the lighter man a blood alcohol level at the legal threshold, which establishes presumptive impairment, would occur with fewer drinks than for the heavier man.

## Toxicity Rating

A relative rating of chemical toxicity has been developed based on a single oral dose of a chemical standardized to weight, which would likely be lethal to an "average" adult (Table 6.2).

**Table 6.2**    Lethal Single Oral Dose

| Toxicity Rating | Probable Lethal Oral Dose For "Average" Adult |
| --- | --- |
| Practically nontoxic | >15 g/kg |
| Slight | 5–15 g/kg |
| Moderate | 0.5–5 g/kg |
| Very | 50–500 mg/kg |
| Extremely | 5–50 mg/kg |
| Supertoxic | <5 mg/kg |

# Referencing Dose to Environmental Media

A dose may be represented as an "exposure dose," or the concentration of a chemical present in a medium, and would be expressed as a gram unit of a chemical per cubic meter of air, liter of water, kilogram of soil, or kilogram of a consumable (e.g., vegetable, fruit, fish). For inhaled chemicals we typically discuss exposure concentration in parts per million (ppm) or milligrams per cubic meter of air ($mg/m^3$); however, this is not equivalent to the actual dose because it does not tell us how much of the chemical has entered the body. A chemical present in the air at 3 $mg/m^3$, for example, may represent an exposure concentration, but the actual absorbed dose depends on factors such as the amount of time spent breathing the air containing this chemical, body weight, pulmonary retention, and the breathing requirements while sitting or walking or exercising. It is possible to estimate the inhaled dose using equations that incorporate these factors. As an example, the dose of an inhaled aerosol may be described by the following formula:

$$D = \frac{\alpha \times (V_T \times f \times C) \times t}{M}$$

where $D$ represents the dose (mg/kg), $\alpha$ is the fraction of aerosol deposited in the lungs (% retained), $V_T$ represents the tidal volume (ml of air moved with each breath), $f$ is the ventilation frequency (breaths per minute), $C$ is the exposure concentration of the chemical ($mg/m^3$), $t$ is the exposure duration (minutes), and $M$ represents body weight (kg).

The total dose of any chemical may be the result of combined individual doses, from different media, over a specified period of time. Consider a family outing for a day of camping, hiking, and fishing for mom, dad, and their 3-year-old. The campsite has well water for drinking, bass in the lake for the angler of the family, and lots of dirt for junior to play in. At the end of the day, dad has brought back enough fish for dinner. Unknown to our campers, some recent environmental sampling data show concentrations of benzene present in the different media: 5 µg/l of well water, 3 mg/kg of soil, and 2 mg/kg in the flesh of lake bass. The amount of a chemical present can also be expressed in parts per million (ppm), parts per billion (ppb), or parts per trillion (ppt). Using an example from above, a concentration of 3 mg benzene/kg of soil can also be expressed as 3 ppm (3 mg/kg = 3 mg/1,000,000 mg = 3 ppm). Based on the above discussion, the total oral dose of benzene for each member of the family can be determined for that day (Table 6.3).

The next morning, Junior complains that his stomach hurts, and dad has learned that the campsite has just been closed due to test results from the State indicating benzene contamination. The family is now extremely concerned that Junior may have become ill from benzene and wants to know how toxic benzene is and how it got to the campsite in the first place. How would you as a State Toxicologist comfort them in light of the fact that information concerning the acute effects from benzene consumption might be limited to animal lethality data and some published incidents of human poisonings that are associated with gastrointestinal disturbances?

Animal lethality data indicate that benzene is of moderate toxicity after acute oral intake (about 1–6 g/kg or 1,000–6,000 mg/kg), whereas in humans it is probably less than 150 mg/kg (150,000 µg/kg), thus falling within the very toxic class. Should the family be alarmed about the consumption of benzene, having learned that it is "very toxic" orally? Although clearly each family member received a different dose, their consumptions were about 10,000 times less than the amount known to be acutely toxic in humans. You would advise the family that acute stomach disturbances are common, especially in children, and may indeed be linked to any food consumed as not agreeing with them; however, you would also advise the family that there is no basis to link their child's stomachache to the small amount of benzene consumed, despite the temporal relationship. You explain that although it may be unclear at this time why the benzene levels at the campsite are higher than normal, its presence there and in other places is to be expected in light of the fact that it is one of the world's major commodity chemicals. The higher than normal levels may have resulted from recent discharges into the atmosphere, seepage from a landfill, improper disposal of hazardous wastes, or leakage of an underground storage tank. Your office will continue to investigate and monitor the levels.

As a responsible public health official, however, you recognize that the story does not end here. You recognize that benzene is a known human carcinogen, and you are obligated to disclose that information to the family. This is where you need to merge your knowledge base and interpersonal skills with relating to what the public might view as a black-and-white situation in which persons may be convinced that cancer will result from this exposure. As a toxicologist you would disclose that benzene is a carcinogen and has been associated with the development of certain

**Table 6.3    Benzene Consumption and Oral Daily Dose**

|  | Body Weight (kg) | Amount of Media Consumed | | | Amount of Benzene Consumed | | | Consumed (µg) | Total Benzene Dose (µg/kg/day) |
|---|---|---|---|---|---|---|---|---|---|
|  |  | Water (l) | Fish (mg) | Soil (mg) | Water (µg) | Fish (mg) | Soil (mg) |  |  |
| Dad | 80 | 3 | 500 | 50 | 15 | 1 | 0.00015 | 1015.15 | 12.7 |
| Mom | 60 | 2 | 300 | 10 | 10 | 0.6 | 0.00003 | 610.03 | 10.2 |
| Child | 25 | 1 | 200 | 200 | 5 | 0.4 | 0.0006 | 405.6 | 16.2 |

types of leukemias. You would further discuss the process of chemical-induced carcinogenesis as not a single exposure event that will result in the disease. You point out that benzene-induced cancer, although documented in workers that have been exposed to large amounts of benzene, is not applicable in this instance. For one thing, this exposure was minimal and to be of real concern would require continued exposures on a daily basis year after year. The family's perceived risk is not consistent with what is known about benzene exposures that have been causally linked to cancer. Additionally, you point out to the family that the process of carcinogenesis goes well beyond aspects related only to the exposure. You might even compare their risk with the risk of being struck by lightning immediately after the winning of the biggest lottery payoff in the state!

## Bibliography

Agency for Toxic Substances and Disease Registry (ATSDR). Retrieved November 2005 from http://www.atsdr.cdc.gov/.

Andersen, M. E., Thomas, R. S., Gaido, K. W., & Conolly, R. B. (2005). Dose-response modeling in reproductive toxicology in the systems biology era. *Reproductive Toxicology, 19*(3), 327–337.

Arts, J. H., Mommers, C., & de Heer, C. (2006). Dose-response relationships and threshold levels in skin and respiratory allergy. *Critical Review of Toxicology, 36*(3), 219–251.

Calabrese, E. J., & Blain, R. (2005). The occurrence of hormetic dose responses in the toxicological literature, the hormesis database: An overview. *Toxicology and Applied Pharmacology, 202*(3), 289–301.

Csajka, C., & Verotta, D. (2006). Pharmacokinetic-pharmacodynamic modelling: History and perspectives. *Journal of Pharmacokinetics and Pharmacodynamics, 33*(3), 227–279.

Extension Toxicology Network. Retrieved November 2005 from http://extoxnet.orst.edu/tibs/doseresp.htm.

Hall, E. J., & Henry, S. (2004). The crooked shall be made straight: Dose-response relationships for carcinogenesis. *International Journal of Radiation Biology, 80*(5), 327–337.

Klaassen, C. D. (2001). *Casarett & Doull's toxicology. The basic science of poisons.* New York: McGraw-Hill.

Klaassen, C. D., & Watkins, J. B. (2003). *Casarett & Doull's essentials of toxicology.* New York: McGraw-Hill.

Ott, M. G., Diller, W. F., & Jolly, A. T. (2003). Respiratory effects of toluene diisocyanate in the workplace: A discussion of exposure-response relationships. *Critical Review of Toxicology, 33*(1), 1–59.

Rosenbaum, P. R. (2003). Does a dose-response relationship reduce sensitivity to hidden bias? *Biostatistics, 4*(1), 1–10.

Tardiff, R. G., & Rodricks, J. Y. (1988). *Toxic substances and human risk: Principles of data interpretation.* New York: Plenum Publishing.

U.S. National Library of Medicine, National Institutes of Health, Environmental Health, and Toxicology Specialized Information Services (SIS). (2005). *Toxicology tutorial I.* Retrieved November 2005 from http://www.sis.nlm.nih.gov/enviro/toxtutor.html.

Weed, D. L. (2004). Methodologic implications of the Precautionary Principle: Causal criteria. *International Journal of Occupational Medicine and Environmental Health, 17*(1), 77–81.

# Absorption of Toxicants and Models of Disposition

## Toxicant Entry into the Body

To produce a systemic effect, a toxicant has to defeat barriers to absorption and enter into the internal compartments of the body; otherwise, all effects are confined to the site of exposure, that is, all toxicity will be local (e.g., irritation to skin or respiratory tract). An orally consumed toxicant, or one that enters into the respiratory system, is not considered to be "internal" until it moves across the epithelial cellular membranes that line the respective systems, thus gaining entry into the internal fluid compartments of the body (Figure 7.1).

Principally, toxicants enter the body through one of three systems:

1. *The respiratory system:* The lungs are an important entry point for toxic gases, solvents, aerosols, and particulates. Pulmonary tissue is highly vascularized and has a large surface area (approximately 100 m$^2$ in adults) for toxicant absorption.
2. *The gastrointestinal system:* The gastrointestinal tract has a large surface area (approximately 300 m$^2$ in adults). The pH, which can influence the absorption of many chemicals, is variable, ranging from approximately 1–3 in the stomach to approximately 6 in the small intestine.
3. *The integumentary system:* The skin, with its surface area of approximately 2 m$^2$, is not highly permeable to most water-soluble chemicals, but lipid-soluble compounds are well absorbed via passive diffusion. Damage to the integrity of the skin increases absorption and may lead to greater systemic toxicity.

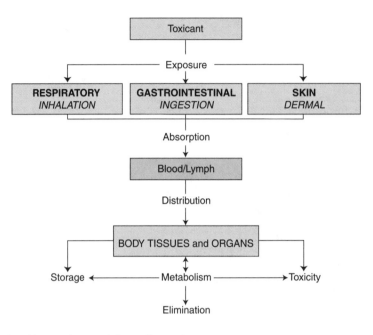

**FIGURE 7.1** Absorption and fate of a toxicant.

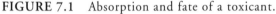

More than one exposure pathway may occur for a chemical. Consider, for example, a situation in which there is aerial spraying of the organophosphate pesticide malathion during a time when an individual might be outside and exposed to the spray. Some skin and respiratory exposure would be anticipated to occur, and depending on the nature of the aerosol produced, pesticide absorption may occur from the mucosa of the nose, upper airways, and perhaps lower airways if the size of the aerosol is sufficiently small to reach it. However, this does not imply that any significant systemic toxicity would result.

It is not the intent in this chapter to discuss the toxicology of each of these systems in detail; this will occur in other chapters. The intent here is to briefly discuss these systems in the context of their importance for the absorption of toxicants.

## Cell Membranes

Cell membranes (also referred to as plasma membranes) are similar in all cells in that they are composed of a phospholipid bilayer approximately 7–9 nm thick and contain proteins that have structural, receptor, or enzymatic function. The bilayer is oriented in a way such that the polar phosphate heads, which are hydrophilic, extend into the aqueous phases (extracellular fluid or intracellular fluid) and the hydrophobic (lipophilic) lipid tails toward each other. Contained within the phospholipid bilayer are proteins that may assist in the movement of chemicals (e.g., some proteins form aqueous pores, whereas others serve as transport proteins for chemicals).

For a toxicant to enter into the internal body fluid compartments or to enter, leave, or move to other cells requires passage across several cell membranes (Figure 7.2).

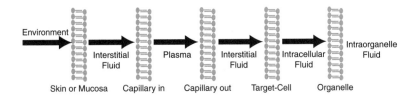

**FIGURE 7.2**    Cell membrane crossings for a toxicant from exposure site to target.

## Movement of Toxicants Across Cell Membranes

Cell membranes are selectively permeable. The degree of toxicant movement across the cell membrane depends on toxicant shape and molecular size, lipid solubility, structural similarity to endogenous molecules, charge and polarity, and its concentration difference across the bilayer. Toxicants can cross a membrane in a variety of ways (Figure 7.3).

Toxicants move across cell membranes by either simple diffusion or specialized transport. Specialized transport mechanisms included active transport, special transport (facilitated or carrier-mediated diffusion and active transport), and endocytosis.

The primary mechanism that moves toxicants into and out of cell membranes is by simple diffusion. Several primary factors determine net diffusion (amount of chemical moved) and the diffusion rate:

- Size of the molecule
- Molecular charge and degree of ionization
- Water solubility
- Concentration differences across the cell membrane

Chemicals that are lipophilic readily diffuse across the phospholipid bilayer, whereas for water-soluble molecules passage across the membrane occurs through aqueous channels. The charge and molecular size are important determinants for net diffusion: large molecular size and the presence of molecular charge would tend to impede diffusion. Water-soluble molecules of several hundred molecular weight would be the upper limit for net movement across cell membranes by diffusion. There are exceptions to this, including the endothelium of blood capillaries and the glomeruli of the kidneys, which have relatively large aqueous pores. A special type of diffusion, known as facilitated diffusion, allows larger molecules such as amino acids and sugars to move across the cell membrane along their concentration gradient with the help of a membrane carrier molecule (generally a specialized protein).

The degree of ionization is an important limiting factor for diffusion across cellular membranes; generally, uncharged toxicant molecules can more easily cross cellular membranes than toxicants that possess a charge, and thus the pH of the environment affects the rate of diffusion

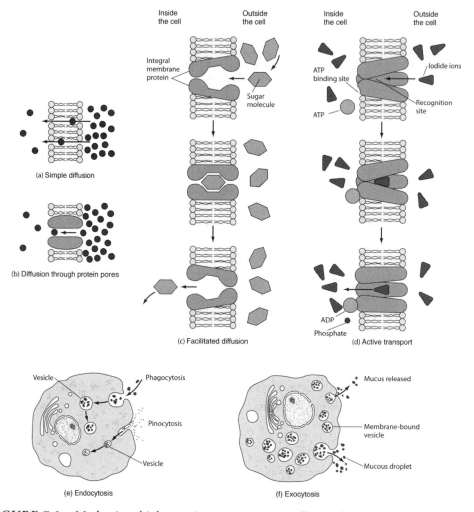

**FIGURE 7.3**   Modes in which a toxicant can cross a cell membrane.

across cell membranes. The pH is very important in determining the possible site of absorption of chemicals that carry acidic or basic functional groups.

The Henderson-Hasselbalch equation defines the amount of a compound that will be in its nonionized form and is useful for estimating the percentage of absorption by passive diffusion. This equation can be summarized as follows:

For acids:

$$pK_a - pH = \log [\text{nonionized}]/[\text{ionized}]$$

For bases:

$$pK_a + pH = \log [\text{ionized}]/[\text{nonionized}]$$

The dissociation constant ($pK_a$) is a type of equilibrium constant that indicates the extent of dissociation of hydrogen ions from an acid. The smaller the $pK_a$ value, the stronger the dissociation of hydrogen ions.

As an example, the high acidity of the stomach provides an important absorption site for weak organic acids (e.g., benzoic acid) that remain primarily in the nonionized form, thus facilitating their diffusion across the gastric mucosa. A weak organic base such as aniline, in contrast, would be highly ionized in the acidic environment of the stomach and therefore would be poorly absorbed across the stomach mucosa but would be well absorbed across the intestinal mucosa, where pH is basic. The clinically important drug aspirin ($C_9H_8O_4$) is better absorbed from the acid environment of the stomach compared with the basic pH of the intestine, where it exists primarily in the ionized form ($C_9H_7O_4^-$).

In some instances the cell may need to expend energy to move substances into or out of the cell. The process of active transport may be important in the transport of some toxicants into and out of the tissues of the body and for maintaining normal electrolyte gradients across the cell membrane. Some heavy metals, such as lead and the herbicide paraquat, may be transported across the intestinal mucosa by active transport mechanisms. Particulates may get into cells by the process of endocytosis, such as the accumulation of particulates by alveolar macrophages in the lungs. This process engulfs the particulate by surrounding it with the cell membrane and then moving the engulfed membrane-enclosed particulate into the cell interior.

## Skin Absorption

The skin can be a significant route of exposure for toxicants, especially at the workplace. The handling of chemicals without personal protective equipment is very common, and contact with the hands or spills to other parts of the body are relatively commonplace, as has occurred, for example, for highly toxic and lipophilic pesticides such as parathion and nicotine because of handling a leaky container, an accidental spill, or spraying into the wind.

The outer layer of the skin (stratum corneum) is the first line of defense between dermal exposure and systemic toxicity. The term *percutaneous absorption* refers to absorption from the surface of the skin into the blood of the cutaneous vessels, which reside in the dermis. In general the skin is relatively impermeable to aqueous solutions and ions; however, it can be a significant route of exposure for chemicals that are lipophilic in nature. As an example, poisonings have occurred through dermal exposure to certain pesticides. Solvents such as n-hexane and carbon hydrochloride can penetrate the skin to produce systemic toxicities such as neurotoxicity and hepatotoxicity, respectively.

The skin or integument consists of an outer epidermis, a middle dermis, and a layer of subcutaneous connective tissue. The toxicology of the skin is discussed in some detail in Chapter 13, but it needs to be emphasized here that the epidermis represents the barrier between a chemical in the outside environment. Once that barrier has been breached and the chemical diffuses into the dermis, it can gain entry into the cutaneous blood vessels where it can be distributed to internal tissues and organs, thus producing systemic effects. Toxicants move across the epidermis by simple diffusion. The stratum corneum generally contains some water (less than 10%), and water-soluble substances can diffuse across the epidermis more effectively when the stratum corneum is wet or well hydrated. The integrity of the epidermis and especially the stratum corneum is important in maintaining cutaneous defense. Cuts, scratches, abrasions, burns, and inflammatory skin conditions enhance the penetration of a chemical across the epidermis and into the dermis. For lipophilic chemicals, diffusion across the stratum corneum and into the dermis readily occurs.

## Gastrointestinal Absorption

Chemicals entering the gastrointestinal tract must first cross the mucosa somewhere along the tract before gaining entry into the blood. Only by absorption from the gastrointestinal tract can a chemical exert a toxic effect that could be considered as systemic. The degree of absorption across the mucosa of the gastrointestinal tract is site, pH, and time dependent, and dependent on the physicochemical properties of the chemical as well. Toxicant absorption in the oral cavity and the esophagus is generally poor for many chemicals because of the relatively short time that they remain there, compared to the slower transport through the stomach and the gastrointestinal tract, which provides for a longer time for absorption. Clearly, for some substances, such as the sublingual form of nitroglycerin, absorption is very quick due to the well-vascularized nature of this portion of the mouth and the physiochemical properties of the drug. This form of absorption is also referred to as buccal absorption, and chemicals that enter the bloodstream this way do not first pass through the liver. This is also true for chemicals that are absorbed from the rectum, where some of the venous blood leads directly into the inferior vena cava, thus escaping the first pass through the liver. With these exceptions, the absorption of chemicals from the stomach and intestinal tract first pass through the liver circulation before entering into the general circulation of the body, and therefore they cannot escape hepatic metabolism. It is in the liver where a significant amount of toxicant is removed from the venous blood and excreted into the bile, metabolically converted (first-pass metabolism), or stored. Unchanged toxicant or its metabolite can be excreted into the bile and back into the small intestine where they may be absorbed (in the case of the first-pass metabolite) or reabsorbed (in the case of the unmetabolized toxicant). This process may continue once again and would tend to reduce the rate of elimination of toxicant from the body. This is referred to as the enterohepatic circulation (Figure 7.4).

Another factor that determines the amount of a chemical that may be absorbed across the gastrointestinal tract is the presence or absence of food in the stomach. This factor has been shown to affect the acute toxicity for many chemicals, resulting in either a lower amount of net absorption from the gastrointestinal tract or a lower peak blood level reached due to a greater amount of time to reach complete absorption. The small intestine, with its large surface area to facilitate diffusion across the mucosa, is the site where the greatest amount of absorption occurs.

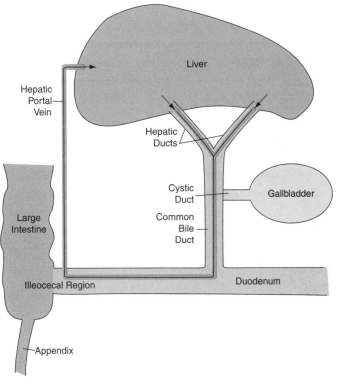

**FIGURE 7.4** Enterohepatic circulation.

Although the gastrointestinal tract proper does little in way of toxicant metabolism, the resident microflora are capable of toxicant biotransformation in some instances. For example, some precarcinogenic chemicals (e.g., certain amines) can be transformed into ones that are carcinogenic (e.g., nitrosamines). Although the large intestine and rectum are generally not of significance for absorption of toxicants, certain medications can be administered in suppository form with significant absorption occurring.

## Respiratory Absorption

The respiratory system constitutes a very important route of exposure for airborne contaminants (e.g., toxic gases, particulates, aerosols, volatile organic solvents). Toxicants that are contained within our breathing zone may be absorbed in the nasopharyngeal, tracheobronchial, or pulmonary exchange surfaces of the lungs, depending on the physical and chemical properties of the toxicant (Figure 7.5). They may also produce local effects in the respiratory system as well (e.g., irritation). With their large surface area for gas exchange and high blood perfusion, the lung alveoli and the terminal bronchioles are one of the most effective surfaces in the body for absorption and are responsible for most of the resultant systemic toxicity that may occur during respiratory exposures.

A rapidly absorbed toxicant is quickly distributed throughout the body. Consider, for example, the rapidity of poisonings that can occur from respiratory exposure to nitrous oxide (laughing gas), hydrocyanic acid (HCN), ether, or chloroform. Lipophilic and low-molecular-weight gases are quickly absorbed. The greater the degree of lipophilicity, the greater the potential rate of absorption. For hydrophilic chemicals the rate of absorption decreases with increasing molecular size. For a large percentage of the gases that readily dissolve in water, removal has already occurred in the upper portions of the tracheobronchial region. For volatile chemicals one can experimentally measure the retention of the chemical in the body by measuring the difference in the concentration between inspired and expired air (see Figure 7.5).

Particles are also taken into the respiratory system during breathing; depending on the characteristics of the particulates and their interaction with the cells in the lungs, this determines the extent of their retention, absorption, and potential to produce local or systemic toxicity.

In the lungs pulmonary macrophages can engulf particulates, some of which may be cleared into the lymphatic system, or may remain within the lungs for an indefinite period of time, as is the case for asbestos and coal dust. Material that remains within the respiratory system may produce local toxicity in which they take the form of lung cancer, chronic bronchitis, lung fibrosis, and emphysema.

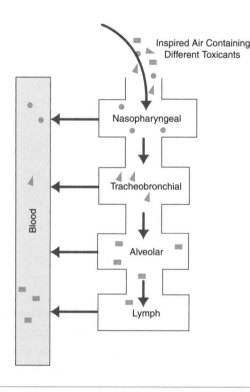

FIGURE 7.5    Toxicant absorption from the respiratory system depending on their physical and chemical properties.

## Other Exposure Routes

Other routes of exposure that have use clinically and experimentally for the delivery of chemicals are summarized as follows:

- Intravenous and intraarterial routes provide direct entry of chemicals into the blood vascular system. This is important clinically when rapid action must be taken to stabilize a patient. This exposure pathway results in 100% of the dose being absorbed.
- Injection of a chemical into the skin is a method to facilitate its systemic absorption. Both intradermal and subcutaneous injections are common clinical routes for the delivery of chemicals. Systemic absorption via intradermal injection is generally much slower than by subcutaneous injection because the tissue here is very well vascularized, thus facilitating rapid absorption into the systemic circulation.
- Injection directly into the muscle is referred to as intramuscular and is a common route for the delivery of many pharmaceuticals and vaccines. Skeletal muscle is well vascularized, and absorption via this route of administration is comparable with the subcutaneous route.
- The direct injection of chemicals into the body by any route is referred to as a parenteral route of delivery. In laboratory studies, animals are often injected with chemicals directly into either the abdominal cavity or into the chest cavity, and these methods are referred to as intraperitoneal and intrapleural injections, respectively. These exposure routes, rarely used clinically, generally result in a relatively slow absorption of chemicals into the blood.

## Chemical Disposition and Toxicokinetics

Chemical disposition and toxicokinetic studies are necessary to determine how a chemical can be absorbed, distributed to the tissues and organs of the body, stored (bioaccumulation), metabolized, and eliminated. The disposition and biological reactivity of a toxicant (its toxicodynamics) are the determining factors in the severity of toxicity. There are specific aspects of disposition that are of primary importance:

- The duration and concentration of the substance at the site of entry
- The rate of absorption (determined by the ability of the substance to pass through cell membranes)
- The total amount of toxicant absorbed
- The distribution within the body and presence at specific sites
- The efficiency of biotransformation
- The toxicity of the metabolites
- The storage of the toxicant and its metabolites within the body
- The rate and sites of elimination

The rate of absorption of the chemical into the body depends on its physical and chemical properties and the route of administration. The interspecific and intraspecific differences in many aspects of chemical disposition and toxicokinetics are important to recognize. Considering humans only, differences, for example, related to age, sex, nutritional status, and preexisting health conditions can impact the toxicity of a chemical. As an example, neonates and young children have an immature gastrointestinal tract, including a high microbial population, lower intestinal enzyme activity, lower gastric acid secretion, and lower surface area for absorption. These differences can greatly impact upon the toxicity of chemicals that are orally consumed in a young adult versus a child. Consider the well-known difference in the toxicity of dietary iron in adults and children.

The role of health and nutrition is also an important consideration in assessing the toxicity of some chemicals. As an example, consider the difference in the toxicity of warfarin, which is clinically used as an antithrombotic and anticoagulant. Like many drugs, a significant amount of the dose is bound to plasma proteins. Pharmaceutical efficacy involves the proper amount of free (unbound) versus bound drug. Too much free warfarin can result in internal bleeding. An individual who is poorly nourished or who may have significant liver disease could be at greater risk for toxicity from this chemical due to differences in the ability of the liver to produce adequate levels of plasma-binding proteins.

Toxicokinetic/disposition studies determine changes in the blood concentration of a chemical in the blood, plasma, or other tissue over time. Toxicokinetic studies consider this for the chemical and a limited number of its metabolites, whereas disposition involves the parent compound and all of the metabolites. Chemical disposition studies measure absorption, distribution, metabolism, and elimination of the chemical, generally following an intravenous administration to ensure a "100% absorption" of the administered dose. To facilitate the tracking of the chemical after its administration, a radioactive version of the chemical is used that generally contains radioactive carbon or hydrogen. This permits easy detection of the chemical and its presence in body fluids, tissues, expired breath, urine, and feces; however, it does not identify whether a radioactive recovery is due to the parent compound or to one of its metabolites. Further analytical methodology is required to determine whether the radioactivity is from the parent compound or a metabolite. Toxicokinetic studies are designed to determine concentration changes of the chemical and its metabolites over time in blood or plasma and other tissues. Toxicokinetic studies are generally conducted using a nonradioactive chemical and an analytical method for the specific detection of that chemical. These studies are useful for determining the bioavailability of the parent compound under consideration. Bioavailability is a measure between an intravenous dose (100% bioavailable) and the same amount of chemical administered by another route of exposure (inhalation, oral, topical).

## Models of Disposition

The movement of toxicants throughout the body, over time, has been described by the use of models of disposition. Models of disposition integrate the processes of distribution, metabolism, and elimination. The body is considered to contain a number of compartments or areas (e.g., blood, liver, adipose tissue) where the administered toxicant can be found at any time. Kinetic modeling is empiric, and there is flexibility in fitting model parameters to the observed data. The minimum number of compartments that adequately describe the data is used. Several different theoretical models have been described:

- One-compartment model
- Two-compartment model
- Multicompartment model
- Physiologically based model

In the one-compartment model, a toxicant when introduced into the body would be distributed evenly and instantaneously into a single homogeneous compartment. In this simple model, the body is depicted as a single homogeneous compartment (Figure 7.6).

This is not to imply that the concentration of the toxicant is the same everywhere in the body, but rather it assumes that the plasma concentration proportionately reflects the changes in tissue concentrations. The rate of elimination is proportional to the amount of the toxicant left in the plasma as measured over time and is referred to as *first-order elimination*. When graphically displayed, it would show a decrease in blood concentration as a linear function of time (see Figure 7.7).

Most toxicants, however, follow a theoretical two- or greater compartment model of disposition. In the two-compartment model the toxicant is distributed from the blood (central compartment) into a peripheral compartment (e.g., the kidney) where it can be eliminated or returned back to the blood (Figure 7.8).

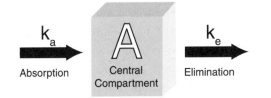

**FIGURE 7.6**   One-compartment model.

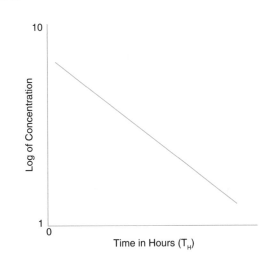

**FIGURE 7.7**   One-compartment model of disposition.

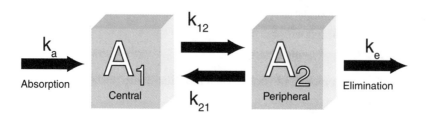

**FIGURE 7.8**    Two-compartment model.

As the concentration in the first compartment declines, the concentration in the second compartment increases, reaches a maximum level, and then declines following the time course for elimination from the body (Figure 7.9). In addition, the plasma concentration over time yields a curved line in the two-compartment model rather than a straight line, thus implying more than a single dispositional phrase.

In these models a *half-life* is described as the time required to reduce the blood or plasma concentration by 50%. This "removal" of toxicant from the blood is complex and should not be viewed as reflecting solely the elimination of toxicant from the body. It is important to recognize that a half-life of a toxicant needs to be referenced to the specific tissue (e.g., blood) that is being analyzed for its presence because it may remain in some tissues for longer or shorter periods of time. Blood or plasma is a convenient way to monitor the body's concentration of a toxicant; however, its disappearance may represent its uptake from the blood into a second compartment (an organ or tissue), its storage, metabolism, and/or its elimination from the body.

Physiologically based kinetic models attempt to simulate the distribution of toxicants in the body. The body is viewed as a multicompartment of tissues that are interconnected by blood flows (Figure 7.10).

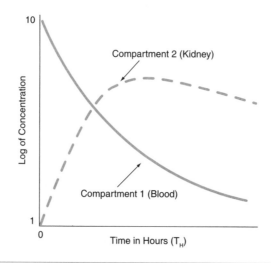

**FIGURE 7.9**    Two-compartment model of disposition.

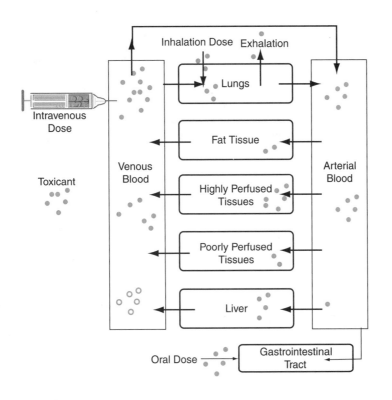

**FIGURE 7.10**    Physiologically based kinetic model.

These models are defined by physiological volumes, blood flows, partition coefficients, metabolic rate, age, sex, body weight, percentage of body fat, ventilation rate, and cardiac output. Thus they can be very complex in nature.

## Bibliography

Beringer, P. M., & Slaughter, R. L. (2005). Transporters and their impact. *Annals of Pharmacotherapy, 39,* 1097–1108. (Erratum in *Annals of Pharmacotherapy,* 2006 Jan;40(1):159.)

Bronaugh, R. L., & Maibach, H. I. (1999). Percutaneous absorption. In *Drugs and the pharmaceutical sciences* (Vol. 97). New York: Marcel Dekkar.

Houston, J. B. (1988). Kinetics of disposition of xenobiotics and their metabolites. *Drug Metabolism and Drug Interactions, 6,* 47–83.

Illing, H. P. A. (1989). *Xenobiotic metabolism and disposition.* Boca Raton, FL: CRC Press.

Klaassen, C. D. (2001). *Casarett & Doull's toxicology. The basic science of poisons.* New York: McGraw-Hill.

Klaassen, C. D., & Watkins, J. B. (2003). *Casarett & Doull's essentials of toxicology.* New York: McGraw-Hill.

Krüse, J., de Raat, W. K., & Verhaar, H. J. (Eds.) (2002). *The practical applicability of toxicokinetic models in the risk assessment of chemicals.* Norwell, MA: Kluwer Academic Publishers.

Lipscomb, J. C., & Lipscomb, C. (2006). *Toxicokinetics and risk assessment.* Boca Raton, FL: CRC Press.

Ramesh, A., Walker, S. A., Hood, D. B., Guillen, M. D., Schneider, K., & Weyand, E. H. (2004). Bioavailability and risk assessment of orally ingested polycyclic aromatic hydrocarbons. *International Journal of Toxicology, 23,* 301–333.

Subramanian, K. (2005). truPK—human pharmacokinetic models for quantitative ADME prediction. *Expert Opinion on Drug Metabolism and Toxicology, 1,* 555–564.

Sun, J., He, Z. G., Cheng, G., Wang, S. J., Hao, X. H., & Zou, M. J. (2004). Multidrug resistance P-glycoprotein: crucial significance in drug disposition and interaction. *Medical Science Monitor, 10,* RA5–RA14.

U.S. National Library of Medicine, National Institutes of Health, Environmental Health, and Toxicology Specialized Information Services (SIS). (2005). *Toxicology tutorial I.* Retrieved October 2, 2005 from http://www.sis.nlm.nih.gov/enviro/toxtutor.html.

U.S. National Library of Medicine, National Institutes of Health, Environmental Health and Toxicology Specialized Information Services (SIS). (2005). *Toxicology tutorial II.* Retrieved October 2, 2005 from http://www.sis.nlm.nih.gov/enviro/toxtutor.html.

Welling, P. G., & De La Inglesia, F. (Eds.) (1993). Drug toxicokinetics series. In *Drug and chemical toxicology* (Vol. 9). New York: Marcel Dekkar.

Wu, C. Y., & Benet, L. Z. (2005). Predicting drug disposition via application of BCS: transport/absorption/elimination interplay and development of a biopharmaceutics drug disposition classification system. *Pharmaceutical Research, 22,* 11–23.

Xu, C., Li, C. Y., & Kong, A. N. (2005). Induction of phase I, II and III drug metabolism/transport by xenobiotics. *Archives of Pharmacal Research, 28,* 249–268.

# CHAPTER 8

# Distribution, Storage, and Elimination of Toxicants

Distribution is the process in which a chemical agent, after first gaining entry into the internal body fluid (usually the blood), translocates throughout the fluid compartments of the body. The blood carries the toxicant to its sites of biotransformation, site(s) of action, storage, and elimination.

A number of factors can affect the distribution of a toxicant in the body:

- Lipid solubility
- Ease of crossing cell membranes
- Blood flow to the tissue or organ
- Extent of plasma protein binding

There are a number of concerns regarding the movement and distribution of toxicants throughout the body. These concerns involve the rate of distribution, the role of exposure route on distribution outcome, and determinants of equal or unequal distribution to the cells and tissues of the body.

## Body Water and Volume of Distribution

The process of toxicant distribution results in the movement of the chemical from the exposure site to internal areas of the body. Toxicant distribution depends on many factors, including what is referred to as the *apparent volume of distribution* ($V_D$), which is a concept that is related to the concentration of the toxicant in different fluid compartments within the body. It is the theoretical total volume of water required to equally distribute the toxicant throughout the body, expressed in liters/kg. This is important to know because it indicates the extent of the distribution of a toxicant within the body fluids. Water, as we all recognize, comprises most of the weight of the body and is distributed into primarily three fluid compartments:

- *Blood plasma water,* simply referred to here as the plasma, accounts for about 4–5% of total body weight.
- *Interstitial water* is referred to as interstitial fluid, which is the fluid surrounding the cells of the tissues of the body, and represents approximately 15% of total body weight.
- *Intracellular water,* or intracellular fluid, is a fluid contained within the cells and represents approximately 40% of total body weight (approximately 28 liters of water).

The blood plasma and the interstitial fluid are collectively referred to as the extracellular fluid, contain approximately 14 liters of water, and represent approximately 20% of the total body weight (Figure 8.1).

A toxicant with a low $V_D$ is distributed to all compartments and therefore is present at a lower concentration than one with a high $V_D$ that may be primarily contained in blood plasma, because of plasma protein binding, which would tend to reduce the concentration of "free or unbound" toxicant. A very high apparent $V_D$ may also indicate that the toxicant has been distributed primarily to and accumulated at a particular site, such as a storage area (e.g., fat tissue). The volume of distribution for a toxicant can be approximated using the following formula:

$$V_D = D/[C_P]$$

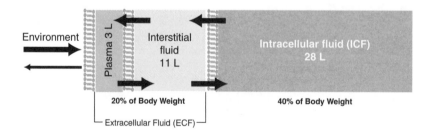

**FIGURE 8.1**   Distribution of body water and movement of toxicant between compartments.

where $D$ is the dose of the toxicant in milligrams and $[C_p]$ is the plasma concentration of the toxicant in milligrams per liter of plasma(mg/l). The total amount of a toxicant that is contained in the body can be estimated if the volume of distribution is known by multiplying it with the plasma concentration:

$$\text{Plasma concentration (mg/l)} \times V_D \text{ (l)} = \text{total amount of toxicant in the body (mg)}$$

## Plasma Binding, Blood Flow, and Barriers to Distribution

A toxicant upon gaining entry into the blood will move in the plasma either in the unbound or bound form to be distributed to the tissues and organs of the body. The distribution of toxicants from the blood to the tissues and organs of the body may not be uniform. Based on specializations of the blood vessels and other factors, certain parts of the body such as the placenta, the testes, and brain may serve as "barriers" to the diffusion of certain chemicals in the blood, thereby restricting their entry and reducing potential toxicity. These barriers should not be viewed as completely restricting the entry of toxicants; instead, they should be viewed as slowing down the rate of entry.

Once the toxicant has gained entry into the blood, it can be stored, eliminated, and metabolized. Unbound and bound toxicants tend to be in equilibrium in the plasma. Plasma proteins, especially albumin, may act to bind to the toxicant, thereby reducing its potential to enter the cells of the body, because generally only the unbound toxicant is able to cross cell membranes. Plasma protein binding therefore affects the distribution of toxicant, the "effective" dose of the toxicant, and its time within the body. Lymph generally plays only a minor role in the distribution of toxicants.

The amount of blood flow to the tissues and organs of the body may be important in the accumulation of a toxicant. Some tissues and organs that have relatively low perfusion rates are often important in the storage of toxicant and not as the target for toxicity. For example, the bones, which have a relatively low blood perfusion, can serve as storage area for some heavy metals and is essentially unaffected, whereas the kidneys with a relatively high perfusion rate, stores metals also and is also a target for toxicity. The storage of toxicants in the body can be viewed as beneficial to some extent, if accumulation is occurring in the tissue or organ that is not the target for toxicity.

## Toxicant Storage

The storage of toxicants occurs in connective tissues, primarily fat and bone, and in the kidneys and liver. Fat or adipose tissue is located in many parts of the body and is especially accumulated in the subcutaneous tissue. It is here where lipophilic toxicants are stored and are mobilized back into the blood for further distribution, metabolism, elimination, or redeposition.

Bone or osseous tissue is also an important site for the deposition of lead, strontium, and fluoride. Although bone has a relatively poor blood supply, mobilization of elements out of the bone matrix does occur, especially during times of extensive bone remodeling (e.g., repair of a broken bone) or during pregnancy when minerals are mobilized from maternal to fetal compartments. For example, lead may be substituted for calcium, and fluoride may be substituted for hydroxyl ions. Heavy metals stored in the bone may reside there for decades.

The liver and kidneys, with their relatively high blood flow, may store toxicants in amounts greater than other organs. The liver has the greatest capacity of all the tissues for metabolism, which may make it especially vulnerable to injury.

## Toxicant Elimination

The processes of toxicant elimination are critical to the reduction of toxicity or potential toxicity in the body. The term *elimination* encompasses all of the processes that are used by the body that lead to a decrease in the amount of toxicant. These processes are as follows:

- Renal elimination
- Fecal elimination
- Pulmonary elimination
- Biotransformation
- Elimination via minor routes (e.g., sweat, milk, hair, and nails)

The more rapid the elimination from the body, the less likely there will be a concentration of toxicant over time that has the potential to produce injury to the cells and tissues of the body. One needs only to think about the potential for toxicity from consuming large amounts of vitamin supplements. A water-soluble vitamin such as vitamin C, for example, is rapidly eliminated with the urine, and other than some potential to produce irritation to the gastrointestinal mucosa, systemic toxicity is unlikely to occur even with the oral consumption of large amounts. This is in contrast to a fat-soluble vitamin such as vitamin K, where because of its much slower elimination from the body the potential exists to reach concentrations over time that may result in toxicity.

Elimination refers to the removal of an absorbed toxicant through both excretion and metabolism. Excretion is the removal of systemic toxicants through specific excretory processes, such as urinary elimination. It is through the excretory processes that most of the elimination of toxicants takes place. The kidneys (through urine), the gastrointestinal tract (through the feces and bile), and the lungs for volatile substances are the most important excretory routes for the elimination of toxicants.

The processes of metabolism (biotransformation), which results in the chemical alteration of the toxicant, occur primarily in the liver; however, metabolism by other tissues (extrahepatic metabolism) may be important as well. Often, only minor chemical alteration of the toxicant molecule and subsequent conjugation with an endogenous molecule (which is most often the case), such as an amino acid or sugar, is required to facilitate elimination.

# Urinary Excretion

Elimination of toxicants by renal excretion is one of the most important routes available to the body. The kidneys are composed of approximately 1 million functional units referred to as *nephrons.* Each nephron (Figure 8.2) is composed of a capillary ball called a glomerulus and a capsule surrounding the glomerulus (Bowman's capsule), leading to the proximal tubule, loop of Henle, distal tubule, and, finally, collecting tubule. The processes of glomerular filtration, tubular secretion, and tubular reabsorption are responsible for getting toxicant from the blood into the urine, which has been produced along the nephron, and delivering it to the collecting tubules. The urine contained within the collecting tubules of the nephrons of each kidney empties into the renal pelvis and exits by the ureter, which leads to the urinary bladder.

The urinary excretion of toxicant is influenced by factors that are related to the properties of the toxicant:

- Molecular size
- Water solubility
- Degree of ionization

For most toxicants, whether they are lipophilic or hydrophilic, size is generally not a problem, and they are filtered across the glomerulus with relative ease if they are not protein bound in the plasma. Ionized toxicants tend to remain within the urine and thus exit when the urine is eliminated from the body. Toxicants that are more lipophilic can reenter into the renal circulation through reabsorption, thus increasing their resident time within the body.

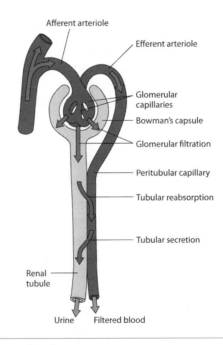

**FIGURE 8.2**    The nephron and toxicant movement.

## Filtration

The kidneys have a very well-developed arterial blood supply. The process of toxicant removal from the blood occurs at the glomerulus of the nephron, where a large amount of blood plasma filters through the large pores of the glomeruli and into the beginning of the nephron tube, Bowman's capsule. The pores are so large that normally the only chemicals that do not filter through are large macromolecules, such as blood cells and proteins. The presence of significant amounts of protein such as albumin in urine may be an indication of injury to the nephron.

Binding of toxicant to proteins in the plasma would reduce its elimination. Both lipid-soluble and water-soluble toxicants pass through the glomerulus to form the glomerular filtrate, which is the first step in the production of urine. The glomerular of the nephron allows for virtually complete passage of chemicals with molecular weights up to about 5 kDa, and therefore the glomerular filtration and the blood plasma are essentially mirror images of each other with respect to these chemicals. The selective nature of the glomerular membrane is essentially related only to the size of a chemical, excluding molecular weights of approximately 40 kDa and higher. Indeed, because of the high blood flow to the kidneys, a positive hydrostatic blood pressure, and osmotic pressure differences across glomerulus coupled with the large glomerular pores, the average adult can produce approximately 40 to 50 gallons of filtrate per day. This filtrate, referred to as the glomerular filtrate or ultrafiltrate, is concentrated within the nephron tubules. About 99% is reabsorbed (the consequences would be dire if it was not) by the capillaries surrounding the nephron tubules, and the remaining 1% is further modified as it moves through the nephron tubules into the collecting ducts as urine.

The concentration gradient, which emerges between forming urine and the blood plasma, can result in the diffusion of some substances out of the tubule cells and back into the blood. In particular, lipophilic substances can rapidly diffuse across the membranes of the tubular cells and return back to the blood, thus causing difficulty in elimination, as for example in the case of polychlorinated biphenyls and dichlorodiphenyltrichloroethane. The process of biotransformation, however, which generally produces a much more polar metabolite, facilitates in the elimination of the toxicant from the body.

## Reabsorption

It is through the process of reabsorption that most of the water, electrolytes, amino acids, glucose, and other low-molecular-weight chemicals are returned back to the blood from the glomerular filtrate. The process occurs primarily in the proximal convoluted tubule and is driven primarily by simple diffusion, which is driven by the difference between the relatively higher concentration or osmotic pressure in the proximal convoluted tubule of the nephron and the relatively lower concentration or osmotic pressure in the blood plasma of the capillaries that surround the tubules of the nephron. Although there are active transport mechanisms for reabsorption, they are generally restricted to normal endogenous compounds such as amino acids and sugars and are thus relatively transport specific. Unless the toxicant is very closely related structurally to the endogenous compound, active transport mechanisms are of little significance because reabsorption of almost all xenobiotics occurs through passive diffusion.

The pH of the urine can be an important factor in determining the extent of reabsorption, and clinically this is exploited in the acute management of patients who have ingested chemicals that are capable of ionizing in the blood. Alkaline urine facilitates the ionization of weak acids and thus their elimination from the body in the urine. Acidic urine results in less ionization of weak acids, thus resulting in decreased elimination and increased reabsorption such as is the case with weak acids such as sulfate and glucuronide conjugates.

Clinically, treatment for poisonings from drugs such as aspirin or phenobarbital (acidic drugs) or amphetamine (basic drugs) can be facilitated by appropriately altering the pH of the urine, which is variable and influenced by numerous factors normally, such as diet. Alkalinization of the urine for phenobarbital and acidification for amphetamine facilitates the elimination of the respective drugs in the urine. The clinical administration of something as simple as sodium bicarbonate can be a life-saving intervention.

### Secretion

The process of renal secretion involves the active transport of chemicals from the blood into the proximal tubule of the nephron and is of importance in the conservation of important body ions such as potassium. Two separate transport systems exist that have a relatively low degree of chemical specificity. These tubular systems are responsible for the transport of weak acids (anions) and bases (cations):

- Anionic system: transports organic acids such as penicillins and aminosalicylic acid, sulfonic acids and acidic metabolites such as glycine and sulfate conjugates, and glucuronides
- Cationic system: transports organic bases such as histamine, morphine, and ammonium compounds

Because secretion involves the expenditure of energy by the proximal tubule cells, the transport systems are not restricted to the molecular size limitations involved in passive transport mechanisms, such as diffusion. Chemicals that are plasma protein bound can be secreted into the proximal tubule, where dissociation of the plasma protein takes place, thereby restoring it back to the blood while incorporating the chemical into the tubule to facilitate its elimination.

## Fecal Elimination

Toxicants can be eliminated in the feces through their direct discharge into the lumen of the gastrointestinal tract or through excretion in the bile. Toxicants and their metabolites may also be reabsorbed and returned to the liver. Biliary excretion is the main route of gastrointestinal elimination of toxicants and their metabolites. Some chemicals are removed from the body primarily by biliary excretion, which is an active secretory process with specific transporters for organic acids and bases, heavy metals such as lead and mercury, as well as nonionized chemicals. In general, however, it is the relatively large ionized molecules that are excreted into the bile for elimination. Disorders of the liver that may compromise bile secretion could intensify or prolong the effects of some chemicals that would normally be eliminated through this route.

Toxicants in the bile are transported to the intestinal tract where they are eliminated with the feces or reabsorbed. Excretion of toxicants from the liver generally is accompanied by their biotransformation.

The enterohepatic circulation is a way in which toxicants can be reabsorbed from the bile that has entered into the gastrointestinal tract at the duodenum and returned to the liver by way of the hepatic portal circulation. The recycling of toxicant between intestine and liver has the effect of prolonging its time in the body. This is of particular concern because biotransformation in the liver may have produced a metabolite that is more toxic than the parent compound.

Toxicants can also be eliminated with the feces through their direct diffusion across the intestinal capillaries of the submucosa to the intestinal lumen where they can be eliminated with the feces. Although this relatively slow elimination pathway is not the primary route of toxicant elimination by way of the gastrointestinal tract, it can be important under conditions where urinary or biliary excretion have become less effective.

## Pulmonary Elimination

The lungs have a large surface area and receive the entire cardiac output, thus making them an important route for the elimination of volatile liquids and gases. Important factors that determine elimination of chemicals from the lungs include concentration differences between alveolar air and blood plasma, vapor pressure, and plasma solubility. Elimination is by simple diffusion from blood to alveolus, following a concentration gradient if the concentration in capillary blood is greater than the concentration of the chemical in the alveolar air.

For those gases that have a relatively low solubility in blood, elimination is generally much more rapid than for those that are more soluble. As an example, chloroform and ethylene are greatly different in their blood solubilities. Ethylene does not dissolve well in the blood and is therefore eliminated much more rapidly than chloroform, which has greater blood solubility. Lipophilic gases such as halothane have the potential to accumulate in the body's adipose tissue, and trace amounts in exhaled breath may be present for a long time after the administration of the gas.

## Minor Routes of Elimination

Minor routes of elimination include

- Saliva
- Milk
- Sweat
- Tears
- Semen
- Hair
- Nails
- Eggs (for birds)
- Placenta

Toxicants can be transferred from mother's milk to the nursing infant as well as from cow milk to people. Of special concern are those chemicals that are lipophilic, because milk contains a relatively high percentage of fat and therefore these chemicals would diffuse from body fat to plasma to mammary gland and be excreted into milk. In addition, chemicals that behave in the body similar to calcium (e.g., lead) can also be excreted along with calcium into the milk. Toxicant transport into milk occurs primarily by diffusion of the nonionized chemical. The pH difference between blood plasma and milk, about 7.4 and 6.5, respectively, would favor higher concentrations of organic bases in milk compared with organic acids.

Some toxicants that are eliminated via sweat may, if present in sufficient quantities, cause skin irritation. Toxicants that are eliminated to some extent in saliva are usually swallowed, thus prolonging residence time in the body.

Although there is negligible elimination of toxicants via the hair and nails, some chemicals such as mercury and arsenic may be found there using detection methods that have been developed primarily for forensic purposes.

The placenta, although not traditionally viewed as an excretory organ for toxicants, does move toxicants from maternal compartment to fetal compartment. At the end of a pregnancy, it has a surface area of approximately 10 m$^2$. It normally functions as an interface, providing oxygen and nutrients to the fetus while eliminating fetal metabolites and carbon dioxide. This occurs by diffusion and active transport. Maternal elimination of toxicants via the placental route can result in a redistribution of chemicals from maternal tissues to fetal tissues. Simple diffusion provides the mechanism to drive lipophilic and low-molecular-weight chemicals across the placenta. The placenta is relatively nonprotective to the fetus for lipophilic chemicals, and maternal and fetal tissue levels may be comparable.

As history has shown, for some birds the elimination of toxicants via the eggs, while posing little hazard to the mother, may result in greatly endangering the chances of survival of the young.

## Bibliography

Balani, S. K., Miwa, G. T., Gan, L. S., Wu, J. T., & Lee, F. W. (2005). Strategy of utilizing in vitro and in vivo ADME tools for lead optimization and drug candidate selection. *Current Topics in Medicinal Chemistry, 5,* 1033–1038.

Barton, H. A., Pastoor, T. P., Baetcke, K., Chambers, J. E., Diliberto, J., Doerrer, N. G., Driver, J. H., Hastings, C. E., Iyengar, S., Krieger, R., Stahl, B., & Timchalk, C. (2006). The acquisition and application of absorption, distribution, metabolism, and excretion (ADME) data in agricultural chemical safety assessments. *Critical Reviews in Toxicology, 36,* 9–35.

Caldwell, J., Gardner, I., & Swales, N. (1995). An introduction to drug disposition: the basic principles of absorption, distribution, metabolism, and excretion. *Toxicologic Pathology, 23,* 102–114.

Ekins, S. (2006). Systems-ADME/Tox: resources and network approaches. *Journal of Pharmacological and Toxicological Methods, 53,* 38–66.

Ekins, S., Nikolsky, Y., & Nikolskaya, T. (2005). Techniques: application of systems biology to absorption, distribution, metabolism, excretion and toxicity. *Trends in Pharmacological Sciences, 26,* 202–209.

Klaassen, C. D. (2001). *Casarett & Doull's toxicology. The basic science of poisons.* New York: McGraw-Hill.

Klaassen, C. D., & Watkins, J. B. (2003). *Casarett & Doull's essentials of toxicology.* New York: McGraw-Hill.

Shitara, Y., Horie, T., & Sugiyama, Y. (2006). Transporters as a determinant of drug clearance and tissue distribution. *European Journal of Pharmaceutical Sciences, 27,* 425–446.

Tsatsaris, V., Cabrol, D., & Carbonne, B. (2004). Pharmacokinetics of tocolytic agents. *Clin Pharmacokinet, 43,* 833–844.

U.S. National Library of Medicine, National Institutes of Health, Environmental Health, and Toxicology Specialized Information Services (SIS). (2005). *Toxicology tutorial III.* Retrieved October 2, 2005 from http://www.sis.nlm.nih.gov/enviro/toxtutor.html.

Welling, P. G., & de la Iglesia, F. A. (Ed.) (1993). Drug toxicokinetics. In *drug and chemical toxicology series* (Vol. 9). New York: Marcel Dekkar.

# CHAPTER 9

# Biotransformation

The term *biotransformation*, which for our purposes can be used synonymously with metabolism, is the sum of all chemical processes of the body that modify endogenous or exogenous chemicals. Biotransformation is one of the focus areas of toxicokinetics; the others are absorption, distribution, storage, and elimination. Biotransformation is affected by factors pertaining to the toxicant as well as the host. Host factors include, for example, age, sex, existing disease, genetic variability (toxicogenetics), enzyme induction, and nutritional status.

The ability to metabolize a toxicant can vary greatly with age and sex, for example. The developing fetus and the very young may have limited biotransformation capability primarily due to a lack of important enzymes. These enzymes generally reach their optimal capacity for biotransformation by the time young adulthood is reached. Similarly, the elderly can also have difficulties with biotransformation due to functional loss with aging. Enzyme fluctuations are at their lowest in early adulthood, which corresponds to the most efficient time in our lives for biotransformation (metabolism).

Differences in hormones account for gender-specific variability in the biotransformation of some toxicants. Nutritional status can impact biotransformation because specific vitamin, mineral, and protein deficiencies can decrease the body's ability to synthesize essential enzymes. Nutritional status can have an effect on the body's ability to metabolize chemicals, because biotransforming enzymes cannot be synthesized or function efficiently in the absence of a dietary supply of important chemicals, such as amino acids; carbohydrates; and cofactors, such as essential vitamins and minerals.

Diseases that affect the liver can be particularly detrimental to biotransformation because the liver is the principal organ for these reactions. Hepatitis, for example, can significantly reduce the biotransformation capacity of the liver, thus further contributing to a decline in the health of the affected individual. Marked species differences must also be taken into consideration, especially because animals are used for toxicity studies that often form the basis for predicting human health effects.

As students of public health, we therefore need to be acutely aware and sensitive to these and other differences that exist within populations, because this may account for great variations in the tolerance to environmental and occupational exposures to chemicals as well as to chemicals intended to produce benefit.

## Enzymes

Enzymes are biological catalysts and high-molecular-weight proteins, which allow for biotransformation reactions to proceed at rates that are consistent with life. Enzyme defects can result in altered body biochemistry and may result in injury to the body, especially if the enzyme is the catalyst for a biotransformation reaction that is essential to the body and for which no or less efficient alternative enzymatic pathways are available. For example, some individuals are born with a genetic condition in which the enzyme that converts the amino acid phenylalanine to another amino acid, tyrosine, is defective, resulting in a condition known as phenylketonuria. These individuals must be maintained on a diet that restricts their intake of foods containing phenylalanine, including the use of some artificial sweeteners during infancy and childhood; otherwise, mental retardation may result.

Enzymes provide the molecular surface for a chemical reaction to proceed for substrates (reactants) that have the correct molecular architecture to fit onto the anchoring and reaction sites of the enzyme. This is sometimes referred to as enzyme specificity, or a "lock and key" arrangement (Figure 9.1). In the absence of "proper fit," biotransformation of the substrate(s) may not proceed. The degree of enzyme specificity for substrates determines the extent of its involvement with different chemicals.

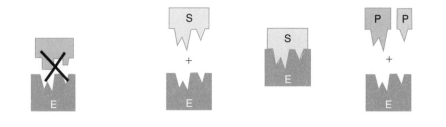

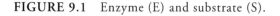

FIGURE 9.1   Enzyme (E) and substrate (S).

The degree of specificity for an enzyme may be absolute in the sense that it will catalyze only one specific reaction, or specificity may be less restrictive and overlapping for many different chemicals that share enough structural similarity with each other to allow for different reactions to proceed with the same enzyme. In the latter case an enzyme may catalyze chemicals that have a particular type of chemical bond or functional group.

As examples, consider the biotransformation of alcohols. These chemicals share a common hydroxyl group and can be metabolized by the nonmicrosomal enzyme alcohol dehydrogenase, which can produce metabolites that differ in their toxicity, depending on which alcohol is metabolized. In the case of ethanol, the metabolite produced, acetaldehyde, is more toxic than ethanol and thus needs to be eliminated from the body as quickly as possible. It is the acetaldehyde that is believed to be responsible for the alcohol hangover. A second enzyme, acetaldehyde dehydrogenase, catalyzes the conversion of acetaldehyde to acetates and other chemicals that the body can use. Some individuals of Asian descent have less capacity to produce acetaldehyde dehydrogenase, thus making them less tolerant to the effects of alcohol due to acetaldehyde accumulation. Clinically, the drug disulfiram (Antabuse) has been used to treat alcoholics by blocking the activity of this enzyme, thus producing a very unpleasant experience if the individual decides to consume any alcohol. In the case of consumption of the alcohol methanol, the same enzyme, alcohol dehydrogenase, produces formaldehyde, which is further metabolized by the aldehyde dehydrogenase to formic acid and formate. These substances can profoundly affect the optic nerve, causing blindness and even death with as little as the consumption of 1 ounce of liquid containing 40% methanol. Because alcohol dehydrogenase is not only present in the liver but occurs in other tissues of the body as well, including the retina of the eye where it is present in relatively high concentration, it is understandable that blindness may result from methanol consumption.

A number of enzymes are important for the biotransformation of toxicants. The resulting modification of the parent compound is a product that we refer to as *the metabolite,* and for any particular chemical it may be one that is used by the body to facilitate, improve, or impede physiological function, elimination, or storage.

For toxicants the "wisdom" of the process is essentially one whereby chemicals are ideally "detoxified" by

- Rendering them *less* harmful through enzymatic modifications
- Rendering them *more* water soluble to facilitate their elimination from the body

Unfortunately, depending on the chemical, biotransformation can result in the production of a metabolite(s) that may be more toxic than the parent compound. When this occurs, we refer to the process as *bioactivation,* as would occur, for example, in the bioactivation of chloroform to the more toxic chemical phosgene (Figure 9.2).

Different enzymes of the body may compete for the same toxicant, producing different metabolites that may greatly vary in their toxicity. Consider the organophosphate pesticide malathion; it can be metabolized by enzymes known as carboxylesterases, producing relatively nontoxic metabolites. Also competing for the pesticide is another enzyme known as cytochrome P450, which produces metabolites that are far more toxic than the parent compound. Under normal circumstances most of the malathion to which we are exposed is

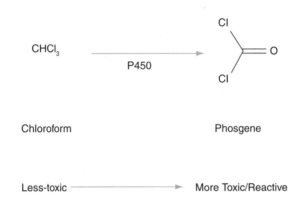

CHCl₃ → P450 → Phosgene

Chloroform                    Phosgene

Less-toxic ─────────→ More Toxic/Reactive

**FIGURE 9.2**    Bioactivation of chloroform to phosgene.

detoxified; however, situations can arise where individuals are "overexposed" to more pesticide than can be handled by the carboxylesterases. This may result in clinically significant nervous system effects through the interference of the body's normal neuromuscular transmission by the bioactivated metabolite that was produced. Malathion is also a good example to illustrate the differences in biotransformation in different species. The pesticide is relatively safe in humans due to our ability to enzymatically hydrolyze it; however, insects have little capacity to hydrolyze this pesticide and instead oxidize it to malaoxon, which is highly toxic to insects (also highly toxic to humans as well).

As a further example, the dye aniline is metabolized by the enzymes P450 and N-hydroxylase. Two very different metabolites are produced that greatly differ in their toxicities (Figure 9.3).

Metabolic reactions can be significantly influenced by the dose of the chemical to be metabolized; at low doses detoxification reactions may proceed at maximum efficiency, whereas at higher dose levels detoxification enzymes may become saturated with substrate, resulting in its accumulation and/or entering into reactions with other enzymes that may produce a metabolite that is more toxic than the parent compound. Enzyme systems normally function to protect us from the toxic effects of small to moderate doses of many of the xenobiotics to which we are exposed. When protection breaks down, toxicity can result, often from essentially overwhelming the body with doses too large to process through the normal detoxification pathways. As an example, con-

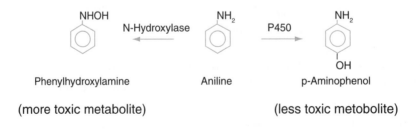

Phenylhydroxylamine ← N-Hydroxylase ← Aniline → P450 → p-Aminophenol

Phenylhydroxylamine          Aniline          p-Aminophenol

(more toxic metabolite)                    (less toxic metobolite)

**FIGURE 9.3**    Metabolism of aniline by two different enzymes.

sider the biotransformation of the pain and fever reducer acetaminophen (Tylenol) under conditions of normal use and overdose. Large amounts of acetaminophen can produce serious liver injury. Normally, this drug undergoes rapid hepatic metabolism and elimination of metabolites through the urine and feces. High doses can deplete detoxification enzymes, resulting in alternate pathways for unmetabolized acetaminophen, which is toxic to the liver.

Our protective biochemicals, including our enzymes, under certain conditions can be essentially depleted when rates exceed the ability of the body to replenish them. The metabolism of many toxicants proceeds through two general phases in the biotransformation process. Phase 1 enzymes catalyze reactions such as oxidation, hydrolysis, and reduction, and phase 2 enzymes catalyze conjugation reactions. Phase 1 enzymes either expose or attach a functional group onto the parent molecule for the "purpose" of making it more hydrophilic. Phase 1 thus facilitates toxicant elimination and makes it more likely to enter into a phase 2 reaction, which further increases hydrophilicity through the attachment of endogenous chemicals, such as carbohydrates, or amino acids onto the phase 1 metabolite.

Some chemicals may undergo only phase 2 metabolism. For example, the chemical phenol already possesses a functional group that can be conjugated without proceeding through a phase 1 reaction. Phenol is sulfated in a phase 2 reaction to yield the chemical phenyl sulfate. Phenol is also obtained from a phase 1 biotransformation of benzene (Figure 9.4).

## Tissues Where Biotransformation Proceeds

The enzymes for biotransformation reactions are found in many tissues of the body. It is the liver, however, that has the highest capacity for entering into reactions because of its high concentration of enzymes. This makes it highly susceptible to toxicity from many chemicals that are bioactivated there. This susceptibility is further enhanced because the venous blood of the liver has a relatively high concentration of toxicants obtained from the oral route of exposure when compared with the systemic circulation, due to the "first-pass" effect.

Other tissues of importance include the lungs, kidneys, intestines, placenta, and skin. The lungs and kidneys have about a fifth of the biotransformation capacity of the liver. Phase 1 enzymes are found in the endoplasmic reticulum. They are microsomal (membrane bound) and lipophilic. The term *microsome* refers to a mixture of fragmented endoplasmic reticulum vesicles present in a cell homogenate after mechanical breakage (homogenization) of tissues such as

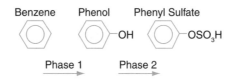

**FIGURE 9.4**    The biotransformations of benzene and phenol. *Source:* Courtesy of the Toxicology and Environmental Health Information Program of the National Library of Medicine, U.S. Department of Health and Human Services.

liver. Microsomes can be concentrated and separated from the other cellular components by means of differential centrifugation, which is based on the principle that different cellular organelles possess different and unique sedimentations and sediment out of an aqueous solution at different centrifugal forces. Unbroken cells, nuclei, and mitochondria sediment out at ~10,000$g$, whereas at 100,000$g$ the endoplasmic reticulum sediments out of solution as a pellet and the soluble cytosolic enzymes stay in the supernatant. The P450 enzymes in microsomes are concentrated and collected for experimental use. Microsomes appear as a reddish brown color due to the presence of heme in P450s and are most concentrated in liver tissue.

Cytochrome P450, a key enzyme in the biotransformation of many toxicants, derives its name from the fact that it has maximum absorbance of 450 nm light when the enzyme is bound to carbon monoxide. Other enzymes are also of importance in the biotransformation of toxicants, including hydrolases, reductases, and carboxylesterases.

In the liver, liver cells (hepatocytes) are arranged in cords of cells associated with blood vascular elements and hepatic ducts in discrete zones. Within the endoplasmic reticulum of the hepatocyte as well as other cell types that are capable of biotransformation are enzymes for phase 1 and some phase 2 reactions. The cytoplasm and to a lesser extent other cellular organelles also contain important biotransforming enzymes that can be referred to as cytosolic in that they are not membrane associated.

## Phase 1 Reactions and Cytochrome P450

Phase 1 biotransformation reactions can be either microsomal or nonmicrosomal. The three main types of phase 1 reactions are oxidation, reduction, and hydrolysis. Oxidation reactions result in the loss of electrons from the parent compound (substrate) and can proceed via the removal of hydrogen from the molecule (dehydrogenation), the transfer of electrons from the substrate to electron acceptor, or the addition of oxygen to the substrate. Depending on the substrate, oxidation reactions may involve the addition of a hydroxyl group onto the substrate (a hydroxylation reaction), removal from the substrate of nitrogen (e.g., deamination), sulfur (desulfuration), or a methyl group (demethylation). The process of chemical reduction is one whereby the substrate gains electrons. Examples of reduction reactions include disulfide, nitro, sulfoxide, and azo reductions. Reduction reactions frequently result in the bioactivation of the substrate rather than its detoxification. The reduction of nitrobenzene to the animal carcinogen, aniline, serves as an example (Figure 9.5).

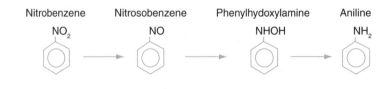

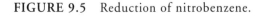

FIGURE 9.5    Reduction of nitrobenzene.

Hydrolysis of toxicants is the common form of biotransformation that results in the splitting of the toxicant molecule into smaller molecules through the addition of water: A hydroxyl group is incorporated into one of the fragments and a proton into the other. Many pesticides, amines, and esters enter into hydrolysis reactions. As examples, the hydroxylation of the pesticide methylparathion and the drug procaine are illustrated (Figure 9.6).

Most xenobiotic metabolism is mediated by cytochrome in P450. Cytochrome P450 is a heme thiolate enzyme that plays a key role in the metabolism of toxicants as well as endogenous chemicals. These enzymes are involved in a wide range of chemical reactions in the body, including oxidation, reduction, hydroxylation, dealkylation, and deamination reactions (Table 9.1). Phase 1 enzymes are capable of making a direct attack on xenobiotics by exposing or attaching a polar group. Cytochrome P450 is a multigene family of isozymes that catalyzes many biotransformations of chemicals, including pesticides, organic solvents, fatty acids, and pharmaceuticals. They demonstrate broad substrate specificity and are especially concentrated in hepatocytes, nasal mucosa, and Clara cells.

When bound to carbon monoxide, these enzymes absorb light of wavelengths near 450 nm, giving the complex a pink hue. An example of this would be biotransformation of the pesticide parathion to paraoxon (Figure 9.7). In this simple biotransformation reaction, conversion of the P=S to the P=O by P450 results in a chemical that is a hundred to a thousand times more toxic than the parent compound. These enzymes incorporate one atom of molecular oxygen (the oxidizing agent monooxygenase) into the substrate (RH), and one atom is reduced to water.

Cytochrome P450 enzymes are termed *isoforms* because they are each the product of a single gene. For example, CYP3A4 is an isoform of the 450 superfamily. It can be used to either

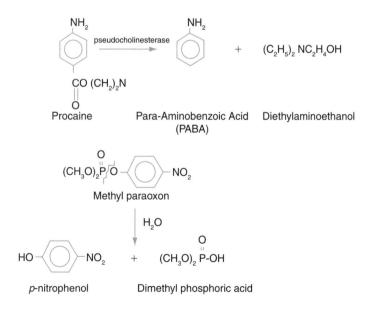

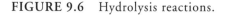

**FIGURE 9.6**  Hydrolysis reactions.

**Table 9.1    Types of P450 Reactions**

| Reaction | Examples of Substrates |
| --- | --- |
| Epoxidation, hydroxylation | Aldrin, nicotine, benzo(a)pyrene |
| S-Oxidation | Thiobenzamide, endosulfan methiocarb |
| N-Oxidation | 2-Acetylaminofluorene |
| P-Oxidation | Diethylphenylphosphine |
| O-Dealkylation | p-Nitroanisole |
| S-Dealkylation | Methylmercaptan |
| N-Dealkylation | Ethylmorphine, atrazine |
| Desulfuration | Parathion, chlorpyrifos |
| Dehalogenation | CCl4, chloroform |
| Nitro reduction | Nitrobenzene |
| Azo reduction | O-Aminoazotoluene |

designate the gene or its product, the P450 enzyme. Over 700 different forms of this enzyme (isoforms) have been characterized in terms of the gene or protein sequence data for many different species of animals. The P450 enzymes and their genes are abbreviated as "CYP." The abbreviation "CYP" is followed by a number to indicate the gene family. This is followed by a capital letter indicating the gene subfamily, which in turn is followed by a number indicating the gene. When referring to the gene and not the enzyme, the name should be italicized; thus CYP3A4 refers to the enzyme and *CYP3A4* refers to the gene.

These enzymes are heme-containing monooxygenases comprised of families and subfamilies of the enzyme as determined on the basis of sequence similarities of amino acids. In humans and other mammals, several families containing numerous P45 isoforms are responsible for xenobiotic metabolism. Other families of P450s are involved in the critical role of steroid, bile, and other endogenous substance metabolism. Mutations in, for example, the *CYP21A2* gene have been associated with birth defects; it is therefore understandable why these enzymes are so well conserved in nature because variation in their activities could be deleterious or even fatal to individuals. Thus these aberrant genotypes would be less likely to be propagated in the popula-

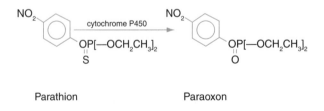

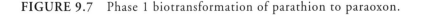

FIGURE 9.7    Phase 1 biotransformation of parathion to paraoxon.

tion. Human cytochrome P450s are a group of enzymes sharing strong structural similarities with each other but divided into 18 families of enzymes. The most important enzymes for metabolism are in the CYP1, CYP 2, CYP3, and CYP4 families. The CYP1 family is made up of three members, 1A1, 1A2, and 1B1. CYP1A2, for example, metabolizes many drugs and carcinogens. The CYP2 family contains nine subfamilies, including 2E1 and 2C, which is involved in the metabolism of many precarcinogens and pharmaceuticals. The CYP3 family, which contains the subfamily 3A4, is important both toxicologically and pharmacologically and makes up approximately 50–60% of the cytochrome P450s that are contained in the liver.

Cytochrome P450s are hemoproteins; the iron at the active site responsible for substrate binding is $Fe^{3+}$. The enzyme-substrate is reduced using nicotamide adenine dinucleotide phosphae-oxadase (NADPH), and the reduced enzyme-substrate complex binds $O_2$. The complex then splits into water, an oxidized substrate, and an oxidized P450 (Figure 9.8).

### Enzyme Induction

The process of enzyme induction is one that results in an increased ability to metabolize toxicants. Cytochrome P450 is the most common type of enzyme induction. The process is complex and generally is stimulated by exposures to the toxicant with the resulting production of greater levels of enzymes being produced to biotransform the chemical to which we are exposed (Figure 9.9). This process has been particularly well studied for chemicals such as the polycyclic aromatic hydrocarbons, phenobarbital, isoniazid, and alcohol. These inducers can alter the rate of biotransformation of other important chemicals, such as pharmaceutical agents, which may lead to an increased tolerance to the pharmaceutical. Additionally, the process of induction may facilitate the transformation of chemicals that are precarcinogens to the ones that are carcinogens.

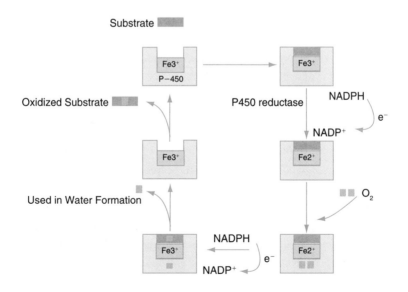

**FIGURE 9.8**    Toxicant biotransformation in phase 1 by cytochrome P450.

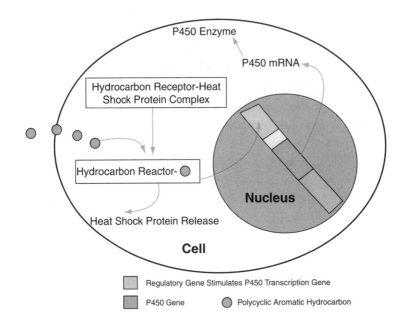

**FIGURE 9.9**    Induction of P450 by a polycyclic aromatic hydrocarbon.

## Examples of Other Phase 1 Enzymes

Epoxide hydrolases, as you would anticipate from the name, catalyze the addition of water to an epoxide to produce a dihydrodiol (two OH groups present). Dihydrodiols are much less likely to enter into chemical bonds with cellular macromolecules and are readily conjugated to facilitate their elimination. Further oxidative metabolism of the dihydrodiol by P450 can result in a more reactive metabolite that can enter into reaction with cellular macromolecules, as is the case for benz[a]pyrene (Figure 9.10).

The flavin-containing monooxygenases represent a group of enzymes that play a more limited role in the metabolism of xenobiotics. They catalyze N-, S-, and P-oxidation reactions on substrates such as nicotine, thiobenzamide, and dethylphenylphosphine, respectively. Broadly, they metabolize certain pesticides, drugs, and other chemicals similar to P450. An example would be the N-oxidation of nicotine (Figure 9.11).

Amidases and esterases are important in the metabolism of amides and esters, producing carboxylic acid and ammonia metabolites and alcohol and carboxylic acid metabolites, respectively (Figure 9.12).

Lipoxygenase is one of the arachidonic acid cascade enzymes and dioxygenates (inserts two oxygen atoms) into polyenoic fatty acids to produce a variety of important cell mediators. Lipoxygenases also contribute to *in vivo* metabolism of xenobiotics. Polyunsaturated fatty acids, fatty acid hydroperoxides, hydrogen peroxide, and synthetic organic hydroperoxides support lipoxygenase-mediated xenobiotic oxidation. The types of catalytic reactions include oxidation, epoxidation, hydroxylation, sulfoxidation, desulfuration, and N-dealkylation.

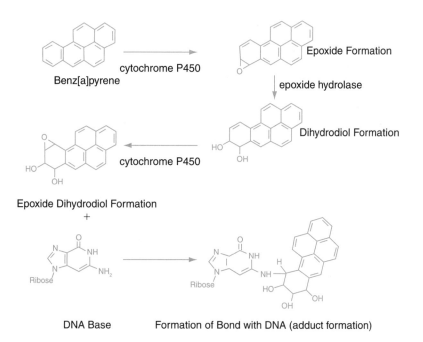

**FIGURE 9.10**    Metabolism of benz[a]pyrene by P450 and epoxide hydrolase.

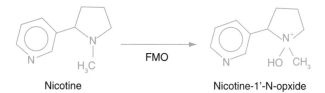

**FIGURE 9.11**    Metabolism of nicotine by flavin-containing monooxygenases.

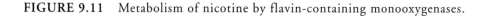

**FIGURE 9.12**    General reactions of amidases and esterases.

## Enzymes and Oxidative Stress

The metabolism of xenobiotics, particularly by the mixed function oxidases in phase 1 biotransformations, generates free radicals and thus increases oxidative stress, which can result in cellular damage. The term *free radical* can be used to designate any molecule that contains one or more unpaired electrons. These entities are usually short lived and include the reactive oxygen species such as superoxide anion radical, hydroxyl radical, and nitric oxide, as well as some nonradical oxygen derivatives such as hypochlorous acid (HOCL). The body's defense mechanisms generally provide for adequate antioxidants; however, we are often faced with oxidative stress, especially during certain times (e.g., illness). The diet provides further important antioxidants such as vitamin C and vitamin E, and the body manufactures important antioxidant enzymes such as superoxide dismutase, glutathione S-transferase, glutathione reductase, glutathione peroxidase, catalase, and epoxide hydrolase. Severe oxidative stress has been associated with, at least experimentally, alterations in DNA, cell membrane damage, depletion of important cellular reserves such as adenosine triphosphate, and metabolic abnormalities. Although reactive oxygen species have certainly been linked to certain diseases and disease pathology, it still remains to be fully elucidated whether oxidative stress is the cause of disease, a contributing factor in disease pathophysiology, or a manifestation whose clinical significance is unclear.

# Phase 2 Reactions

Xenobiotics that have undergone a phase 1 biotransformation reaction produce an intermediate metabolite. This metabolite has been slightly modified from the parent compound and now contains a "polar handle" such as a carboxyl (–COOH), amino ($NH_2$), or hydroxyl (OH) functional group. Although the metabolite is more hydrophilic in nature, it most often requires additional biotransformation to further increase hydrophilicity sufficient to permit significant elimination from the body. It is in these phase 2 reactions where this is accomplished. Phase 2 reactions are also referred to as *conjugation reactions* and result in the addition of an endogenous chemical to the functional group produced during phase 1 biotransformation. Examples of phase 2 reactions and the enzymes that catalyze the transfer of the endogenous chemical include the following:

- Glutathione conjugation       (glutathione S-transferase)
- Glucuronide conjugation       (UDP-glucuronosyltransferase)
- Amino acid conjugation        (aminotransferase)
- Sulfate conjugation           (sulphotransferase)
- Acetylation                   (acetyltransferase)
- Methylation                   (methyltransferase)

Glucuronide conjugation is an important phase 2 reaction whereby the glucose-derived chemical glucuronic acid is added onto the phase 1 metabolite via the enzyme UDP-glucuronosyltransferase (uridine 5'-diphosphate-glucuronyltransferase). These enzymes are found in membrane bound in the cell and play an important role in the detoxification of a wide range of xenobiotics in addition to endogenous compounds such as steroids and bilirubin. Through the action of these enzymes, a more polar metabolite is produced that can be readily excreted in the urine or bile. Although conjugation via this pathway generally produces metabolites of decreased toxicity, bioactivation of carcinogenic substances may occur. The glucuronide conjugation of aniline is illustrated in Figure 9.13.

Sulfate conjugation results in highly hydrophilic conjugates that are readily eliminated in the urine. Sulfation and glucuronidation are often competing pathways, with the former being the principal pathway at lower substrate levels. Conjugation by sulfate is the major phase 2 pathway for phenols.

Acetylation of aromatic amines and sulfamides is mediated by the enzyme *N*-acetyltransferase, which requires the cofactor acetyl Coenzyme A. This phase 2 reaction occurs primarily in Kupffer cells of the liver and to a lesser extent in the reticuloendothelial cells of the lung, gut, and spleen.

Glutathione-S-transferase is the enzyme responsible for conjugating glutathione, an endogenous tripeptide. The conjugates are typically less toxic than the parent compounds. The substrates are highly electrophilic products of phase 1 metabolism. Glutathione-S-transferase is widely distributed in the cytosol of the lung, liver, and kidney, and the conjugates are excreted in the bile and kidney. Glutathione-S-transferase is very important in drug metabolism, and genetic regulation of glutathione-S-transferases is complex and inducible by drugs and xenobiotics.

Xenobiotics are chemicals not normally produced by the body, and they do not have any benefit. The metabolism of these chemicals continues to be an important area of toxicological investigation to understand the mechanisms of toxicity, their fate and transport in the environment, effects on plant and animal species, and rational management approaches in dealing with both the poisoned individual and environmental remediation.

Acetaminophen toxicity can serve as a good example of the importance of a proper balance between phase 1 and phase 2 reactions. Under normal circumstances most acetaminophen that is consumed enters directly into a phase 2 reaction with the enzymes sulfotransferase and glucuronyl transferase to form the sulfate and glucuronide conjugation products that can be readily eliminated by the body. Approximately 4–5% of the clinical dose of acetaminophen is processed via phase 1 biotransformation mediated by cytochrome CYP2E1, producing a hepatotoxic metabolite, called *N*-acetyl-benzoquinoneimine (NAPQI). This metabolite also enters into a phase 2 reaction mediated by glutathione-S-transferase, thereby conjugating it to glutathione for elimination. When the liver's reserves of glutathione are depleted, hepatotoxicity results.

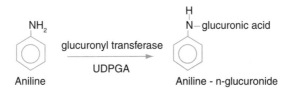

FIGURE 9.13   Glucuronide conjugation of aniline. *Source:* Courtesy of the Toxicology and Environmental Health Information Program of the National Library of Medicine, U.S. Department of Health and Human Services.

Although consumption of clinically appropriate amounts of acetaminophen is generally of little toxicological significance to the liver, large doses or doses taken too frequently can overwhelm the conjugating enzymes and result in toxicity. Toxicity is the result of acetaminophen entering into reaction with CYP2E1; therefore, the production of high levels of NAPQI can produce liver cell destruction and possibly liver failure, depending on the dose.

Elevated levels of cytochrome P450 enzymes, as a result of their induction by certain drugs and xenobiotics, can result in a facilitated competition for acetaminophen substrate and preferential formation of NAPQI even with therapeutic doses. The inhibition of enzymes or their induction can account for the toxicity or ineffectiveness of certain medications. Additionally, our diet may supply ingredients that can modify the activity of our enzymes. An example of this would be the effect of grapefruit juice on certain isoforms of cytochrome P450 that are important in metabolizing some medications and steroids.

Genetic differences are sometimes responsible for significant variations in an individual's response to chemicals. The drug isoniazid, for example, is used in the treatment of tuberculosis and is detoxified through the addition of an acetyl group onto the molecule (acetylation reaction) mediated via the enzyme *N*-acetyl-transferase. Individuals that have the normal form of this enzyme can eliminate a dose by 50% in approximately 1 hour. These individuals are referred to as "fast acetylators." Individuals who possess a mutation that codes for this enzyme possess one that is less effective, requiring about 3 hours to eliminate half of the dose. These individuals are referred to as "slow acetylators" and are at greater risk for developing isoniazid toxicity, which is characterized by numbness, tingling, and pain in the extremities (a form of peripheral neuropathy). This enzyme also plays a role in the detoxification of aromatic amines that one may be exposed to, for example, from tobacco smoke. Some research has suggested that slow acetylators may be at greater risk for the development of certain types of cancers than fast acetylators, although no clear picture at this time has emerged.

## Bibliography

Amacher, D. E. (2006). Reactive intermediates and the pathogenesis of adverse drug reactions: the toxicology perspective. *Current Drug Metabolism, 7,* 219–229.

Baer, B. R., & Rettie, A. E. (2006). CYP4B1: an enigmatic P450 at the interface between xenobiotic and endobiotics metabolism. *Drug Metabolism Reviews, 38,* 451–476.

Crowley, L. V. (2001). *An introduction to human disease: pathology and pathophysiology correlations.* Sudbury, MA: Jones and Bartlett Publishers.

Deeley, R. G., Westlake, C., & Cole, S. P. (2006). Transmembrane transport of endo- and xenobiotics by mammalian ATP-binding cassette multidrug resistance proteins. *Physiological Reviews, 86,* 849–899.

Ekins, S., Andreyev, S., Ryabov, A., Kirillov, E., Rakhmatulin, E. A., Bugrim, A., & Nikolskaya, T. (2005). Computational prediction of human drug metabolism. *Expert Opinion on Drug Metabolism and Toxicology, 1,* 303–324.

Gong, B., & Boor, P. J. (2006). The role of amine oxidases in xenobiotic metabolism. *Expert Opinion on Drug Metabolism and Toxicology, 2,* 559–571.

Ioannides, C. (2006). Cytochrome p450 expression in the liver of food-producing animals. *Current Drug Metabolism, 7,* 335–348.

Klaassen, C. D. (2001). *Casarett & Doull's toxicology. The basic science of poisons.* New York: McGraw-Hill.

Klaassen, C. D., & Watkins, J. B. (2003). *Casarett & Doull's essentials of toxicology.* New York: McGraw-Hill.

Lewis, D. F. (2005). Human P450s in the metabolism of drugs: molecular modelling of enzyme-substrate interactions. *Expert Opinion on Drug Metabolism and Toxicology, 1,* 5–8.

Ramadoss, P., Marcus, C., & Perdew, G. H. (2005). Role of the aryl hydrocarbon receptor in drug metabolism. *Expert Opinion on Drug Metabolism and Toxicology, 1,* 9–21.

Stanley, L. A., Horsburgh, B. C., Ross, J., Scheer, N., & Wolf, C. R. (2006). PXR and CAR: nuclear receptors which play a pivotal role in drug disposition and chemical toxicity. *Drug Metabolism Reviews, 38,* 515–597.

U.S. National Library of Medicine, National Institutes of Health, Environmental Health, and Toxicology Specialized Information Services (SIS). (2005). *Toxicology tutorial III.* Retrieved October 2, 2005 from http://www.sis.nlm.nih.gov/enviro/toxtutor.html.

Yamada, H., Ishii, Y., Yamamoto, M., & Oguri, K. (2006). Induction of the hepatic cytochrome P450 2B subfamily by xenobiotics: research history, evolutionary aspect, relation to tumorigenesis, and mechanism. *Current Drug Metabolism, 7,* 397–409.

# CHAPTER 10

# Chemical-Induced Mutagenesis

## DNA and Mutations

A mutation is a permanent change in the DNA, the informational molecule that is the chemical basis of heredity. It is contained within our chromosomes and codes for all the information that makes us uniquely different from each other, as well as the similarities we share as a species. It codes for all cellular proteins (e.g., enzymes) that are critical to life (Figure 10.1). Human DNA is packaged in 23 pairs of chromosomes: 22 homologous pairs and 2 sex chromosomes (XX in females and XY in males). Each chromosome is composed of a DNA molecule that is complexed with numerous proteins. It must be able to replicate, segregate, and maintain its integrity from replication to replication.

DNA is organized into genes, of which 30,000 or so encode information that is critical to maintain human life. The DNA is a base sequence that codes the information necessary for cellular growth, differentiation, and replication. DNA is composed of the following bases:

- Purines: adenine (A), guanine (G)
- Pyrimidines: cytosine (C), thymine (T)

Bases are organized into the DNA nucleotide, which contains a purine or pyrimidine base + sugar (deoxyribose) + a phosphate group (Figure 10.2).

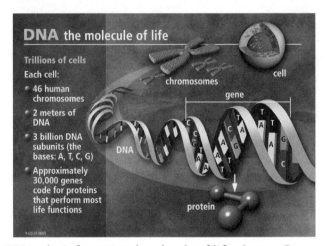

**FIGURE 10.1**    DNA: the informational molecule of life. *Source:* Courtesy of Genome Management Information System, Oak Ridge National Laboratory.

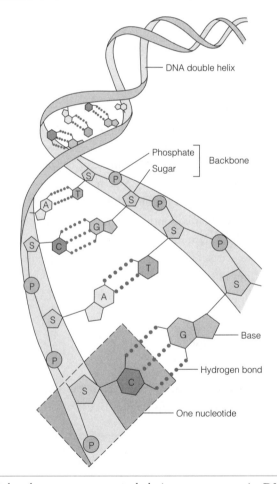

**FIGURE 10.2**    Molecular components and their arrangement in DNA.

The pairing of bases is A-T and C-G. Incorrect base pairing can result in the potential alteration of information that may be important to the normal physiology of the individual. The deletion or replacement of a single nucleotide can result, for example, in an altered protein, such as an enzyme. If these changes occur in an informational portion of the DNA, then an abnormal protein may result (Figure 10.3).

The nucleotides make up the genes, which are the fundamental physical and functional units of heredity and represent an orderly sequence within a particular region on a specific chromosome. All the component nucleotides of genes are transcribed into messenger RNA, but much "information" is discarded because genes contain coding (exons) and noncoding (introns) regions. RNA is similar to DNA (Figure 10.4) and is also composed of purine bases (adenine, guanine) and pyrimidine bases (cytosine, uracil). In RNA, however, uracil is paired with adenine during transcription. The messenger RNA is the transcription product of DNA and is the cytoplasmic informational molecule used to assemble all the necessary proteins required by the cell to function normally (Figure 10.5).

The failure of DNA to maintain its integrity or to repair errors may lead to mutations that may be critical to the survival of the cell or to those that, over time, may result in disease or impairment (Figure 10.6). Fortunately, most mutations are "silent" and produce no effect, especially if they occur in a noncoding region of the DNA.

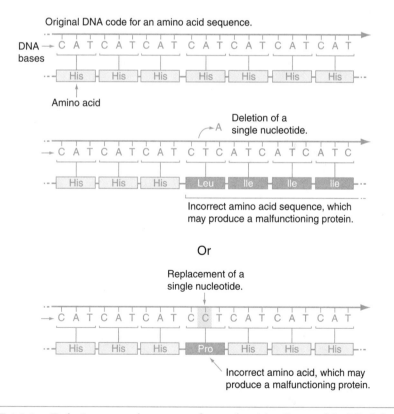

FIGURE 10.3   Deletion or replacement of a nucleotide. *Source:* Modified from *Help me understand genetics.* Courtesy of National Library of Medicine.

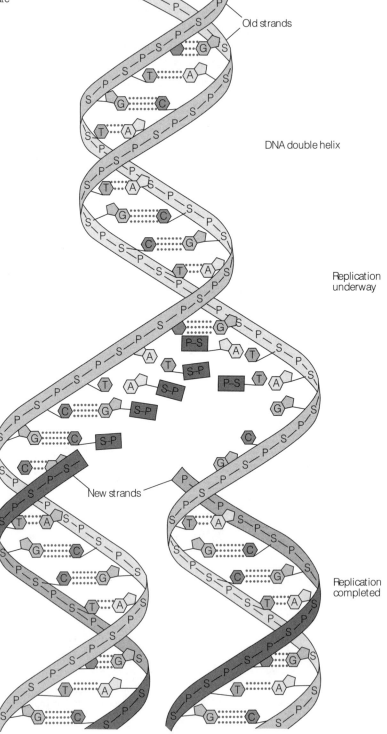

P = phosphate

S = sugar

A = adenine

G = guanine

C = cytosine

T = thymine

FIGURE 10.4a   Comparison of DNA and RNA.

Damage to DNA occurs both spontaneously and as a result of exposures to environmental agents. Fortunately, we have the capacity to both recognize and repair mutated DNA, and this may well be the only biological macromolecule that can be repaired.

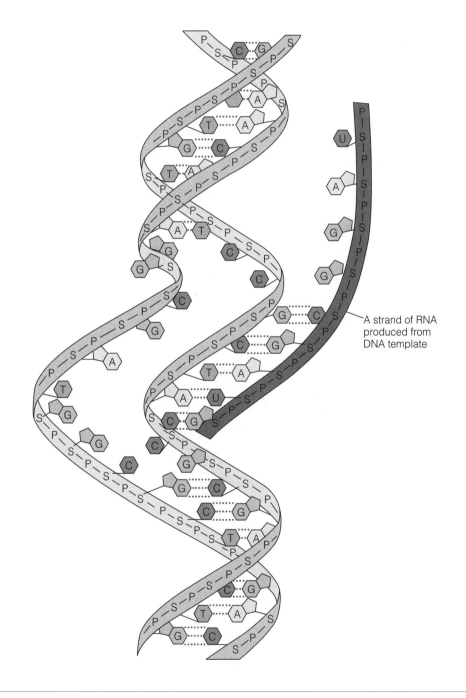

A strand of RNA produced from DNA template

**FIGURE 10.4b**    Comparison of DNA and RNA.

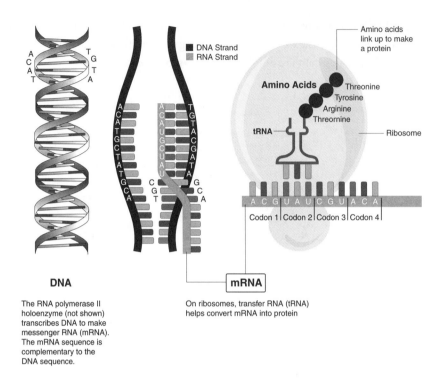

DNA

DNA Strand
RNA Strand

Amino acids link up to make a protein

Amino Acids

Threonine
Tyrosine
Arginine
Threornine

tRNA

Ribosome

A C G U A U C G U A C A

Codon 1 | Codon 2 | Codon 3 | Codon 4

mRNA

The RNA polymerase II holoenzyme (not shown) transcribes DNA to make messenger RNA (mRNA). The mRNA sequence is complementary to the DNA sequence.

On ribosomes, transfer RNA (tRNA) helps convert mRNA into protein

**FIGURE 10.5**    Messenger RNA is the cytoplasmic informational molecule transcribed from DNA. *Source:* Accessed at: http://publications.nigms.nih.gov/thenewgenetics/ images/ch_trans.jpg.

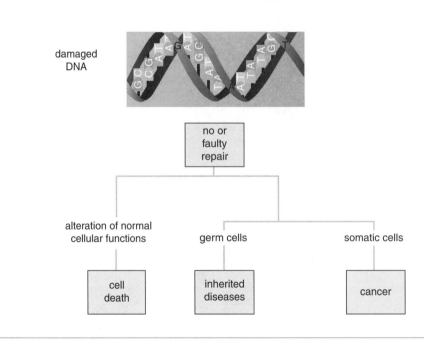

damaged DNA

no or faulty repair

alteration of normal cellular functions

germ cells

somatic cells

cell death

inherited diseases

cancer

**FIGURE 10.6**    Consequences of damaged DNA.

Mutations are acquired at some time during a person's life, or they can be inherited from a parent. Mutations can be

- Induced as a result of exposure of the DNA to environmental mutagens.
- Spontaneous as a result of "normal" cellular processes.
- Acquired (= somatic) some time during the life of an individual. Unless these occur in the gametes, they cannot be passed onto offspring.
- Hereditary (= germline) acquired from a parent through the union of the gametes at fertilization and can be present in all the cells of the offspring.

## Mutations and Apoptosis

Apoptosis is a form of planned or programmed cell death and is a normal process that occurs during embryological development, normal cellular replacement, and in response to physical, biological, or chemical stressors. Normal cell turnover occurs, without necrosis and inflammation. Apoptosis is also an important way that genetically altered cells can be removed from the body if DNA repair does not occur (Figure 10.7). Unlike necrosis, in which large numbers of

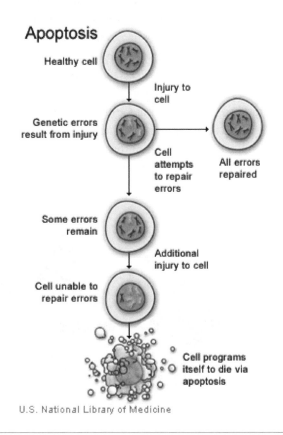

FIGURE 10.7  Apoptosis. *Source:* Accessed from: http://ghr.nlm.nih.gov/handbook/illustrations/apoptosisprocess.

cells have died and which is frequently accompanied by inflammation and cellular replacement by connective tissue, the programmed cell death of apoptosis is a selective destruction of the cell. As the cell dies, one can observe "apoptotic bodies" that in the final stage of apoptosis are digested by phagocytic cells (Figure 10.8). The triggering of apoptosis is complex and involves the cell receiving chemical messengers to "turn on" those genes involved in the self-destruction process. If these genes become mutated and apoptosis is compromised, then the cell is at greater risk of becoming one that may transform into a cancerous cell.

## Tests for DNA Damage and Mutagenicity

A number of toxicological tests can evaluate the effects of a chemical agent as being deleterious to DNA: the Ames test, tests for chromosome aberrations, micronuclei assays, sister chromatid exchanges in populations of proliferating cells, DNA repair studies (unscheduled DNA synthesis assay), and others that detect "changes" in the DNA. The Ames mutagenicity assay was developed in the early 1970s by Dr. Bruce Ames and has been used for many years as a screen for chemicals that may have mutagenic potential as determined by the frequency of mutations produced in strains of bacteria (e.g., *Salmonella typhimurium, Escherichia coli,* and *Bacillus subtilis*). A strain of *Salmonella* or *E. coli* may be used where a DNA base pair mutation has resulted in the inability to produce histidine or tryptophan, respectively, and therefore they must be provided with these amino acids in the culture medium to survive. The assay is based on a reverse mutation occurring that permits the respective bacterium to survive and grow in the absence of these essential amino acids.

Let's look at the basics for testing a chemical for mutagenicity with the bacterium *Salmonella typhimurium.* Bacteria that are deficient in the synthesis of the amino acid histidine (His–), and therefore histidine dependent, are cultured on bacterial medium that does not contain the amino acid or other amino acid supplements (minimal medium). Growth on this medium is

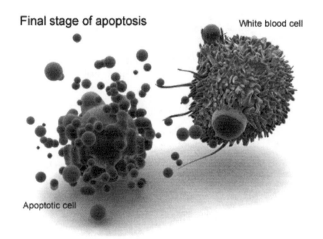

FIGURE 10.8    Final stage of apoptosis. *Source:* From *Help me understand genetics.* Courtesy of National Library of Medicine.

poor as judged by colony formation. The growth of these controls is compared with the growth of the same bacteria but cultured with the chemical of interest to be tested for mutagenic potential. If the chemical is mutagenic, then some of the bacteria undergoes a reversion mutation (His+) and forms colonies in the absence of histidine. If there is little difference in growth between the experimental and control, then the chemical is considered to be one that is not mutagenic. Because many chemicals must be metabolized and bioactivated in humans and other animals before they are capable of producing mutations, the Ames test is made more relevant by considering this and by preincubating the chemical of interest with a standardized extract (S9) of liver. This provides a source of enzymes for bioactivation should biotransformation be required to produce a mutagen (Figure 10.9).

Many chemical agents have tested positive as mutagens in the Ames test. Occasionally, the public has interpreted this test to be predictive for chemicals that may produce cancer in humans. This, of course, is not so. For one thing, to extrapolate from a bacterium to a human directly is absurd! Additionally, this test has relevance only as a screening test, not for carcinogenicity but for mutagenicity. Although it is true that many mutagens are also carcinogens, we must recognize that not all carcinogens are mutagenic (Table 10.1). As public health professionals, we must understand the values and limitations of these types of tests, although it is true that many chemicals that have tested positive in this assay have also been demonstrated to be mutagenic in laboratory tests using mammalian cells, including humans *in vitro* (Table 10.1).

The mammalian cell gene mutation test is an *in vitro* test used to detect possible mutagens by means of gene mutations induced in cell lines such as L5178Y mouse lymphoma cells, Chinese Hamster ovary cells, and TK6 human lymphoblastoid cells. For example, the cell line L5178Y, which is deficient in thymidine kinase, may be used. This is the result of a mutation, which also makes the cells resistant to the cytotoxic effects of trifluorothymidine (a pyrimidine analogue). This chemical inhibits cellular metabolism and cell division in nonmutated cells. The mutated

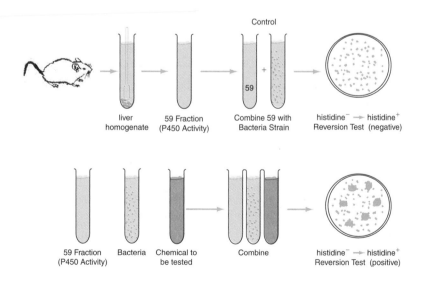

**FIGURE 10.9**    The Ames mutagenicity test.

**Table 10.1**   Not All Carcinogens Are Mutagens

| Known Human Carcinogens | Mutagen | Suspected Human Carcinogens | Mutagen |
|---|---|---|---|
| Aflatoxins | + | Acrylamide | + |
| Arsenic and arsenic compounds | – | Benz[a]anthracene | + |
| Asbestos | – | Benzidine-based dyes | + |
| Azathioprine | – | Benzo[a]pyrene | + |
| Benzene | – | Carbazole | – |
| Benzidine | + | Chlordane | – |
| Beryllium | + | Ethylene dibromide | + |
| Cadmium compounds | + | Glycidol | – |
| Chromium [VI] compounds | + | Lead | + |
| Cyclophosphamide | – | Styrene-7,8-oxide | – |
| Diethylstilbestrol | + | Tetrachloroethylene | – |
| Ethylene oxide | + | Benzofuran | – |
| Formaldehyde | + | Tris(2,3-dibromopropyl) phosphate | – |
| Gallium arsenide | + | Vinyl bromide | + |
| Vinyl chloride | + | Vinyl fluoride | + |

cells, however, are able to proliferate in the presence of the chemical, whereas normal cells, which contain the enzyme thymidine kinase, are not. Experimental (with suspected mutagen added to culture medium) and control (without suspected mutagen added to culture medium) samples are established both with and without prior bioactivation of the chemical by S9. Mutant frequency is derived from the comparison of the number of colonies formed in the various media.

## Examples of Chemical Mutagens

Some chemical mutagens directly react to disrupt the base pairing within the DNA macromolecule. Nitrous acid can, for example, deaminate (remove an amino group) the pyrimidine and purine bases. If this occurs in the base adenine, for example, it is converted to hypoxanthine, which now pairs with cytosine.

The scientific literature contains numerous examples of chemical agents that have been shown to be mutagenic. Some of these chemicals resemble the purine and pyrimidines bases of DNA, such as bromouracil. This chemical was synthetically created and has been used extensively in research because it resembles the pyrimidine thymine but has a bromium atom instead of a methyl group. It is an example of a DNA base analogue. It is incorporated into the DNA and pairs with adenine during DNA replication. These types of chemicals may be of some value to the chemotherapy of certain cancers because it is anticipated that the rapidly dividing cancerous cells preferentially incorporate this chemical into the DNA, producing defects that may lead to cellular death. Unfortunately, the chemical is not specific for cancerous cells, and other dividing cells (e.g., those of the hair follicle and the mucosa of the gastrointestinal tract) result in side effects. Some chemical agents are referred to as intercalating agents in that they tend to wedge in between the bases along the DNA molecule, thus preventing the functions of DNA polymerase and other normally present chemicals (e.g., binding proteins). This results in the inability of the DNA to properly transcribe information or prevent DNA synthesis. The dyes ethidium bromide and acridine orange are examples of this type of chemical mutagen. These chemicals can produce base frameshifts by molecular stretching of the DNA double helix and may trick the DNA polymerase into placing an additional base into the DNA macromolecule.

Other chemicals, such as methyl or ethyl methanesulfonate, mustard gas, and nitrosoguanidine, can add methyl or ethyl groups onto the bases. These types of chemicals are referred to as alkylating agents and can cause, for example, the replacement of a pyrimidine base with a purine base.

Some large molecules can bind to the DNA bases, such as benzo[a]pyrene and *N*-acetoxy-2-acetylaminofluorene, causing chemical adducts. They may form noncoding regions within the affected DNA, whereas others such as peroxides may actually cause breaks within the DNA strand.

## Bibliography

Chemical information from the Environmental Health Information Program of the National Library. Retrieved October 2, 2005 from http://chem.sis.nlm.nih.gov/chemindex.html.

Cooper, C. S. (Ed.) (1990). *Chemical carcinogenesis and mutagenesis II.* Berlin: Springer-Verlag.

Cooper, C. S., & Grover, P. L. (Ed.) (1990). *Chemical carcinogenesis and mutagenesis I.* Berlin: Springer-Verlag.

Frickel, S. (2004). *Chemical consequences: environmental mutagens, scientist activism, and the rise of genetic toxicology.* New Brunswick, NJ: Rutgers University Press.

Guengerich, F. P. (2006). Interactions of carcinogen-bound DNA with individual DNA polymerases. *Chemical Review, 106,* 420–452.

Hemminki, K., Dipple, A., Shuker, D. E. G., Kadlubar, F. F., Segerback, D., & Bartsch, H. (1994). DNA adducts: identification and biological significance. IaRC Scientific Publication [MSOffice1].

Klaassen, C. D. (2001). *Casarett & Doull's toxicology. The basic science of poisons.* New York: McGraw-Hill.

Klaassen, C. D., & Watkins, J. B. (2003). *Casarett & Doull's essentials of toxicology.* New York: McGraw-Hill.

Mathews, C. K. (2006). DNA precursor metabolism and genomic stability. *FASEB J, 20,* 1300–1314.

Mortelmans, Z. (2000). The Ames salmonella microsome mutagenicity assay. *Mutation Research: Fundamental and Molecular Mechanisms of Mutagenesis, 455,* 29–60.

Shim, J. S., & Kwon, H. J. (2004). Chemical genetics for therapeutic target mining. *Expert Opinion on Therapeutic Targets, 8,* 653–661.

Singer, B., & Grunberger, D. (1983). *Molecular biology of mutagens and carcinogens.* New York: Plenum Press.

Snyder, R. D., & Smith, M. D. (2005). Computational prediction of genotoxicity: room for improvement. *Drug Discovery Today, 10,* 1119–1124.

U.S. National Library of Medicine, National Institutes of Health, Environmental Health, and Toxicology Specialized Information Services (SIS). (2005). *Toxicology tutorial II.* Retrieved October 2, 2005 from http://www.sis.nlm.nih.gov/enviro/toxtutor.html.

Valko, M., Izakovic, M., Mazur, M., Rhodes, C. J., & Telser, J. (2004). Role of oxygen radicals in DNA damage and cancer incidence. *Molecular and Cellular Biochemistry, 266,* 37–56.

# CHAPTER 11

# Chemicals and Cancer

The etiology and pathophysiology of cancer is extremely complex. Cancer is a collection of diseases that share common aspects of cellular pathophysiology, primarily related to their lack of confirmation to the usual constraints of growth and cell proliferation that is typical to that tissue.

Cells, through a series of changes, may lose the normal regulatory control mechanisms that keep growth and replication in check with each other. In the absence of regulatory controls, chaos ensues. Although cancerous cells are clearly abnormal by all measures of physiology, biochemistry, and behavior, other patterns of growth are recognized to be associated with changes in normal cellular physiology. For example, hyperplastic growth results in the production of more cells than one would expect to see in a particular tissue. Pregnancy induces hormone-dependent hyperplasia in the breast. The end of gestation and cessation of lactation return the tissue to its normal state. Metaplasia refers to a change in growth that is not necessarily concomitant with a change in mass. It can also be induced environmentally. The columnar ciliated respiratory epithelia of the airways, for example, can become nonciliated and squamous from smoking. The epithelia may revert over time back to the normal ciliated morphology given enough time away from cigarettes and depending on the extent of the exposure. Unlike metaplasia and hyperplasia, neoplastic growth generally persists or progresses.

# Mutations in Genes That Regulate Cell Growth and Differentiation

Molecular biology is not new to the area of toxicology and has been an integral part of the science for some time. Its application as applied to the discipline of toxicology (molecular toxicology) has yielded much information concerning mutations and cancer development. Among the contributions to public health from molecular toxicology include novel models for the testing of chemicals (e.g., transgenic models for carcinogen testing), mutagenicity testing of potential carcinogens, and better understanding of relationships between chemical exposures and the development and progression of disease. Today we clearly see relationships between lifestyle factors and disease. An important concern is the relationship between chemical exposures early in life and health outcomes as we grow older. The idea that "environment imprinting" early in life may influence an individual's susceptibility to disease in the future is an important area for investigation. The modern technologies that are available today and others that may be developed in the future are important tools for understanding the control of gene expression that may be brought to bear on these issues.

Molecular biology has been instrumental in understanding the mechanisms of DNA action and repair, and its application in toxicology has shed light on understanding at the molecular level responses to chemical exposures. Molecular toxicology has been important in understanding the malignant disease process and the role that DNA plays. Thus we now recognize the presence of genes that "encourage" cellular changes that lead to cancer formation and progression as well as genetic expressions that tend to restrict the process and progression of cancer.

Over the last decade a revolution in our understanding of genetics has occurred, giving rise to an area of study called *genomics*. Genomics studies individual genes and multiple gene interactions and the effect of environmental stressors on them. The importance of this has led to the formation of the Centers for Disease Control and Prevention (CDC) Office of Genomics. In 2004 the CDC and Institute of Medicine formed a Committee on Genomics and the Public Health in the 21st Century, which included experts in the fields of genetics, public health law, toxicology and pharmacology, health care delivery, and others. The following topics were included in the discussions:

- Bridging genomics and public health
- Genomics as a science
- The clinical use of genomic information
- Gene–environment interactions

Because a great deal of genomic information is basic science, an important outcome of the science is to understand the potential benefit that it has to the health of the public. This can be accomplished only through understanding that the potential contributions of the science must be translated so they are useful in the formulation of public health strategies.

One of the areas where genomics has contributed greatly to our understanding is in the area of DNA interactions with environmental stressors, including physical, biological, and chemical agents. Exposure to certain chemicals has clearly been shown to be causally related to adverse effects in human DNA and the DNA of other species. Some chemicals have been shown to produce mutations. The chemical mutations have additionally been shown to be associated with many forms of neoplasms or tumors. Some clarification of these and other commonly used terms may be necessary:

- **Tumor:** A mass of cells whose growth is atypical when referenced to the normal surrounding tissue structure. Tumors may be benign or malignant.
- **Neoplasm:** Literally means "new growth" and is a term commonly used the same way that the term tumor is used.
- **New formation:** A mass whose growth is incoordinate with the surrounding normal tissue and that persists in the absence of an inciting stimulus.
- **Benign tumor:** A noncancerous tumor or growth that remains confined to the growth site and may increase in size over time but does not invade into distant tissues. Benign tumors are generally innocuous, slow growing, well organized, and well differentiated (more normal-like than cancerous). Cells may closely resemble normal parenchymal cells of the organ and may produce proteins/substances characteristic of the normal tissue.
- **Malignant tumor:** Any cancerous tumor that may, depending on the type of cancer, spread from its primary growth site to potentially distant sites by its ability to metastasize. Latin for "crab"; named for streaks of tissue that extend from tumor into normal tissue. Malignant tumors contain numerous mitotic figures, large vesicular nuclei, large nucleoli, increased nucleus-to-cytoplasm ratio, and poorly differentiated (more cancer-like than normal) cells that can invade and destroy normal organ architecture. Malignant tumors have an intrinsic ability to kill the organism by invading normal tissues and spreading throughout the body (metastasis).
- **Cancer:** The general term to designate any tumor or cells that have departed far from what is recognized as normal with respect to structure, growth, and replication.

That genetic mechanisms and exposure to certain chemicals are both involved in the process of carcinogenesis is supported by the following:

- The malignant genotype is one that is stable and heritable.
- Many chemical mutagens are also carcinogens.
- The malignant phenotype from cells of the tumor can be transferred by DNA transfer (DNA transfection) to nontumorous cells, thus producing similar phenotypic characteristics.
- Chromosomal abnormalities are common to many cancers.
- The growth of malignant tumors is generally by clonal expansion.
- Many carcinogens can bond to the DNA of cells, thus forming DNA adducts, either directly or after metabolic activation.
- A greater incidence of certain types of cancers is the result of inheritance.
- In individuals that have a family history of certain types of mutations, cancer tends to develop at a much earlier age than cancers that result from acquired mutations.

As an example, a small percentage of individuals that have developed colon cancer do so as an inherited condition known as familial adenomatous polyposis. These individuals have inherited a mutation in a gene that regulates apoptosis (adenomatous polyposis coli gene); at a relatively early age they tend to have more benign polyps of the colon than the general population and a greater likelihood that cancer of the colon will develop. Occasionally benign polyps develop in the colon of many individuals; however, in these individuals hundreds of them develop. Because many forms of cancer develop from benign tumors during the process of transformation, the chances of developing cancer is greatly magnified in these individuals.

Exposure to some chemicals can "promote" the transformation process. We further know that exposure to dietary chemicals has been implicated in colon cancer, thus providing a link to the pathobiology of the process.

Normal cell growth and division is a regulated process unique to the particular tissue in question. Chemical messengers such as growth factors may initiate the process by stimulating cell surface receptors that then transduce those events so they ultimately reach the nucleus of the cell. It is here where transcription factors bind to DNA, resulting in the production of proteins and other regulatory chemicals that control cellular growth and division. Genes involved in cell growth and division are the most important in regards to cancer. It is the genes within the DNA that regulate the process, and if they become mutated or damaged, this may be expressed in atypical growth and division in what is clinically recognized as a tumor or neoplasm. These regulatory genes include oncogenes, tumor suppressor genes, DNA repair genes, and genes that regulate the process of apoptosis. Cancer results from an accumulated series of genetic mutations in the cells of the body often over a period of decades (Figure 11.1); however, it is the accumulated mutations in regulatory genes for cellular growth and division that are necessary to produce what is clinically recognized as a malignant tumor.

Genetic mutation and cancer development

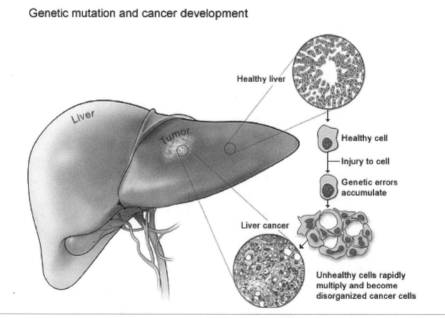

**FIGURE 11.1**   Accumulated mutations and cancer development. *Source:* From *Help me understand genetics.* Courtesy of National Library of Medicine.

## Oncogenes

Oncogenes are mutated forms of proto-oncogenes. Proto-oncogenes are the normal regulatory genes that code for cellular growth factors, chemical messengers, and other cellular mediators that orchestrate growth and differentiation. A number of these genes have already been identified in mammals, including humans. Mutations in these genes can result in the uncoupling of their normal cellular responses. These mutated genes have now become oncogenes and can be accompanied by a loss of normal function that is largely due to their inability to respond in an appropriate fashion to normal cellular cues such as cytokines and other chemical messengers, which normally would be transduced into appropriate cellular responses (e.g., cell division).

Oncogenes can result from a single point mutation of the DNA of the proto-oncogene. The mutated DNA can result in the production of abnormal proteins or altered levels of proteins that are necessary for growth and differentiation. They encode for proteins that are essential for the initiation, promotion, and progression to the malignant state. There are more than 100 different oncogenes whose products include

- Growth factors
- Receptors
- Cytoplasmic kinases
- Survival proteins
- Transcription factors
- Other proteins for signal transduction

Signal transduction is an important process of communication between the cell and its outside environment. Many signaling molecules are too large to gain entry into the cell across the cell membrane and must therefore interact with a cell membrane receptor, which in turn transduces that event via postreceptor signal transduction pathways into an appropriate cellular response. *Myc* is an example of a transcription factor mutated in lung cancer.

It is doubtful that a single oncogene alone is sufficient for the growth and progression of cells toward neoplasia; however, this is a beginning step in the process of carcinogenesis.

Over 100 oncogenes have been identified. Cancerous cells often have very different levels and types of receptors, growth, and other factors involved in their signal transduction. The K-*ras* oncogene codes for an abnormal signal transduction protein associated with cancers such as lung and colon. Another oncogene is the *HER2/neu* oncogene, which codes for an abnormal cell membrane receptor that has been linked to breast cancer.

## Tumor Suppressor Genes

Tumor suppressor genes play an important role in maintaining a balance in the response of the cell to positive and negative regulators of cellular growth. The gene codes for

- Inducers of differentiation
- Cell adhesion molecules
- Inhibitors of cellular proliferation
- Transcription factors
- Inhibitors of angiogenesis

These genes are sometimes referred to as antioncogenes. The importance of the tumor suppressor gene is to limit the proliferation of mutated cells. If these genes malfunction, there may be no "braking" mechanism to prevent the mutated cells from replicating their damaged DNA; thus it will be incorporated into daughter cells during mitosis. This may be an increased risk factor for cancer development and is supported by observations in humans where there is a family history of certain types of cancers, that is, a mutated tumor suppressor gene has been inherited. Examples of mutated tumor suppressor genes include

- *BRCA-1* associated with breast cancer
- *APC* associated with colon cancer
- *p53* associated with over 50% of human cancers

The *p53* tumor suppressor gene is important for the coding of enzymes that are important in DNA repair, apoptosis, and regulation of cell division:

- *p53* senses DNA damage and induces cell division arrest and DNA repair.
- Unrepairable DNA is directed to apoptosis by the *p53* gene.

*p53* is a guardian of the genome. Its homozygous loss leads to accumulation of damaged DNA, which may lead to malignancy. A mutation of the *p53* gene could, for example, result in a cell escaping apoptosis. This becomes especially important for cells with unrepaired DNA because they may continue to divide. If they continue to divide in an unregulated manner, the pool of mutated DNA in a tissue may be increased. Further mutations of these types of cells can result in unregulated cell growth and division, the hallmark of cancer. Some studies suggest that the mutated *p53* gene can be inherited, thus posing an additional risk factor for the development of cancer.

Experimental studies with rodents have been traditionally used to help in the identification of potential human carcinogens. Experimental animals that have been genetically altered, referred to as *transgenic*, may greatly increase the promise for providing mechanistic information on chemical carcinogenesis, thus improving our basis for making reliable inferences to corresponding human effects. Laboratory animals that have modified genomes (e.g., altered oncogenes or tumor suppressor genes) have traits that enable detection of neoplastic processes more effectively and earlier in the testing to chemicals than conventional rodent strains, which need to be tested over a period of 2 years, during which the incidence of spontaneous tumors may increase as these animals age.

## History of Chemical Carcinogenesis

The area of chemical carcinogenesis today is one of intense research that has led to a rich scientific literature on the relationship between chemical exposures and the development and mechanisms that underlie the process of carcinogenesis. Early recognition of a relationship between chemicals and an increased incidence of cancer include the observations of

- John Hill, who in 1761 observed a causal relationship between nasal cancer in snuff users
- Sir Percival Pott, who in 1775 observed a relationship between scrotal cancer in chimney sweeps and poor personal hygiene (fairly common at the time). Pott recognized that soot and coal tar were the likely causal agents.

The first experimental studies on chemical carcinogenesis are probably those of Yamagiwa and Ichikawa in 1918. They observed that coal tar applied to the skin of rabbit ears resulted in skin carcinomas. This required multiple applications and confirmed Pott's observations.

Early recognition of a relationship between cancer and genetics can be attributed to the following researchers:

- Theodore Bovari in 1914 hypothesized that alterations in the genetic material of the cells of the body are somehow involved in the process that produces cancer. This idea has been referred to as the *somatic mutation theory*. He hypothesized that this involved the production of some type of abnormalities in the chromosomes of the somatic cells of the body.
- Furthand Kahn in 1934 experimentally used animal tumors to test cells for their ability to produce tumors in a tumor-free animal. It was observed that when the cells were introduced into a tumor-free host animal, similar tumors could be produced.
- James and Elizabeth Miller in the 1950s recognized the relationship between metabolism and the bioactivation of carcinogens to produce metabolites that could bind to the macromolecules of the cell. The process of metabolism was recognized to produce electrophilic products, more reactive than the unmetabolized parent chemicals, thus establishing what has been referred to as the *electrophilic theory of carcinogenesis.*

## Characteristics of Cancer Cells

The malignant phenotype refers to the structural, functional, and behavioral differences in the cells of malignant neoplasms, including

- Loss of contact growth inhibition
- Autonomy of proliferation
- Avoidance of apoptosis
- Aberrant differentiation
- Induction of angiogenesis

Although cancerous cells are clearly abnormal by all measures of physiology, biochemistry, and behavior, other patterns of growth are recognized to be associated with changes in normal cellular physiology. For example, hyperplastic growth results in the production of more cells than one would expect to see in a particular tissue. Pregnancy induces hormone-dependent hyperplasia in the breast. The end of gestation and cessation of lactation return the tissue to its normal state. Metaplasia refers to a change in growth that is not necessarily concomitant with a change in the mass of the tissue. The pseudostratified columnar ciliated epithelium of the respiratory tract (airways), for example, can become nonciliated and squamous (flattened in appearance) from smoking. The epithelia may revert back to the normal, given enough time away from cigarettes and depending on the extent of the damage. The other possibility is that they begin to show signs of dysplasia, a hallmark feature of cells that will become malignant.

When malignant cells are viewed through the microscope, there are very noticeable differences in their cytology when compared with the normal tissue of origin. These differences form the basis for assessing whether a biopsy is deemed malignant. The malignant cell has a large nucleus, prominent nucleoli, and frequently irregularities of the chromosomes. The malignant cell also appears more immature or more embryonic in appearance when compared with normal cells and may produce embryonic proteins such as carcinoembryonic antigen and alpha-feto-protein, for example, which serve as tumor markers that may be of clinical diagnostic value. This lack of differentiation or dedifferentiation is characteristic. Whereas normal adult cells can be recognized by the specific type of cell that it is, malignant cells have lost their normal specialized functions and cellular appearance as well.

A pathologist can assign the tumor a grade from 1 to 4 that corresponds to its degree of malignancy, with 4 being the most malignant and 1 being benign (Figure 11.2). The more malignant the tumor, the less organized the cells of the tissue are and the more anaplastic or dedifferentiated they appear. The prognosis worsens as cells become less differentiated, that is, a well-differentiated cancer carries a better prognosis than one that is poorly differentiated.

The growth rate of tumors is complex and determined by numerous factors. In cell culture normal cells require the supplementation of their culture medium with a number of growth factors, whereas malignant cells are much less demanding, perhaps because they make many of the factors they need and are therefore more tolerant to their environment. This is perhaps the case for malignant cells *in vivo* as well. Malignant cells *in vivo* form an increasing mass, not because the cells necessarily divide faster than the normal cells of the tissue but rather because they probably produce more cells that are capable of division. In the laboratory malignant cells not only look different from normal ones but behave in cell culture differently as well. When grown in cell culture, normal cells divide and grow until they form a confluent monolayer of cells. Malignant cells, on the other hand, do not recognize their neighbor's space, and rather than stopping their growth and division they continue even to the extent of growing on top of the cells that are attached to the substrate of the cell culture vessel. Malignant cells do not respond to the normal cues that should turn division off. They typically lack what is known as "contact inhibition" and continue to grow and divide, piling up on each other and forming a mass of growing cells that resembles a tumor *in vivo*.

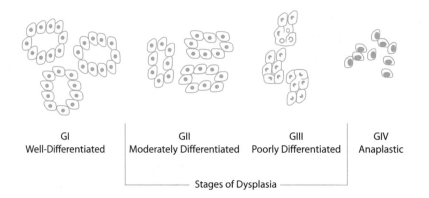

| GI | GII | GIII | GIV |
| Well-Differentiated | Moderately Differentiated | Poorly Differentiated | Anaplastic |

———————— Stages of Dysplasia ————————

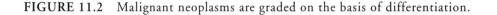

FIGURE 11.2    Malignant neoplasms are graded on the basis of differentiation.

# Benign and Malignant Tumors

The tissues that make up the organs of our body may consist of numerous cell types. Two terms to denote the "division of labor" in the tissue are the *parenchyma* and the *stroma*. Parenchymal cells are the functional cells that are recognized as being unique to that organ. For example, in the liver we can recognize the parenchyma as consisting of the hepatocyte, which is the cell type that we associate with liver function. Stromal cells, which are important to the tissue, may be viewed as supportive in nature. The hepatocytes within the liver require connective tissue and blood vessels to support their function. Similarly, a neoplasm consists of both parenchymal and stromal components. In benign neoplasms the parenchymal and stromal cells may closely resemble those of the normal surrounding tissue. Benign neoplasms are named for the tissue of origin (Table 11.1).

The benign neoplasm is characterized by its encapsulation by connective tissue. As it grows in size, it pushes against the normal surrounding tissue, which may result in the atrophy and death of the surrounding parenchyma and formation of a surrounding capsule by the remaining connective tissue. Benign tumors can be life threatening, depending on their size and location. Consider, for example, a benign tumor of the cells of the adrenal gland, which produces catecholamines (pheochromocytoma), or of the islets of Langerhans of the pancreas, which produce insulin.

Malignant tumors are similarly named for the tissue from which the tumor is derived; one of three suffixes is generally attached to create the name of the cancer (Table 11.2):

- Carcinomas: epithelia tissue origin and the most common of all human malignancies (approximately 90%). This cancer spreads primarily through the lymphatic system.
- Sarcomas: connective tissue origin.
- Blastomas: derived from (or resembling) embryonic tissue

Some cancers are inconsistent with this nomenclature, such as malignant liver tumors (hepatomas), leukemia (a sarcoma of the blood-forming tissues), and melanoma (cancer of the melanocyte). A cancer classified as a bronchiogenic carcinoma *in situ* is of epithelial cell origin, from the bronchial tubes of the airways, and, because it is *in situ,* it is presently confined there.

**Table 11.1** Examples of Benign Tumors and Their Tissues of Origin

| Prefix | Tissue | Benign Tumor Name |
|--------|--------|-------------------|
| Adeno- | Gland | Adenoma |
| Chondro- | Cartilage | Chondroma |
| Hemangio- | Blood vessels | Hemangioma |
| Hepato- | Liver | Hepatoma |
| Lipo- | Fat | Lipoma |
| Myo- | Muscle | Myoma |
| Osteo- | Bone | Osteoma |
| Fibro- | Fibrous connective tissue | Fibroma |
| Neuro- | Neural tissue | Neuroma |

**Table 11.2**  Examples of Malignant Tumors and Their Tissue of Origin

| Malignant Tumor Name | Tissue of Origin |
| --- | --- |
| Adenocarcinomas | Glandular epithelium |
| Squamous cell carcinoma | Squamous epithelium |
| Osteosarcoma | Bone |
| Chondrosarcoma | Cartilage |
| Lymphosarcoma | Lymph node |
| Liposarcoma | Adipose tissue |
| Retinoblastoma | Retinal tissue |
| Neuroblastoma | Neural tissue |
| Nephroblastoma | Renal tissue |

## Tumor Angiogenesis, Metastasis, and Staging

The malignant tumor grows within its tissue of origin; however, it may spread beyond these local confines. Malignant tumor cells can invade into deeper layers of tissue (invasion) and are capable of metastasis as well. Consider the growth of a carcinoma as an example. Carcinomas are of epithelial cell origin and are the most common types of malignancies. Epithelial tissue covers the external surface of the body and lines the hollow organs (e.g., urinary bladder, heart, gastrointestinal tract, blood vessels). In some areas of the body, epithelial tissue is referred to as mucosa. A mucosa lines the respiratory and gastrointestinal tracts. Although these tissues produce mucus, hence the name mucosa (sometimes referred to as the mucous membrane), and although they share similarities, the epithelial cells that make up the respective tissues are very much different in both their histology and function. The cells rest on a basement membrane, below which is connective tissue containing blood and lymphatic vessels. If our tumor remains confined to the epithelial tissue, it can be referred to as an *in situ* tumor. A bronchiogenic carcinoma can grow into and partially occlude a bronchial tube as well as grow into the underlying connective tissue. As the mass of the tumor increases beyond about a millimeter or so, it needs to establish circulatory support for its continued survival. At this point cells within the core of the tumor have died and necrosis is occurring, due to lack of vascular support. Like any other tissue, malignant tissue has requirements for adequate levels of oxygen, the removal of metabolic wastes, and a supply of nutrients and other factors.

Tumors release a number of factors that collectively can be referred to as *angiogenic factors*. Vascular endothelial growth factor is one such factor that stimulates the growth of capillaries into the tumor. This is the process of angiogenesis, which serves a dual role in that it provides the vascular support for the tumor proper and provides close access of blood vessels for metastasis. Another management approach in treating patients with cancer is to use drugs such as endostatin that inhibit the angiogenesis process.

Cancer cells can breach the basement membrane and produce chemicals that can break down the membrane, thus facilitating their entry into the deeper tissue. Malignant cells that gain entry into the lymphatic and blood vessels can travel within the circulation until such time as they receive appropriate signals to attach to the vessel wall and move into new tissue. This process is referred to as *metastasis,* and it results in a secondary tumor. Common locations for metastasis in tumors are the lungs, liver, and bone. Chemotherapeutic approaches to the management of cancer attempt to use the immunological system and the fact that malignant cells express unique antigens on their cell surface. The development of monoclonal antibodies is an area of important research. It is hoped that these antibodies can recognize and attach onto the specific antigens found on circulating cancer cells, thereby targeting them for destruction.

Staging is a way of describing the extent or severity of the cancer based on the metastasis of the original tumor. It is one way of determining the prognosis of the patient. The staging of cancer is a way to clinically judge how extensive the cancer is and can be used to judge the prognosis of the patient. Staging considers the location, size, metastasis, and involvement of the lymph nodes. The TNM (tumor, node, and metastasis) staging system is one of the most widely used systems (Table 11.3).

To protect public health, it is important for us to know whether a chemical is carcinogenic or not to humans. This is an easy question to ask but frequently difficult to answer. Chemicals are classified as to whether or not they are carcinogens based on human data, which have come primarily from retrospective epidemiological studies in industrial workers. A number of chemicals have been shown to be human carcinogens from such studies (Table 11.4). Chemicals are also classified as to whether or not they are carcinogens, based on laboratory studies. Great confusion can arise, however, when the two words *human* and *carcinogen* are used together, because there is often limited information available. Different agencies, both regulatory and nonregulatory, have developed classification systems for carcinogens, and confusion can result in trying to

**Table 11.3  TNM System of Tumor Grading**

| **Primary Tumor (T)** | |
|---|---|
| TX | The primary tumor cannot be evaluated |
| T0 | No evidence of primary tumor |
| Tis | Carcinoma *in situ* |
| T1, T2, T3, T4 | Refers to the size and/or extent of the primary tumor |
| **Regional Lymph Nodes (N)** | |
| NX | Regional lymph nodes cannot be evaluated |
| N0 | No regional lymph node involvement |
| N1, N2, N3 | Involvement of regional lymph nodes (number and/or extent of spread) |
| **Distant Metastasis (M)** | |
| MX | Distant metastasis cannot be evaluated |
| M0 | No distant metastasis |
| M1 | Distant metastasis |

**Table 11.4    Examples of Occupational Carcinogens**

| Carcinogen | Occupation | Cancer Type |
| --- | --- | --- |
| 4-Aminobiphenyl | Chemical and dye workers | Bladder |
| Arsenic | Mining, pesticides | Lung, skin, liver |
| Asbestos | Construction | Lung |
| Benzene | Leather, petroleum, rubber, and chemical | Leukemia |
| Benzidine | Chemical, dye, and rubber | Bladder |
| Chromium | Electroplaters, metal workers | Lung |

place a chemical into a category from one classification system into another. The principal agencies and their classification systems are summarized as follows:

### International Agency for Research on Cancer (IARC)

*Group 1:* carcinogenic to humans

*Group 2A:* probably carcinogenic to humans

*Group 2B:* possibly carcinogenic to humans

*Group 3:* not classifiable as to its carcinogenicity to humans

*Group 4:* probably not carcinogenic to humans

### U.S. Environmental Protection Agency (EPA)

*Group A.* Human Carcinogen

Sufficient evidence from epidemiological studies exists to support a cause-and-effect relationship between the substance and cancer.

*Group B.* Probable Human Carcinogen

*B1*: Sufficient evidence from animal studies, limited epidemiological evidence

*B2*: Sufficient evidence from animal studies, but epidemiological data are inadequate or nonexistent

*Group C.* Possible Human Carcinogen

Limited evidence from animal studies, no epidemiological data

*Group D.* Not Classifiable as to Human Carcinogenicity

Data from human epidemiological and animal studies are inadequate or nonexistent, so assessment is not possible.

*Group E.* Evidence of Noncarcinogenicity for Humans

The chemical tested negative in at least two EPA-approved testing protocols in different species. There are currently no adequate epidemiological or animal studies available.

### National Toxicology Program (NTP)

*Group K:* known to be human carcinogens

*Group R:* reasonably anticipated to be human carcinogens

**American Conference of Governmental Industrial Hygienists**

*Group A1:* confirmed human carcinogen

*Group A2:* suspected human carcinogen

*Group A3:* confirmed animal carcinogen with unknown relevance to humans

**California Environment Protection Agency**

*Known to the state to cause cancer*

For ease of comparison between agencies and by omitting letter and/or number designations, refer to Table 11.5.

# Carcinogen Classification

## Based on Chemistry

Although we recognize a relatively limited number of known human carcinogens, thousands more suspected carcinogens have already been tested for their ability to produce mutations and cancer in laboratory animals and *in vitro* systems. These chemicals fall into many different categories of chemical agents based on shared structural similarities. Some of these categories and examples of representative chemicals are summarized in Table 11.6.

## Based on Mechanism of Action

### Genotoxic

Carcinogens can be classified by their mode of action, genotoxic or nongenotoxic. Genotoxic carcinogens are DNA reactive or DNA-reactive metabolites capable of altering the integrity DNA through direct interaction:

- Proximate or direct-acting carcinogens that act directly without metabolic change, such as the alkylating agents
- Indirect acting after being metabolized into active compounds (procarcinogen → ultimate carcinogen) such as the toxin aflatoxin, aromatic amine benzidine, and the polycyclic hydrocarbon benz[a]pyrene (Figure 11.3).

The mechanism can proceed stepwise from activation of the chemical or its metabolite from the outside of the cell, its transport to the nucleus, formation of a DNA adduct by the activated carcinogen, and "fixing" the mutation by cell proliferation if repair does not occur.

### Nongenotoxic

Nongenotoxic carcinogens do not directly cause DNA mutation. The mechanism of action is poorly understood. They are also difficult to detect, requiring a rodent carcinogen bioassay. Metal–DNA interactions can be genotoxic or nongenotoxic. Platinum-based anticancer drugs are believed to exert their therapeutic action through binding with DNA. The mechanism of metal–DNA interactions is far from complete; carcinogenicity of metal ions such as

**Table 11.5**    Comparison of Human Carcinogen Classification by Agency

| EPA | IARC | NTP | OSHA | ACGIH | CAEPA |
|---|---|---|---|---|---|
| **Human Carcinogen** | **Carcinogenic to Humans** | **Human Carcinogen** | **Known Occupational Carcinogen** | **Confirmed Human Carcinogen** | **Known by the State to Cause Cancer** |
| Evidence of carcinogenicity drawn from epidemiological studies | Sufficient evidence of cancer in humans or (rarely) compelling evidence from animal studies | Sufficient evidence from human studies showing cause and effect | Sufficient evidence of cancer in humans or (rarely) compelling evidence from animal studies | | |
| **Probable Human Carcinogen** | **Probable Human Carcinogen** | **Reasonably Anticipated to be a Human Carcinogen** | **Potential Occupational Carcinogen** | **Suspected Human Carcinogen** | |
| Evidence drawn primarily from animal studies with limited to no epidemiological evidence | Evidence drawn primarily from animal studies with limited to no epidemiological evidence | Evidence drawn primarily from animal studies with limited to no epidemiological evidence | Evidence drawn primarily from animal studies with limited to no epidemiological evidence | | |
| **Possible Human Carcinogen** | **Possible Human Carcinogen** | | | **Confirmed Animal Carcinogen with unknown relevance to humans** | |
| Limited evidence from animal studies, no epidemiological evidence | Limited evidence in humans and insufficient evidence from animal studies | | | | |
| **Not Classifiable as to Human Carcinogenicity** | **Not Classifiable as to Human Carcinogenicity** | | | | |
| Data are inadequate or nonexistent so no assessment is made | Data are inadequate or nonexistent so no assessment is made | | | | |
| **Evidence of Noncarcinogenicity for Humans** | **Probably not Carcinogenic to Humans** | | | | |
| Substance has tested negative in at least two animal cancer tests | Evidence suggests lack of carcinogenicity in humans | | | | |

ACGIH, American Conference of Governmental Industrial Hygienists; CAEPA, California Environmental Protection Agency; OSHA, Occupational Safety and Health Administration.

## Table 11.6    Examples of Chemical Carcinogens Based on Chemistry

**Alkylating agents**
Bis(chloromethyl) ether
α-Halo ethers
Methyl chloromethyl ether

**Sulfonates**
1,4-Butanediol methylsulfonate (myleran)
Diethyl sulfate
Dimethyl sulfate
Ethyl methanesulfonate
Methyl trifluoromethanesulfonate

**Epoxides**
Ethylene oxide
Epichlorohydrin
Propylene oxide

**Azridines**
Ethylenimine
2-methylaziridine

**Electrophylic alkenes and alkynes**
Acrylonitrile
Acrolein
Ethyl acrylate

**Acylating agents**
β-Propiolactone
β-Butyrolactone
Dimethylcarbamyl chloride

**Organic compounds**
Carbon tetrachloride
Chloroform
1,2-Dibromethane
1,4-Dichlorobenzene
Methyl iodide
Mustard gas (bis(2chloroethyl)sulfide)
Tetrachloroethylene
Trichloroethylene
2,4,6-Trichlorophenol
Vinyl chloride

**Hydrazines**
Hydrazine and hydrazine salts
1,2-Diethyl hydrazine
1,1-Dimethyl hydrazine

**N-nitroso coumpounds**
N-Nitrosodimethylamine
N-Nitroso-N-alkyureas

**Aromatic amines**
Aniline
Benzidine (4,4'-diaminobiphenyl)
α-Napthylamine
β-Napthylamine
4-Aminobiphenyl
2,4-Diaminotoluene
o-Toluidine

**Aromatic hydrocarbons**
Benzene
Benz[a]anthracene
Benzo[a]pyrene

**Natural products and antitumor drugs**
Adriamycin
Aflatoxins
Progesterone

**Other organohalogen compounds**
Formaldehyde gas
Acetaldehyde
1,4-Dioxane
Urethane(ethyl carbamate)
Hexamethylphosphoramide
Styrene

**Heavy metals**
Arsenic and certain arsenic compounds
Beryllium and certain Cd compounds
Cadmium and certain Cd compounds
Lead and certain Pb Compounds
Nickel and certain Ni compounds
Selenium sulfide

chromium, nickel, and cadmium are believed to be associated with direct and/or indirect inter-action with DNA.

Genomic information can be classified as genetic or epigenetic. The genetic information is the sequence of bases encoding the proteins, and epigenetic information is the regulation of gene expression by means other than alterations in the DNA sequence. DNA methylation is also involved in DNA repair, regulation of chromatin structure, and genome instability. Epigenetic carcinogens can be defined as solid state, hormonal, immunosuppressant, cocarcino-genic, or promoter (Table 11.7).

The evidence for epigenetic mechanisms for some chemicals includes the following observations:

- Not all carcinogens are mutagens.
- Carcinogenesis is often associated with changes in the methylation of DNA.

Asbestos is an example of a solid-state epigenetic and fibrous carcinogen (Figure 11.4). Six fibrous silicates are characterized: fibrous serpentine mineral chrysotile amphiboles, actinolite, amosite, anthophyllite, crocidolite, and tremolite. Chrysotile is produced in the greatest amounts because it is the most widely used form of asbestos. Consequently, it is ubiquitously present in the environment.

By the 1960s evidence linked asbestos to the development of certain types of cancer. Although it is basically a chemically nonreactive substance to the body, it does produce nonspecific irritant effects believed to somehow encourage certain cells to proliferate. Not all forms of asbestos are

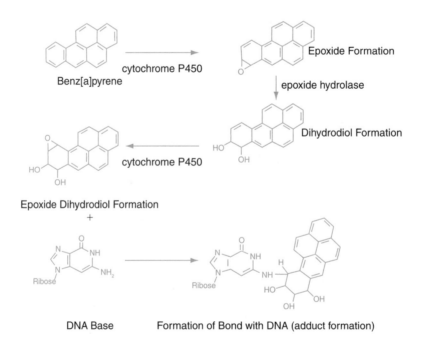

**FIGURE 11.3**    Metabolic activation of benz[a]pyrene.

**Table 11.7**  Epigenetic Carcinogens

| Type | Carcinogen |
|------|-----------|
| Solid state | Asbestos, plastics |
| Hormonal | Estrogenic, androgenic |
| Immunosuppressant | Azathioprine |
| Cocarcinogenic | Ethanol, solvents |
| Promoter | Phorbol esters, ethanol |

equally capable of doing so. Fiber shape and size are crucial to the carcinogenic properties of asbestos. Asbestos-related cancers have been associated with long latency periods, often decades.

Here is an example of how public health early warning breaks down due to the relatively long latency period between human exposures and an adverse health outcome. Because asbestos stays in the lungs for a very long period of time, additional exposure to other carcinogens, such as those contained within cigarettes, greatly increases the likelihood for cancer development. Another example about the long-term effects of chemicals includes the irritant and carcinogenic potential of chemicals that compose medical implants, and this has become an intense area of investigation by the manufacturers of these devices. It is difficult to draw inferences from studies in laboratory rodents that show irritant properties and occasional sarcoma formation with such commonly used materials as titanium, silver, gold, hydrocarbon polymers, silastic, and others.

Another concern that has received a great deal of attention and experimental effort is the relationship between hormones and cancer. Hormones may play a dual role in that they may induce neoplasms that may depend on hormones for their optimal growth. The link between hormones and the development of tumors has been well substantiated in the population (e.g.,

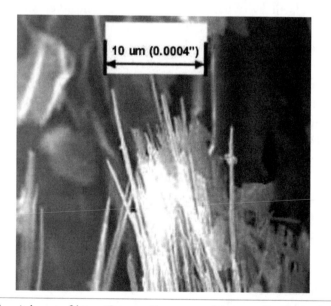

**FIGURE 11.4**  Asbestos fibers. *Source:* Courtesy of Agency for Toxic Substances and Disease Registry/CDC.

diethylstilbestrol and vaginal/uterine carcinomas; estrogen and breast cancer). Prostate, breast, and thyroid carcinomas are stimulated by hormones, and although reduction of their level does not stop growth, it may slow it to some extent.

## Exposure to Carcinogens

We have defined a chemical carcinogen as any substance that can significantly increase the incidence of tumors. The public recognizes the term *carcinogen* as well, perhaps not as something that increases the incidence of tumors but rather as something that causes cancer. The U.S. governmental regulatory definition of a carcinogen is "any substance at any dose, administered by any route, that increases tumor incidence in rats." Because the term *carcinogen* is so frequently used, a great deal of public confusion has and will continue to exist in the absence of information to identify to whom it is carcinogenic and under what conditions. Historically, carcinogenicity testing in laboratory rodents has used the maximum tolerated dose, which often leads to grossly exaggerated risks. In 1986 orange dye no. 17 was banned by the U.S. Food and Drug Administration (FDA) under the Delaney Clause. This clause of the 1958 Food Additive Amendment prohibits the use of any food additive (including food dyes) if it can be demonstrated that tumors result from its use in either humans or laboratory animals. The worse case estimate for this chemical was 1 cancer in approximately 20 billion people! Although almost all human carcinogens are carcinogenic in laboratory rodents, only a small percentage of chemicals carcinogenic to laboratory rodents have been shown to be human carcinogens. In addition, the word *tumor,* as used in the regulatory definition, is not synonymous with cancer because we know that tumors can be either benign or malignant. Although the intentions of the FDA were to protect the American public from cancer-producing agents, a more realistic risk of one cancer per million human lifetimes has been set as a reasonable standard or "virtually safe dose" in the 1996 Food Quality Protection Act (FQPA), which is consistent with the EPA standard for environmental contamination scenarios set about a decade earlier.

We are frequently exposed to chemical carcinogens through the air we breathe and the things we consume. We are exposed to polycyclic aromatic hydrocarbons (PAH), nitrosamines, and many others, both intentionally and unintentionally. We are exposed to the carcinogens called aflatoxins, which are naturally occurring mycotoxins produced by variants of the fungus *Aspergillus.* These peanut and grain contaminants are highly toxic to humans and other animals and are strongly correlated with liver cancer, and yet they are knowingly present in the peanut butter we eat. Considering the amount of peanut butter consumed in the United States on an annual basis, is this then not of great public health concern? After all, doesn't the FDA prohibit carcinogens in our food products? It does, of course, for chemicals that would be intentionally introduced during the manufacturing process. One can say with a great deal of certainly that if you sampled any jar of peanut butter on your supermarket shelf, you would find aflatoxin present. The reason you would find it is because you are looking for it and because you have available sophisticated analytical tools that can find chemicals in the parts per billion/trillion range. This technology is available to the manufacturers of peanut butter as well and would be used not to detect if aflatoxin is present but rather to screen for the possibility of a "highly contaminated" batch of peanut butter as part of their quality control. We are always hopeful that the manufacturers of products used by the American consumer are concerned with high quality and that they too recognize it is always preferable to protect the health of the public when a potential hazard is recognized, especially when there are control measures in place to intervene as early on as is feasibly possible. If that in and of itself is insufficient motivation, then economics would certainly indicate that it is cheaper to use the best control measures available than to have a product recall and along with it the negative image and legal expenses that could be incurred.

Is it a reasonable inference that the presence of liver cancer in the general population may be linked to the consumption of peanut butter? We must all learn to discourage recognizing causation as just identifying the chemical and an exposure pathway in the absence of a great deal of additional information that would rule out other potential causes.

## Chemical-Induced Carcinogenesis Is a Multistep Process

The process of oncogenesis is a progression of events that lead to the formation of a tumor. It is extremely unlikely that a single mutagenic event could result in the production of a malignant neoplasm. The so-called single-hit hypothesis wherein a single mutation is believed to be sufficient to result in cancer development is not widely accepted in the scientific community. A multiple-hit hypothesis, rather, is envisioned to be a more likely process that requires multiple genetic mutations that develop, either spontaneously produced by physical, chemical, and biological agents or as an inherited defect. In the process of chemical carcinogenesis, there are at least three stages of the process: initiation, promotion, and progression (Figure 11.5).

### Initiation

The process of initiation is the genotoxic event that leads to mutations of the DNA and places the affected cells at a greater risk for tumor formation. The interaction between chemical carcinogen and DNA must, however, be within the portions of genome that are involved in regulating processes of cellular growth and differentiation. It is the interaction between chemical

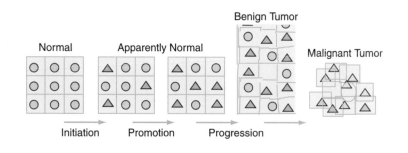
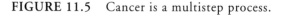

**FIGURE 11.5**    Cancer is a multistep process.

carcinogens and the inactivation of tumor suppressor genes or activation of proto-oncogenes that "initiates" the process. Importantly, the process of initiation alone is insufficient to result in a chemical-induced tumor formation. For the carcinogenic process to continue requires that the mutagenic event escapes detection and DNA repair, thereby allowing it to become "fixed." At this point in the process, however, the cells do not have growth autonomy or other features typically associated with cancerous cells (i.e., they do not possess the "malignant phenotype") and are apparently normal. They are, however, genotypically different from the normal cells, while remaining phenotypically identical, replicating normally, and showing no apparent structural or functional abnormalities. These permanently altered cells, however, may be more resistant to agents that produce cytotoxicity.

## Promotion

The process of promotion is classically considered as the second step in the carcinogenesis process, which moves initiated cells further along their transformation process. Exposure of initiated cells to chemicals that stimulate cell proliferation, such as irritating substances, results in the production of a clone of proliferating cells within the tissue. These chemicals are collectively referred to as *promoters*. Different promoting agents have been used experimentally:

- Skin tumor promoters: 12-O-tetradecanoylphorbol-13-acetate (TPA) (Figure 11.6)
- Hepatic tumor promoters: include chlordane, phenobarbital, 2,3,7,8-Tetrachlorodibenzo-p-dioxin

The potency of promoting agents is measured by their ability to produce proliferation in a population of initiated cells. This population of cells can increase in numbers and at some point may be clinically recognized as a tumor. This is the end point of promotion—the production of a neoplasm. This neoplasm or tumor may never progress to the stage of malignancy.

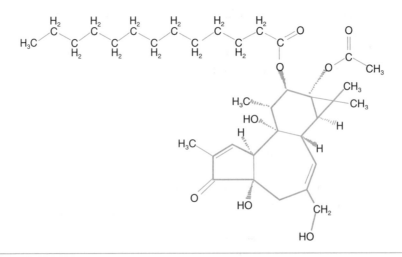

FIGURE 11.6    12-O-tetradecanoylphorbol-13-acetate. *Source:* Accessed from: http://ntp.niehs.nih.gov/ntp/htdocs/structures/2d/TR441(TPA).gif.

The mouse skin initiation-promotion model has been used to elucidate the first two steps in the process of chemical carcinogenesis. In this model an initiator such as a polycyclic aromatic hydrocarbon (PAH) and a promoter such as TPA are used. TPA belongs to a family of compounds called phorbol esters. Phorbol esters stimulate cellular proliferation by activating a transducer protein in the cell membrane known as protein kinase C (Figure 11.7). These esters have been isolated from croton oil and have been used classically in the mouse skin initiation-promotion assay (Figure 11.8).

Results from studies of topical application of initiators and promoters on mouse skin have shown the following:

- Initiation must precede promotion for tumor formation.
- Initiation followed by no promotion does not result in tumor formation.
- Initiation followed by multiple exposures to promoter (chronic exposure) results in tumor formation.
- Promoter by itself does not result in the production of tumors.
- Promotion followed by initiation does not result in the production of tumors.
- Initiation followed by multiple exposures to promoters can result in tumor formation even though a relatively long time has elapsed since the initiator was applied.
- Initiation followed by promotion does not result in tumors if subsequent applications of promoting agents are spaced too far apart temporally.

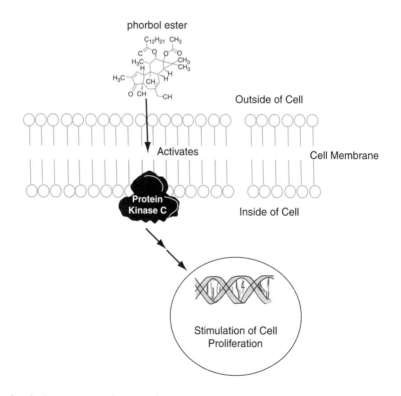

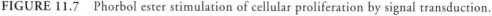

FIGURE 11.7    Phorbol ester stimulation of cellular proliferation by signal transduction.

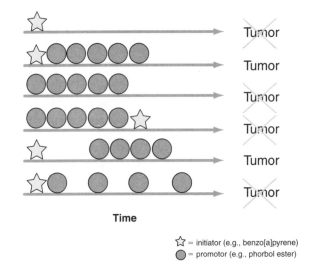

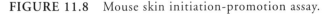

**Time**

☆ = initiator (e.g., benzo[a]pyrene)
⬤ = promotor (e.g., phorbol ester)

**FIGURE 11.8**    Mouse skin initiation-promotion assay.

## Progression

Progression is the next step toward the transformation of cells into a tumor that is malignant. At this stage in the process, and depending on the particular tissue of origin of the cell, a high growth rate and invasion into surrounding tissue may occur. Malignant cells, although autonomous in their growth and division, are nonetheless under the influence of the same types of chemicals that regulate these processes in normal cells. These types of chemicals serve to either stimulate or inhibit mitosis in some cells. It is during this stage that some cells may migrate from the clone to gain entry into lymphatic and blood vessels, a process generally referred to as metastasis. Progression to the malignant state is considered to be an irreversible process. At this stage, chromosomal (karyotypic) aberrations are common.

The process of chemical carcinogenesis is then one of a multistep process where initiation, promotion, and progression to the malignant state results from the stepwise accumulation of mutations in the DNA accompanied by phenotypic changes (Figure 11.9).

## Informing the Public on Carcinogens

The federal government has the obligation to inform the public about known and anticipated human carcinogens. The *Report on Carcinogens* is a document prepared in response to section 301 of the U.S. Public Health Service Act. It is stipulated that the Secretary of the Department of Health and Human Services shall publish a report that contains a list of all substances

- That either are known to be human carcinogens or may reasonably be anticipated to be human carcinogens
- To which a significant number of persons residing in the United States are exposed

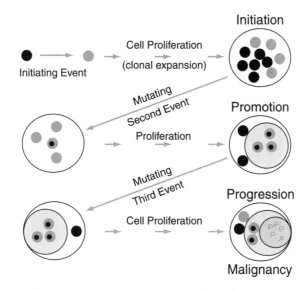

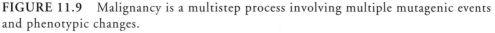

**FIGURE 11.9** Malignancy is a multistep process involving multiple mutagenic events and phenotypic changes.

The responsibility for the preparation of this document has been delegated to the NTP. Agencies represented on the NTP Executive Committee are as follows:

- Department of Health and Human Services
- National Institute of Environmental Health Sciences/NTP
- Agency for Toxic Substances and Disease Registry
- FDA
- Consumer Product Safety Commission
- EPA
- National Center for Environmental Health/CDC
- National Institute for Occupational Safety and Health
- Occupational Safety and Health Administration
- National Institutes of Health and National Cancer Institute

The most recent document is the 11th edition, released in January 2005. The report identifies chemicals as potential carcinogenic hazards and is not a risk assessment document. It is based on the premise that an individual during one's lifetime has an approximately 50% chance of developing cancer. It is further based on the well-documented hypothesis that environmental factors are likely to be the major contributors to cancer development. Environment is loosely defined to include workplace exposures, lifestyle choices, diet, medications, socioeconomic factors, and chemicals in the water, air, and soil. Other important factors to consider are aging, infectious agents, and genetic predisposition.

The report is a listing of chemicals that are known human carcinogens or those that may be reasonably anticipated to be and to which significant numbers of individuals are exposed in the United States. The report contains estimated numbers of individuals as well as information about the nature of the exposures. The report is essentially a compilation of information on chemical carcinogenicity and its mechanisms, the pathways for human exposures, and current federal regulations in place to limit potential exposures. It is not a quantitative risk assessment; however, it can serve as the basis for such by federal and state regulatory agencies.

For a chemical to make the list (or be removed from it) requires that it be nominated. Supporting documentation for any specific chemical comes primarily from peer-reviewed scientific literature and published technical reports from both human and laboratory studies. Epidemiological studies represent the strongest link in the chain of evidence in support of a causal relationship between the chemical and the production of cancer. Frequently, chemicals under consideration for listing have also been reviewed by other organizations such as the IARC in Lyon, France (e.g., the IARC Monographs on the Evaluation of the Carcinogenic Risk of Chemicals to Humans) and the EPA of the State of California. Occasionally, requests for nominations come from the public and are published in the *Federal Register.*

## Bibliography

American Cancer Society. www.cancer.org.

Arcos, J. C., Argus, M. F., & Woo, Y. T. (Eds.) (1995). *Chemical induction of cancer: modulation and combination: effects an inventory of the many factors which influence carcinogenesis.* Boston: Birkhaüser.

Cancer risk assessment: a quantitative approach series. (1990). *Occupational safety and health* (vol. 20). Boca Raton, FL: CRC Press.

Clayson, D. B. (2001). *Toxicological carcinogenesis.* Boca Raton, FL: CRC Press.

Huff, J., Barrett, J. C., & Boyd, J. A. (Eds.) (1996). *Cellular and molecular mechanisms of hormonal carcinogenesis: environmental influences.* New York: John Wiley & Sons.

Humble, M. C., Trempus, C. S., Spalding, J. W., Cannon, R. E., & Tennant, R. W. (2005). Biological, cellular, and molecular characteristics of an inducible transgenic skin tumor model: a review. *Oncogene, 24,* 8217–8228.

Luch, A. (2006). The mode of action of organic carcinogens on cellular structures. *EXS, 96,* 65–95. [MSOffice2]

Monceviciute-Eringiene, E. (2005). Neoplastic growth: the consequence of evolutionary malignant resistance to chronic damage for survival of cells (review of a new theory of the origin of cancer). *Medical Hypotheses, 65,* 595–604.

National Cancer Institute. http://www.cancer.gov/.

Park, B. K., Kitteringham, N. R., Maggs, J. L., Pirmohamed, M., & Williams, D. P. (2002). The role of metabolic activation in drug-induced hepatotoxicity. *Annual Review of Pharmacology and Toxicology, 45,* 177–202.

Shields, P. G. (2005). *Cancer risk assessment series: basic and clinical oncology* (vol. 32). Washington, DC: Georgetown University.

U.S. National Library of Medicine, National Institutes of Health, Environmental Health, and Toxicology Specialized Information Services (SIS). (2005). *Toxicology tutorial III.* Retrieved October 2, 2005 from http://www.sis.nlm.nih.gov/enviro/toxtutor.html.

Valko, M., Rhodes, C. J., Moncol, J., Izakovic, M., & Mazur, M. (2006). Free radicals, metals and antioxidants in oxidative stress-induced cancer. *Chemico-Biological Interactions, 160,* 1–40.

Waalkes, M. P. (1994). *Carcinogenesis series: target organ toxicology series.* New York: Raven Press.

Warshawsky, D., & Landolph, J. R. (Eds.) (2005). *Molecular carcinogenesis and the molecular biology of human cancer.* Boca Raton, FL: CRC Press.

# Role of Immune System

The immune system provides important defensive mechanisms to reduce potential adverse effects from exposures to biological agents (e.g., bacteria, viruses), mutated cells, and certain chemicals to which we are exposed. Its importance to our survival is attested to by the fact that significant immunosuppression (e.g., human immunodeficiency virus [HIV], chemotherapy) can greatly reduce the ability to mount an effective assault against these agents. Its significance, from a toxicological viewpoint, is that it is a target for toxicity from a number of chemicals of clinical and nonclinical importance, which can suppress its function.

Nonspecific immunity is the result of recognition and destruction of pathogens such as bacteria by phagocytic cells. The recruitment of these phagocytic cells results in an inflammatory response at sites of infection. The first cell to arrive on the scene is the neutrophil, which is specialized for ingesting and destroying these microorganisms in the tissues and circulation. Clinically, this inflammatory response is characterized by redness and swelling on visible sites due to increased capillary permeability and blood flow to the area. Circulating monocytes and their tissue correlates, the macrophages, continue the assault on the offending agent. An additional type of nonspecific response is by the action of cytotoxic lymphocytes, which can recognize cell surface markers on some malignant and viral infected cells. Specific immune responses include cell-mediated and humoral-mediated immunity.

There are two basic types of responses between a chemical and the immune system:

- Stimulation: Allergic reactions may occur in response to antigens and other chemicals or autoimmune responses whereby the immune system is stimulated to recognize "self" tissues or cells and mounts a response against them.
- Suppression: Can lead to an increased susceptibility to infectious agents or the enhancement of tumor formation due to a depressed recognition and response to aberrant or mutated cells.

## Organs of the Immune System

The organs of the immune system are positioned throughout the body (Figure 12.1). They are called lymphoid organs or tissues because their primary occupants are lymphocytes, the white blood cells of the immune system. We recognize primary and secondary lymphoid tissues.

Primary lymphoid tissue is composed of

- Bone marrow—the tissue from which immune cells are derived and the source of all blood cells, including those of the immune system
- Thymus—the tissue in which T lymphocytes are differentiated

Secondary lymphoid tissue is composed of

- Spleen—a flattened organ at the upper left quadrant of the abdomen where immune cells are housed

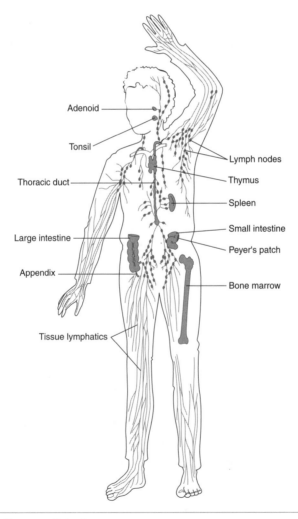

**FIGURE 12.1**    Organs of the immune system.

- Lymph nodes—small bean-shaped structures scattered throughout the body found along the lymphatic vessels, with clusters especially in the armpits, neck, abdomen, and groin. Each lymph node contains specialized compartments where immune cells congregate and encounter antigens.

In addition to these organs, lymphoid tissue is present in the digestive tract, airways, lungs, tonsils, adenoids, and appendix. Movement of cells of the immune system and their communications with each other and with other body tissues are through a network of lymphatic vessels that carry the lymph. Lymph originates as blood plasma that is lost from the circulatory system into the surrounding tissues. The lymphatic system collects this extracellular fluid by diffusion into lymph capillaries and vessels and returns it to the circulatory system. Lymph is of similar composition to the interstitial fluid (the extracellular fluid that bathes the body cells). The lymphatic vessels closely parallel the body's arteries and veins; thus lymphocytes can travel throughout the body through these vessels as well as the blood vessels. Cells and fluids are exchanged between lymphatic vessels and blood, thus providing a way to monitor the internal compartments of the body for bacteria and other pathogens.

## Cells of the Immune System

The functional units of the immune system are the leukocytes (white blood cells) that develop from pluripotent stem cells (Figure 12.2). The stem cells undergo differentiation, maturation, and proliferation into morphologically and functionally distinct cell populations, including:

- Granulocytes
  - Neutrophils (phagocytes, also referred to as PMNs or polymorphonuclear leukocytes)
  - Basophils (granulocytes found in blood; share similarities with the tissue mast cell, e.g., both cell types store histamine and are involved in certain allergic responses)
  - Eosinophils (granulocytes important in certain allergic responses)
  - Mast cells (granulocytes found in tissue; liberate mediators of inflammation, e.g., histamine)
- Monocytes (phagocytic cells found in blood)
- Macrophages (similar to monocytes but found in the tissues)
- Lymphocytes
  - Natural killer cells (large granular lymphocytes)
  - T lymphocytes (T cells)
  - B lymphocytes (B cells)

The myeloid progenitor cells develop from multipotential (pluripotential) stem cells. These cells develop into the adult blood cell types and respond early to infections. The phagocytic neutrophils engulf bacteria, and the monocytes transform in the tissues to the phagocytic macrophages. Basophils and mast cells can degranulate to liberate stored mediators of inflammation such as histamine, leukotrienes, and other chemicals associated with allergy and infection. Eosinophils play a role in fighting viral and parasitic infections and in asthma pathogenesis.

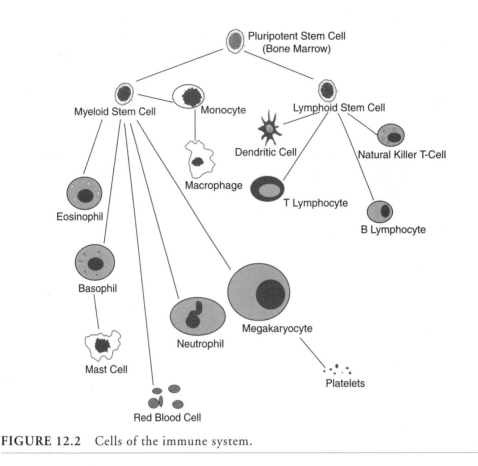

**FIGURE 12.2** Cells of the immune system.

The lymphoid progenitor cells also develop from the multipotential stem cells. The progenitor cells develop into small nongranulated white blood cells, known as *lymphocytes,* that also respond as a second-line defense later on in infection, when they respond to antigens that are presented to them by macrophages and dendritic cells. B lymphocytes, with the assistance of T lymphocytes, transform into plasma cells that produce and release antibodies that attack the offending agent. The T cells, in addition, act to help eliminate viruses contained in infected cells. B cells are concentrated in the lymph nodes, and when stimulated by an antigen-presenting macrophage (antigen binds to cell surface receptors) and then internalized, the B cell becomes a plasma cell producing antibody molecules (Figure 12.3).

This process requires the assistance from special helper T cells that regulate the overall immune response. Other T cells, cytotoxic T cells (also referred to as killer T cells), destroy infected cells and those that have become malignant early on in the malignant transformation process, before the cell develops the capability of evading the immunological surveillance system. The cytotoxic T cells also play a role in tissue rejection.

In addition to cytotoxic T cells, there are also natural killer cells. To mount an effective immunological assault, the former cell needs to detect specific antigen bound to cell surface

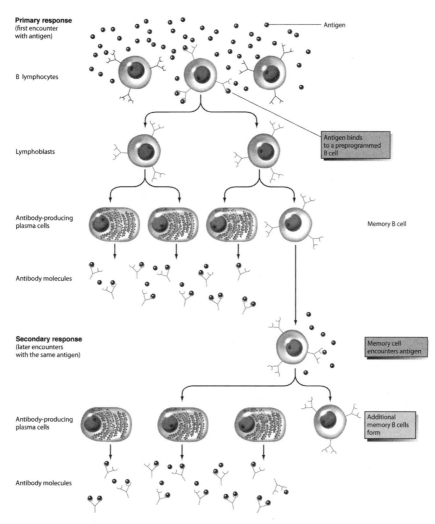

Primary response
(first encounter
with antigen)

Antigen

B lymphocytes

Lymphoblasts

Antigen binds
to a preprogrammed
B cell

Antibody-producing
plasma cells

Memory B cell

Antibody molecules

Secondary response
(later encounters
with the same antigen)

Memory cell
encounters antigen

Antibody-producing
plasma cells

Additional
memory B cells
form

Antibody molecules

**FIGURE 12.3**   Activation of B cells to make antibody.

major histocompatibility (MHC) markers of the infected cell, whereas natural killer T cells do not require their detection to mount an assault against "foreign" cells. Both types contain granules filled with potent cytotoxins (perforin and granulysin) that when released at the target cell's plasma membrane produce pores that result in water and ion deregulation, cell bloating, and eventful lysis.

## Antibodies

Antibodies belong to a group of protein molecules known as immunoglobulins that are produced and secreted into the lymphatic and circulatory systems by the B cells that are stimulated to transform into plasma cells. Some B cells differentiate into memory cells that can provide a more rapid response to an antigen reexposure. The process of antibody production can be divided into several components:

- *Antigen presentation to B cell:* Antibody production requires that a particular antigen or hapten is presented to the B cell by, for example, a macrophage. Haptens are not antigenic by themselves (e.g., a heavy metal such as nickel) but rather must first be linked onto a cellular protein before they can be successfully presented to the B cell.
- *Antigen internalization:* Antigen is internalized in the B cell and then transferred to the MHC II displayed on the cell surface where it is carried to other (uncommitted) B cells. This also results in the activation of helper T cells.
- *B cell commitment:* The B cell begins synthesis of an antigen-specific antibody and then differentiates into memory B cells and plasma (antibody-forming) cells that intensely secrete the specific antibody. IgM is produced early in the process, followed by IgG, the main antibody secreted in response to both the initial insult and later on if memory B cells are reexposed to the antigen.

The five classes of antibodies, designated by the prefix "Ig" for immunoglobulin, are as follows:

- IgG—the major immunoglobulin in the blood that attaches to microorganisms and other cells to facilitate their destruction by other immunological cells
- IgA—found in bodily fluids such as saliva, secretions of the gastrointestinal and respiratory tracts, and tears
- IgM—often forms complex star-like clusters in the bloodstream where it is very effective against bacteria
- IgE—normally present in only trace amounts but is responsible for the symptoms of allergy; fixed on mast cells and responsible for immediate-type hypersensitivity
- IgD—almost exclusively found inserted into the membrane of B cells, where it somehow regulates the cell's activation; functions as an antigen receptor

The basic structure of an immunoglobulin is one that consists of four polypeptide chains; two identical heavy chains and two identical light chains are shaped to form a "Y" and held together by disulfide bonding (Figure 12.4). The constant region of the antibody is identical for all antibodies of the same class and serves as a point of attachment to other immune cells.

Antibodies have a variable region whose specific amino acid sequence differs from antibody to antibody. The antigen binds to the variable region. The region of the antibody that binds antigen is referred to as Fab and contains specific receptors (Figure 12.5) for antigen epitopes (surface antigen molecules that fit antibody receptors).

Antibodies protect the host from infectious agents via several mechanisms:

- *Antibody-dependent cell cytotoxicity:* binding of white blood cells to the target cells via antibody bridges and the subsequent lysis of the target cell
- *Virus neutralization:* specific antibody binds to virus attachment sites on infected cells, thus blocking attachment by virus
- *Opsonization:* antibody coating of bacteria or virus can render them more susceptible to phagocytosis by neutrophils and macrophages that have antibody receptors

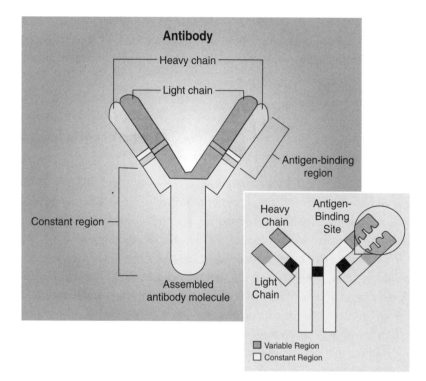

FIGURE 12.4 Antibody. *Source:* Courtesy of National Cancer Institute and courtesy of National Institute of Allergy and Infectious Diseases.

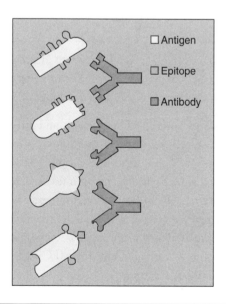

FIGURE 12.5 Specific binding of antigen to antibody. *Source:* Courtesy of National Institute of Allergy and Infectious Diseases.

- *Complement-mediated lysis:* antibody binds to target cell and activates the complement system, a cascade consisting of serum proteins that sequentially interact, resulting in the lysis of the immunological target (bacteria, viruses, neoplastic or transplanted cells)

## Immunological Disorders

A common type of immunological response to certain chemicals is that of hypersensitivity reaction. There are four basic forms of these types of reactions:

- *Type I hypersensitivity* (anaphylactic response) is the result of IgE binding to the receptors of mast and other cells containing granules of inflammatory mediators such as histamine and other cytokines that when liberated result in inflammation, swelling, bronchoconstriction, and decreased blood pressure, which is life threatening.
- *Type II hypersensitivity* (antibody-dependent cellular hypersensitivity) results when antibody (IgM, IgG) or complement is directed against the body's cells, which marks them for attack and destruction by phagocytic cells such as macrophages and neutrophils and other cells, which produce cytotoxic mediators.
- *Type III hypersensitivity* (immune complex deposition) results when complexes of antigen-antibody deposit in the tissues of the body. Common sites of deposition include the kidneys, lungs, and joint capsule. This marks the tissue for assault by phagocytic and cytotoxic cells.
- *Type IV hypersensitivity* (cell-mediated hypersensitivity) results when an individual has become sensitized to an antigen from a prior exposure. Reexposure results in a delayed hypersensitivity, usually in 12–48 hours. This is typically seen for allergic contact dermatitis and photosensitization responses. Requires prior exposure to the antigen.

## Immunosuppression by Toxicants

Many different types of chemicals have been shown to affect immune function, primarily through suppression of specific and nonspecific mechanisms of immunity. Examples that are representative of these chemicals can be placed into a number of categories:

- *Pharmaceutical compounds* such as corticosteroids and antitumor drugs target the bone marrow, thymus, and spleen, resulting in immunosuppression by interfering with cell division and by depression of phagocytosis. Examples of these types of chemicals include cyclophosphamide, analogues of purine and pyrimidine bases such as 6-mercapto-purine, 5-fluorouracil, and folic acid analogues such as aminopterin and methotrexate.
- *Halogenated aromatic hydrocarbons* such as 2,3,7,8-tetrachlorodibenzo-*p*-dioxin (TCDD) has been shown experimentally to produce thymic involution in perinatal animals and lymphoid atrophy and polychlorinated biphenyls (PCBs) and polybrominated biphenyls (PBBs) suppress the antibody response.
- *Polyaromatic hydrocarbons* (PAHs) have been linked to depressed humoral immunity, cell-mediated immunity, and tumor resistance.

- *Nitrosamines* such as dimethylnitrosamine and diethylnitrosamine may inhibit T cell–dependent humoral immune responses.
- *Pesticides* in laboratory studies (many categories) have been demonstrated to be immuno-toxic; however, there is limited evidence in humans.
- *Metals* have been shown to be associated with a number of effects on immune function:
  - As—technically classified as a metalloid is immunosuppressive
  - Be—induces T cell–mediated hypersensitivity and berylliosis
  - Cd—depression of humoral, macrophage, and other immune cell functions
  - Hg—type III hypersensitivity (immune complex deposition) and glomerulonephritis and may augment anaphylaxis by enhancing IgE production
  - Pb—increased susceptibility to upper respiratory infections

## Examples of Chemical-Induced Immunological Disorders

Allergic contact dermatitis has been associated with exposures to a number of different chemicals:

- Metals such as platinum, nickel, and chromium—type IV reactions
- Formaldehyde—types I and IV reactions
- Isocyanates such as toluene diisocyanate—types I and IV reactions

Asthma has been linked to exposures to chemicals both occupationally and nonoccupationally. Perhaps the best studies come from occupational reports that causally implicate a number of occupational chemicals and processes in the etiology and pathophysiology of the disorder, such as

- Bakers exposed to flour
- Clam shuckers
- Bacterial enzymes in laundry detergent
- Toluene diisocyanate in spray paint and polyurethane foam
- Red-cedar wood and wood products

Autoimmune responses can occur whereby a chemical (hapten) stimulates an immune response after it has become associated with an endogenous protein. Later, the protein alone is recognized by the immune system as "non-self" and stimulates a further immune response. An example is glomerular nephritis from exposure to certain heavy metals.

## Experimental Immunological Testing

A number of tests are available experimentally, either *in vivo* or *in vitro*, to study chemicals suspected to have an effect on immunological function. An example of a test for cell-mediated immunity would be to establish experimental and control animals and pretreat each with either the chemical of interest or a control medium (without the chemical present). Lymphocytes from either the spleen or blood would be collected and tested with a mitogen, such as concanavalin

A, phytohemagglutinin for T lymphocytes, and lipopolysaccharides for B lymphocytes, as a test for proliferation capacity. Proliferation would be determined and quantified by DNA synthesis as measured by the incorporation of radioactively labeled bases (e.g., thymidine) into the DNA.

The effects of chemicals on humoral immunity can be performed by challenging experimental animals already pretreated with the chemical of interest to an antigen and measuring specific immunoglobulins in the blood. The spleen is next removed, and a suspension of cells is obtained to which the antigen is added along with complement, and the number of cell plaques formed is determined. A decreased number of plaques are taken as an indicator for immunosuppression. A simple assay for delayed hypersensitivity reactions involves injecting an antigen such as keyhole limpet hemocyanin into the footpad, ear, or subcutaneously, followed by a challenge with the chemical in question several days later at the same site to measure the extent of swelling.

## Bibliography

Burleson, G. R. (2000). Models of respiratory immunotoxicology and host resistance. *Immunopharmacology, 48,* 315–318.

Cederbrant, K., Marcusson-Stahl, M., Condevaux, F., & Descotes, J. (2003). NK-cell activity in immunotoxicity drug evaluation. *Toxicology, 185,* 241–250.

Dean, J. H. (2004). A brief history of immunotoxicology and a review of the pharmaceutical guidelines. *International Journal of Toxicology, 23,* 83–90.

Descotes, J. (1998*). Introduction to immunotoxicology.* Boca Raton, FL: CRC Press.

Holladay, S. D. (2004). *Developmental immunotoxicology.* Boca Raton, FL: CRC Press.

Holsapple, M. P. (2003). Developmental immunotoxicity testing: a review. *Toxicology, 185,* 193–203.

Kimber, I., & Dearman, R. J. (2002). Immune responses: adverse versus non-adverse effects. *Toxicology and Pathology, 30,* 54–58.

Klaassen, C. D. (2001). *Casarett & Doull's toxicology. The basic science of poisons.* New York: McGraw-Hill.

Klaassen, C. D., & Watkins, J. B. (2003). *Casarett & Doull's essentials of toxicology.* New York: McGraw-Hill.

Luebke, R., House, R., & Kimber, I. (2006). *Immunotoxicology and immunopharmacology* (3rd edition series). Target Organ Toxicology Series Volume 23. Boca Raton, FL: CRC Press.

Luster, M. I., Simeonova, P., Gallucci, R., Matheson, J., Yucesoy, B., & Sugawara, T. (2000). Overview of immunotoxicology and current applications to respiratory diseases. *Immunopharmacology, 48,* 311–313.

Merk, H. F., Sachs, B., & Baron, J. (2001). The skin: target organ in immunotoxicology of small-molecular-weight compounds. *Skin Pharmacology and Applied Skin Physiology, 14,* 419–430.

The National Cancer Institute. http://newscenter.cancer.gov/sciencebehind/.

The National Institute of Allergy and Infectious Diseases. http://www.niaid.nih.gov/final/immun/immun.htm#Defense.

Pieters, R., & Albers, R. (1999). Screening tests for autoimmune-related immunotoxicity. *Environmental Health Perspectives, 107*(suppl 5), 673–677.

Selgrade, M. K., Germolec, D. R., Luebke, R. W., Smialowicz, R. J., Ward, M. D., & Sailstad, D. M. (2001). Immunotoxicity. In E. Hodgson and R. C. Smart (Eds.), *Introduction to biochemical toxicology* (pp. 561–598). New York: Wiley-Interscience.

Thomas, P. T. (1998). Immunotoxicology: hazard identification and risk assessment. *Nutrition Reviews, 56*(1 Pt 2), S131–S134.

U.S. National Library of Medicine, National Institutes of Health, Environmental Health, and Toxicology Specialized Information Services (SIS). (2005). *Toxicology tutorial III.* Retrieved October 2, 2005 from http://www.sis.nlm.nih.gov/enviro/toxtutor.html.

# CHAPTER 13

# Skin

The skin (integument) is not a passive structural barrier; rather, it participates actively in a variety of defense strategies designed to prevent widespread internal or cutaneous damage. The skin is the heaviest organ in the body, weighing in at approximately 15% of total body weight, with an average exposure surface area of 1.5–2.0 m$^2$. The skin plays an important role in

- Physical protection from environmental agents
- Hydroregulation through both passive and active mechanisms
- Thermoregulation to maintain core body temperature
- Absorption of clinically important pharmaceutical preparations
- Chemical synthesis of vitamin D
- Immunological surveillance and function
- Sensory reception of pain, temperature, touch, and pressure

From a toxicological viewpoint, the skin is of concern because it is a

- Route of exposure for systemic toxicants
- Direct target for toxicity
- Xenobiotic metabolizing organ
- Minor pathway for the elimination of certain toxicants

The early studies of chemical carcinogenesis involved the topical application of precarcinogens and observation for tumor incidence. The skin possesses cytochrome P450, epoxide hydrolase, and other enzymes for biotransformation reactions. This biotransformation occurs mainly in the epidermis, and cytochrome P450–dependent microsomal monooxygenases are the primary enzyme system involved in the metabolism of lipophilic xenobiotics.

## Structure of the Skin

The skin can be divided into three basic regions; epidermis, dermis, and hypodermis (Figure 13.1). The designation of thin or thick skin is based on the thickness of the epidermal layer. Thin skin covers most of the body and is characterized by a thinner stratum corneum. Thick skin is found on the palms, fingertips, and soles of the feet and lacks hair follicles and sebaceous glands. The epidermis is composed of stratified squamous epithelium. Epidermal thickness varies from 0.06 mm to several millimeters, as does moisture and lipid content in different regions of the body. The principal type of cell, the keratinocyte, comprises greater than 90% of all cells of the epidermis. The stratum basale is the deepest layer of the epidermis and is represented by a single layer of cuboidal to columnar keratinocytes, which are mitotically active. The source of all keratinocytes is the basal layer (also referred to as the stratum germinativum) and to a much lesser degree the cells of hair follicles.

The cells of the basal layer follow an orderly process of cellular division and differentiation. It is this process of differentiation that gives rise to the names of the other epidermal layers. From the skin surface and working toward the basal layer are the stratum corneum, stratum lucidum, stratum granulosum, stratum spinosum, and stratum basale. The progression of differentiation

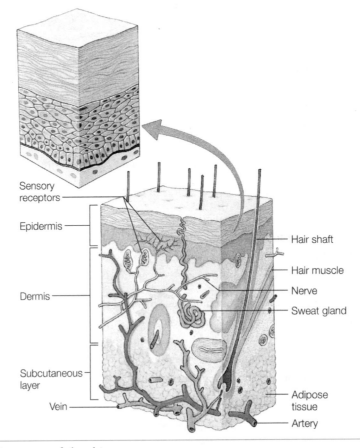

**FIGURE 13.1**    Structure of the skin.

from basal layer to the stratum corneum normally requires approximately 2 weeks (less than a week in individuals with psoriasis). The cells undergo terminal differentiation as they migrate to the surface of the body, accumulate keratin, flatten, and increase in volume. The cells are 80% keratin once they reach the surface.

The stratum spinosum is represented by a layer of cells that are cuboidal, polygonal, and slightly flattened. The stratum spinosum is named for the tonofilaments that terminate with desmosomes in spiny-like projections that hold the cells together and may serve in a protective fashion against tearing of the skin. Psoriasis is a skin disorder in which excessive cell division leads to an increased and irregular thickening of the stratum basale and spinosum.

The stratum granulosum is three to five layers of flattened polygonal cells and derives its name from the accumulated granules of keratohyalin. This layer of cells contains nuclei and other cellular organelles but lacks mitotic activity. These granules contain histidine and cysteine-rich proteins and lipid-rich granules. These materials appear to serve as extracellular "cement" designed to seal the skin from foreign objects and water.

The stratum lucidum is a thin translucent layer of extremely flattened eosinophilic cells. These cells lack nuclei and organelles but retain filaments and desmosomes. The cells of the stratum lucidum contain eleidin, a transformation product of keratohyalin.

The stratum corneum is the outermost layer of the epidermis. It is composed of 15 to 20 layers of flattened non-nucleated keratinized cells. These cells are filled with keratin filaments embedded in lipid-rich material. Between cells there is ceramide-containing material (a type of lipid produced from cholesterol) that contributes as a water permeability barrier. The surface layer of cells is continuously desquamated. The stratum corneum is also commonly referred to as the "horny layer" of the skin.

The epidermis also contains several types of specialized cells:

- *Melanocytes* produce the pigment melanin, which is incorporated in nearby keratinocytes through small cell membrane bound vesicles containing melanin. These vesicles bud off of the melanocyte and are referred to as *melanosomes.*
- *Langerhans cells* are bone marrow–derived monocytes that have become skin macrophages and function in the presentation of antigen to lymphocytes. They are characterized by pale nuclei and granular cytoplasm. Though present in all layers, the cells are predominantly in the stratum spinosum. Their numbers increase in cases of chronic inflammatory skin disease.
- *Merkel's cells* are thought to have sensory mechanoreceptor or neuroendocrine functions. These granule-containing cells are located in the stratum basale, though they are rarely found in thin skin.

The dermis makes up approximately 90% of the skin and is composed of dense fibroelastic connective tissue. It contains hair, hair follicles, sebaceous glands, and eccrine glands that originate in the epidermis and extend into the dermis. Blood vessels are found in the dermis but not the epidermis. Extensive nerve, vascular networks, and other structures are required to support the epidermis. The blood vessels are important in body temperature and blood pressure regulation.

# Skin Absorption of Chemicals

Although exposures to many chemicals can produce toxic effects to the skin directly, systemic toxicity is also an important consideration when dealing with skin exposures. A widely publicized case of systemic toxicity from skin exposure was that of Dr. Karen Wetterhahn, a Dartmouth chemistry professor who in 1996 spilled a small amount of dimethylmercury and weeks later died from progressive neurological toxicity. The chemical penetrates latex and polyvinyl chloride (PVC) gloves. Exposure can occur from skin deposition of a liquid; contact with a vapor, aerosol, or solid; and transfer from a contaminated surface. A skin exposure can be linked to an internal dose through the diffusion of the chemical through the stratum corneum.

Systemic toxicity (Table 13.1) from skin exposure can occur only if the chemical moves from the epidermis into the dermis of the skin, which contains the blood vessels. Movement is by passive diffusion. The term *percutaneous absorption* refers to this transport. The major barrier is the stratum corneum. Conditions that alter the structural integrity of the skin such as lacerations or abrasions can enhance the absorption of xenobiotics. The rate of penetration is largely related to the lipophilicity of the chemical; the more lipophilic a chemical, the greater its rate of penetration. Lipophilic substances (nonpolar substances) essentially diffuse through the nonaqueous lipid matrix of cells and extracellular space. Hydrophilic substances (polar substances) diffuse through any available aqueous channels within the epidermis, including epidermal appendages such as sweat glands. A number of factors affect skin absorption including:

- Applied dose
- Chemical concentration
- Duration of exposure
- Surface area involved

**Table 13.1**  Systemic Effects from Percutaneous Absorption

| Chemicals | System Effects |
|---|---|
| Organophosphates | Cholinesterase inhibition |
| Benzidine | Bladder cancer |
| Carbon tetrachloride | Kidney, liver, central nervous system |
| Hydrofluoric acid | Electrolyte deregulation; kidney |
| Methyl-n-butyl ketone | Peripheral neuropathy |
| Aniline | Methemoglobinuria, bladder cancer |
| Acrylamide | Peripheral neuropathy |
| Carbon disulfide | Coronary artery disease, central and peripheral nervous system effects |
| Glycol ethers | Aplastic anemia |
| Hexachlorophene | Encephalopathy |
| Nitroglycerin | Coronary dilatation |
| Inorganic mercury | Renal toxicity |
| Alkyl lead | Neurotoxicity |
| Boric acid | Gastrointestinal lesions |

- Physical integrity of stratum corneum
- Regional variations of skin
- Degree of hydration
- Temperature
- Presence of other substances
- Circulatory effects chemical–skin binding

The region of skin exposure plays a major role in the relative rate of absorption, especially for lipophilic chemicals. For hydrocortisone, as an example of a clinically useful chemical, the relative rate of absorption from the plantar foot arch is 1, the forehead 43, and the scrotum 300.

## Skin Toxicity: Local Effects

There are a number of effects certain chemicals can have on the skin (e.g., acute irritant dermatitis, chronic irritant dermatitis, corrosion, allergic contact dermatitis). Perhaps the best information comes from occupational reports. The hands, wrists, and forearms are the most common sites of occupational contact dermatitis. Preexisting skin conditions, allergies, age and work experience, temperature, humidity, and seasons are examples of factors that affect the development of skin reactions to chemical exposure.

Contact dermatitis is the most common occupational dermatosis, with more than 90% of reported cases. Dermatitis may be the result of the chemical directly producing a skin inflammatory response (primary irritant response) or indirectly due to the allergic sensitization of the individual upon reexposure to the offending agent. In both cases an inflammatory response results, however; the allergic response is due to the liberation of mediators of inflammation triggered by the immune system and not to the direct damaging effects of the chemical on the skin, as might occur from an exposure to an organic solvent, which dissolves the lipids of the skin. Both the primary irritant response and the allergic response may share a common clinical picture of itching, burning, discomfort, erythema, edema, induration, vesiculation, oozing, and scaling.

Irritant contact dermatitis is responsible for 80% of all contact dermatitis cases. The extent of irritant action of chemicals on the skin is determined by factors such as the duration and repetitiveness of contact, concentration, pH, and temperature. Primary irritants include solvents, surfactants, strong inorganic and organic acids and alkalis, cement, soaps and detergents, and metals such as chromium, antimony, and nickel.

An extreme form of direct skin damage by chemicals is that of skin corrosion, an immediate and irreversible response from a single exposure to an agent that results in epidermal and dermal necrosis. In this case it is largely a difference in the concentration of the chemical that determines whether skin corrosion or a primary irritant response results from an exposure. Examples of corrosives include concentrated acids, bases, ammonia, chlorine, hydrofluoric acid, isocyanates, phenol, phosphorous, ethylene oxide and hydrogen peroxide, and calcium oxide.

Allergic contact dermatitis represents approximately 20% of the cases of contact dermatitis reported. It is a cell-mediated (T-cell) or type IV immunological reaction in individuals who have become sensitized to the offending agent. The key factors include a genetic predisposition to sensitization, a sensitizing event, and contact after the sensitization. The mechanism producing allergic contact dermatitis begins when haptens penetrate the stratum corneum and link to epidermal proteins. Langerhans cells present these allergens to helper T lymphocytes, thereby activating them. This activation results in clonal proliferation in regional lymph nodes. Subsequent exposures stimulate the activated cells to return to the area and cause dermatitis.

The process can be divided into four phases:

1. *Refractory phase:* Periodic or continuous contact with an allergen occurs over the course of days to a lifetime without any apparent response.
2. *Induction phase:* Hapten penetrates skin, conjugates with an epidermal protein, and is presented to T lymphocytes by macrophages. Lymphocytes migrate to regional lymph nodes where they proliferate into effector and memory cells. This occurs over a period of approximately 2–3 weeks.
3. *Eliciting phase:* Recontact with the specific hapten is recognized at the exposure site by effector cells, which trigger the release of mediators of inflammation. This occurs over a period of approximately 12–48 hours.
4. *Persistence phase:* The retention of effector cells that have the capability of specific hapten recognition and ability to trigger another inflammatory response upon reexposure. This capability can last for years to a lifetime in the sensitized individual.

Unlike the primary irritant response, where the extent of injury is proportional to the magnitude of the exposure, in contact allergic dermatitis even a small amount of chemical in the sensitized individual can result in a significant dermatitis. Examples of common occupational sensitizers are summarized in Table 13.2.

Light and chemicals on the skin can interact to produce a phototoxic skin response. We all recognize that ultraviolet (UV) radiation in the 280 to 320 nm range (UVB) penetrates into the dermis and depending on time and intensity can cause a short-term inflammatory response (erythema) as well as long-term changes upon chronic exposures, such as actinic keratosis, basal and squamous carcinomas, and malignant melanoma. It can also lead to a decline in immunocompetence due to a depletion of Langerhans cells. Sunlight also facilitates normal biochemical reactions such as formation of vitamin $D_3$ and the breakdown of bilirubin. It is thought that the combination of UV light and skin exposure to certain chemicals results in the production of free radicals that produce effects that are similar to contact dermatitis. Both natural light and artificial light, as may be encountered by glassblowers, foundry workers, and welders, have the ability to induce skin changes. The minimal erythremic dose refers to the minimum exposure (intensity and time dependent) required to produce skin redness. UVA light (320–400 nm) has greater penetrative power compared with UVB light (280–320 nm). Exposures to certain plant products such as the furocoumarin 8-methoxy psoralen found in limes and polyaromatic hydrocarbons (PAHs) can produce a "phytophotodermatitis." A photoallergic response can result from exposure to sulfanilamide, for example, which is catalyzed by light to p-hydroxylaminobenzene sulfonamide, which is a more potent allergen.

Acne induced by contact with chemicals such as coal tars and chlorinated hydrocarbons is referred to as *acne venenata.* The chemicals capable of producing acne venenata are termed *come-*

**Table 13.2** Examples of Occupational Skin Sensitizers

| Substance | Uses | Occupation |
|---|---|---|
| **Disinfectants** | | |
| Glutaraldehyde | | Health care, cleaners, papermaking |
| **Fragrances** | Cleaning agents | Cleaning personnel, hairdressers |
| **Pharmaceuticals** | | |
| Antibiotics | | Health care |
| **Preservatives** | | |
| Chloracetamide, formaldehyde releasers, isothiazolinones (Kathons), parabens | Metal cutting fluids, cosmetics, wood preservatives, water-based paints, glues | Metal workers, beauticians, masseurs, hairdressers, wood workers |
| **Rubber chemicals** | | |
| Thiuram accelerators phenylenediamine derivatives | | Health care workers, hairdressers, rubber industry |
| **Solvents** | | |
| d-Limonene, Ethylene diamine | Paint cleansers, degreasers | Metal workers, painters, assembly line workers, mechanics, printers |
| **Industrial enzymes** | Amylases in flour, proteases in detergents, etc. | Food and detergents industry, cleaners |
| *Proteins from Natural Materials* | | |
| **Natural rubber latex proteins** | Protective gloves, medical instruments | Health care workers, hairdressers |
| **Animal proteins** | Animal dander, epithelia and urine | Farmers, laboratory animal handlers |
| **Foodstuff Decorative plants** | Vegetables, plants Flour Spices | Farmers, florists, kitchen workers, cooks, food industry, bakers |

*dogenic* for the comedone lesions elicited by exposure. Papules, cysts, pustules, and scars may also result. Hair follicles can become inflamed when compacted keratinocytes are immersed in sebum or by exposure to chemicals or infection. Folliculitis typically presents on the face, neck, forearms, backs of hands and fingers, lower abdomen, buttocks, and thighs. Chloracne is an uncommon refractory form of acne caused by halogenated hydrocarbon exposure. Contact produces persistent yellow or straw-colored cysts along the side of the forehead, lateral eyelids, and behind the ears. The chemicals that produce chloracne are referred to as chloracnegens and include:

- Polychlorinated biphenyls (PCBs)
- Polybrominated biphenyls (PBBs)
- Hexachlorodibenzo-p-dioxin (HCDD)
- Tetrachlorodibenzo-p-dioxin (TCDD)

- Polybrominated dibenzofurans
- Polychlorodibenzofurans
- Tetrachloroazobenzene
- Tetrachloroazoxybenzene
- Polychloronaphthalenes

Other examples of skin effects from chemical exposures are as follows:

- *Urticarial reactions:* Type 1 allergic reactions cause the release of histamines, IgE, and other local inflammatory mediators
- *Cutaneous granulomas:* Inflammatory response to insoluble materials
- *Physical dermatitis:* Fiberglass
- *Hair loss:* Destroy hair-producing cells in the follicle or in the hair matrix due to exposures to depilatories, thallium, ionizing radiation, cancer chemotherapeutic agents
- *Hypopigmentation:* Inhibition/destruction of melanocytes (e.g., phenolic preparations, hydroquinones)
- *Hyperpigmentation:* Heavy metals, acridines
- *Color changes:* for example, orange/yellow from picric acid, green from copper dust, black from osmium trioxide

Many factors have been attributed as causal agents in the etiology of skin cancers, including chemical carcinogens, physical injuries such as burns and trauma, family history, and UV and ionizing radiations. Studies suggest that a sequential application of a carcinogen such as BaP and UVA radiation to the skin causes a synergistic formation of specific BaP-DNA adducts as well as 8-hydroxy-2'-deoxyguanosine, a biomarker of oxidative DNA base damage and oxidative stress. This is likely to be a very important public health issue because both UV radiation and carcinogens are prevalent in the environment, and their interaction is likely to be an important contributor to the development of a significant number of skin cancers.

## Bibliography

Andersen, K. E. (1999). Systemic toxicity from percutaneous absorption. In R. M. Adams (Ed.), *Occupational skin disease* (pp. 69–85). Philadelphia: W.B. Saunders, 1999.

Birmingham, D. J. (1980). Cutaneous absorption and systemic toxicity. In V. A. Drill and P. Lazar (Eds.), *Cutaneous toxicity* (pp. 53–62). New York: Academic Press.

British Association of Dermatologists. Retrieved November 2005 from http://www.bad.org.uk/.

California Pesticide Illness Surveillance Program. (2002). *Summary of illness/injury incidents reported in California as potentially related to pesticide exposure; summarized statewide and by county of occurrence.* Retrieved November 2005 from http://www.cdpr.ca.gov/docs/whs/pdf/2000totalstablecounty.pdf.

Cartotto, R. C., Peters, W. J., Neligan, P. C., Douglas, L. G., & Beeston, J. (1996). Chemical burns. *Canadian Journal of Surgery, 39,* 205–211.

Dermatology Image Atlas. Retrieved November 2005 from http://dermatlas.med.jhmi.edu/derm/.

*The electronic textbook of dermatology.* Retrieved November 2005 from http://www.telemedicine.org/stamford.htm.

Emedicine. Retrieved November 2005 from http://www.emedicine.com/derm/.

European Agency for Safety and Health at Work: Skin Sensitizers. Retrieved November 2005 from http://agency.osha.eu.int/publications/factsheets/40/factsn40-en.pdf.

Freeman, S., & Maibach, H. I. (1991). Systemic toxicity caused by absorption of drugs and chemicals through the skin. In F. N. Marzulli and H. I. Maibach (Eds.), *Dermatotoxicology* (pp. 851–875). New York: Hemisphere Publishing Corporation.

Klaassen, C. D., & Watkins, J. B. (2003). *Casarett and Doull's essentials of toxicology.* New York: McGraw-Hill.

Kulling, P. E. (1992). Dermal toxicology. *Archives of Toxicology, 15*(suppl), 123–129.

Lewis, R. (1997). Researchers' deaths inspire actions to improve safety. *The Scientist, 11,* 1–5.

Loomis, T. A. (1980). Skin as a portal of entry for systemic effects. In V. A. Drill and P. Lazar (Eds.), *Current concepts in cutaneous toxicity* (pp. 153–169). New York: Academic Press.

Maibach, H. I. (2001). *Toxicology of the skin.* Target Organ Toxicology Series. Philadelphia: Taylor & Francis.

National Institute of Arthritis and Musculoskeletal and Skin Diseases. Retrieved November 2005 from http://www.niams.nih.gov/.

Riviere, J. E. (2005). *Dermal absorption models in toxicology and pharmacology.* Philadelphia: Taylor & Francis.

Roberts, M. S., & Walters, K. A. (1998). *Dermal absorption and toxicity assessment.* Drugs and the Pharmaceutical Sciences, Volume 91. Philadelphia: Taylor & Francis.

Skin Cancer Foundation. Retrieved November 2005 from http://www.skincancer.org/.

Stinchcomb, A. L. (2003). Xenobiotic bioconversion in human epidermis models. *Pharmacological Research, 20,* 1113–1118.

Suskind, R. R. (1983). Percutaneous absorption and chemical carcinogenesis. *Journal of Dermatology, 10,* 97–107.

U.S. National Library of Medicine, National Institutes of Health, Environmental Health, and Toxicology Specialized Information Services (SIS). (2005). *Toxicology tutorial III.* Retrieved October 2, 2005 from http://www.sis.nlm.nih.gov/enviro/toxtutor.html.

World Health Organization. (1990). *Public health impact of pesticides used in agriculture.* Geneva, Switzerland: World Health Organization.

Zhai, H., & Maibach, H. I. (2004). *Dermatoxicology.* Philadelphia: Taylor & Francis.

# CHAPTER 14

# The Liver and Kidneys

## The Liver

### *General Considerations*

When one thinks about the effects of chemicals on the liver, one cannot escape the significant public health concern about the abuse of alcohol. Alcoholic liver disease affects tens of millions of Americans, with approximately a quarter of a million deaths annually that can be directly attributed to the abuse of alcohol. Chronic use of alcohol increases the vulnerability of the liver to insult from other chemicals as well. The progression of the disease is complex, beginning with fatty liver, alcoholic hepatitis, and the progression to alcoholic cirrhosis. On the short term, the consumption of approximately six alcoholic drinks a day (a standard drink contains approximately 12 g of ethanol) leads to fatty changes in the liver. At this level of consumption, the individual is considered to be an alcoholic. Higher levels of consumption result in alcoholic cirrhosis in approximately 20% of individuals.

The liver constitutes about 8% of the body mass and is the largest internal organ (Figure 14.1). It has a number of vital functions for our normal physiology including:

- Carbohydrate storage and metabolism
- Storage of vitamins A and D
- Biosynthesis of glycogen, albumin, globulins, steroids, blood-clotting factors, and angiotensinogen

- Biotransformation and excretion of xenobiotics
- Fat metabolism
- Synthesis of bile acids/salts that aid in digestion of fats
- Metabolism of hormones
- Formation of urea from amino acids
- Degradation of hemoglobin (bilirubin) and route of elimination for bile pigments and hemoglobin metabolites
- Transport and storage of lipids, metals such as iron, copper, zinc, and cadmium
- Phagocytosis of microorganisms and other foreign bodies

The liver is often the most vulnerable target for toxicity from orally ingested chemicals. There are many reasons for this, including the fact that the liver is the first organ to be exposed to ingested chemicals following absorption due to its portal blood supply and its high content of xenobiotic metabolizing enzymes which may increase toxicity for certain chemicals.

The liver is the primary organ for biotransformation reactions, the primary goal of which is the metabolic conversion of a xenobiotic from a readily absorbed lipophilic form to an easily excreted hydrophilic form. These biotransformations also have the potential to produce metabolites that are more or less toxic than the original toxicant. When the daughter metabolites are less toxic than the parent compound, the process is called *detoxification.* Conversely, when the daughter substances are more toxic than the original parent compound, the process is referred to as *bioactivation.*

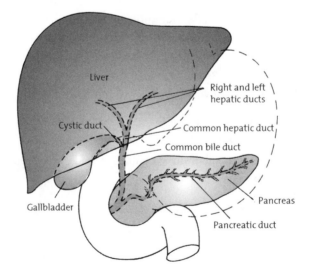

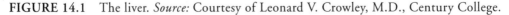

**FIGURE 14.1**   The liver. *Source:* Courtesy of Leonard V. Crowley, M.D., Century College.

Ethanol, vinyl chloride, acetaminophen, arsenic, and carbon tetrachloride are all agents whose metabolites are associated with hepatotoxicity. The metabolites of chemicals transformed by hepatic phase I reactions are often capable of being excreted without further metabolic action. If the intermediates are not readily excreted at this stage, they can, depending on the chemical, go on to further metabolic transformation in phase II reactions. Benzene is an example of a substance that requires both phase I and phase II reactions to complete biotransformation.

The basic structure of the liver is a specialized arrangement of cells into functional units called acini or lobules (Figure 14.2). The blood supply to the liver is mixed. It receives about 80% venous blood and 20% arterial blood with a blood volume between 10% and 15% at any given time. Blood enters the lobules through branches of the portal vein and hepatic artery and then flows through small channels called sinusoids that are lined with primary liver cell type, the hepatocytes. The space between the sinusoids and the hepatocytes is called the space of Disse.

The hepatocytes directly receive chemicals from the venous return of the digestive tract, including toxicants and drugs. Hepatocytes comprise approximately 80% of the mass of the liver and are the primary cell that performs liver functions. The portal vein carries blood from the small intestines, spleen, and pancreas. This portal circulation is responsible for the "first-pass" effect in that the liver is the first organ to receive this blood from the gastrointestinal tract before it enters into the general circulation. The hepatic or portal triad of the lobule represents a branch of the hepatic artery, portal vein, and bile duct, with blood and bile flow in opposite directions: mixed blood flow through the sinusoids into the central vein (hepatic venule) and

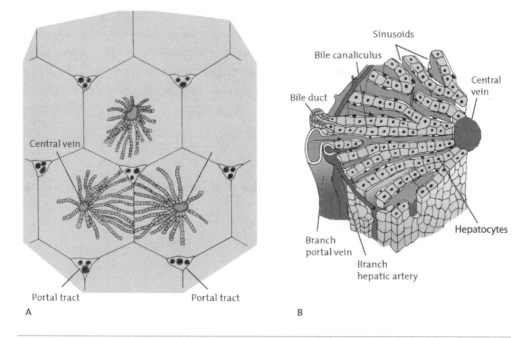

**FIGURE 14.2**  Liver lobule. *Source:* Courtesy of Leonard V. Crowley, M.D., Century College.

bile through the canaliculi into a bile duct. Stored in the gallbladder, bile is an emulsion that contains dissolved substances like conjugated bilirubin, bile salts, lecithin, cholesterol, water, and minerals; it is discharged into the duodenum when food enters the digestive tract.

The reticuloendothelial system consists of Kupffer cells, lipocytes (Ito cells), pit cells, oval or stem cells, and endothelial cells. The Kupffer, Ito, and endothelial cells are all found in the hepatic sinusoids, the channels between the cords of hepatocytes. Hepatocytes are characterized by their abundant endoplasmic reticulum, mitochondria, and secretory organelles. Kupffer cells are macrophages, attached to the endothelium, that are a source of cytokines and can act as antigen-presenting cells. Ito cells are fat-storing cells in the sinusoids that synthesize collagen and are the major site for vitamin A storage. Pit cells, attached to the endothelium, serve as natural killer lymphocytes. Oval cells provide a source for liver regeneration.

## Functional Organization of the Liver

The hepatic lobule or acinus is the structural and functional unit of the liver. Its unique arrangement of cells is recognizable based on landmarks of the portal tract (hepatic triad) and central vein. The central vein drains the mixed venous–arterial blood supply to the liver: The portal vein delivers approximately 60% of the blood supply and the hepatic arteriole, 40%. These two sources mix in the sinusoid and drain toward the central vein.

Regions of the lobule are based on hepatocyte location relative to the hepatic triad and central vein. Zone 1 (periportal) is closest to the input of arterial blood at the triad, and zone 3 (centrilobular) is closest to the central vein. The region between zone 1 and 3 is referred to as the mid-zonal or zone 2 region. The hepatocytes in zone 1 are closest to the oxygenated blood supply and are the youngest cells. They are high in respiratory enzyme activity and glutathione content, take up more bile acids and secrete more biliary constituents, and play the greater role in ammonia detoxification to urea. The hepatocytes in zone 3 receive an oxygen-depleted blood and are often less resistant to hepatotoxicants. The hepatocytes here have high concentrations of P450 enzymes and lower concentrations of glutathione compared with the cells of zone 1. The hepatocytes of the mid-zonal region have the most regenerative activity. There is then a heterogeneity in the acinus that is based on blood supply, nutrient supply, and metabolite gradients.

## Types of Hepatic Injuries Produced by Toxicants

The liver responds to chemical insults in a number of different ways, depending on both the chemical dose and whether exposure is acute or chronic in nature (Figure 14.3).

Examples of hepatic injuries from exposure to toxicants include:

- Necrosis
- Steatosis (lipidosis or fatty liver)
- Cholestasis
- Cirrhosis (fibrosis)
- Vascular injury
- Neoplasia

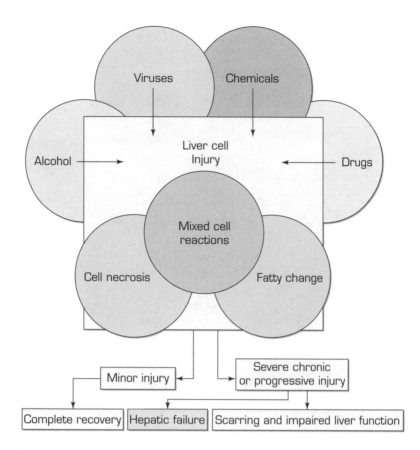

**FIGURE 14.3**    Common causes and effects of hepatic damage. *Source:* Courtesy of Leonard V. Crowley, M.D., Century College.

Many different classes of chemicals have been linked to liver injury. Those that are collectively referred to as the "organic solvents" are especially hepatotoxic by all exposure routes (Table 14.1).

## Hepatocyte Death and Necrosis

Hepatocyte death can be focal and confined to a few cells, zonal (centrilobular, midzonal, periportal), or massive (panlobular) depending on the nature of the toxicant and its dose. As hepatocytes age, they move toward the central vein; the cell's life span is about 6 months. Hepatocytes die by either necrosis or apoptosis. Necrotic cells are characterized by cell swelling, leakage of cellular enzymes, nuclear disintegration, and inflammation. Apoptotic cells are characterized by cell shrinkage, nuclear fragmentation, formation of apoptotic bodies, and digestion by phagocytic cells with no inflammation.

Acute chemical insult of sufficient magnitude and duration can result in functional and structural changes that may be irreversible. Necrosis is an irreversible cell injury and indicates significant acute cellular death. Necrosis is a catastrophic event that may significantly reduce the functional capacity of the organ, especially when a source of replacement cells is absent or limited.

**Table 14.1**   Organic Solvent Hepatotoxicity

| Solvent | Effect |
| --- | --- |
| Xylene | Steatosis<br>Fibrosis<br>Necrosis |
| Toluene | Steatosis<br>Fibrosis<br>Necrosis |
| Styrene | Steatosis<br>Fibrosis<br>Necrosis |
| Acrylonitrile | Necrosis |
| Carbon disulfide | Necrosis |
| Isopropanol | Necrosis |
| Dimethylformamide | Necrosis<br>Steatosis |
| Trichloroethane | Liver tumors<br>Biliary tract tumors |
| Methylene chloride | Liver tumors<br>Biliary tract tumors |
| White spirit (Stoddard solvent) | Steatosis<br>Fibrosis<br>Necrosis |

During necrosis one can detect the leakage from cells of characteristic enzymes such as alanine aminotransferase (ALT) and aspartate aminotransferase (AST). Higher than normal levels appearing in the blood plasma are taken as an indication of irreversible injury. Loss of these enzymes is accompanied by a reduction in specific hepatic functions. Significant loss of AST from hepatocytes, for example, is accompanied by a reduction in the liver's ability to catalyze the reversible transfer of an amino group between aspartic acid and alpha-ketoglutarate to form glutamic acid in the mitochondria. Similarly, a significant loss of ALT results in the reduction of hepatic transfer of an amino group between alanine and alpha-ketoglutarate to form glutamate. Significant necrosis is accompanied by increased levels of these and other hepatic enzymes.

The region of the liver that is most affected from toxic insult is largely dependent on the nature of the chemical and the level and types of toxicant-metabolizing enzymes present in the hepatocytes of the region. For example, carbon tetrachloride and related hydrocarbons cause severe zone 3 (centrilobular) necrosis and fatty infiltration due to their bioactivation by higher concentrations of hepatic cytochrome P450. The generation of reactive metabolites during biotransformation and the depletion of glutathione are responsible for cytotoxicity. The generation of unstable chemical intermediates such as free radicals, oxides, and peroxides contributes significantly toward the breakdown of cellular lipids by their peroxidation. Other examples of chemicals that can produce necrosis are acetaminophen (Tylenol), allyl alcohol, beryllium, furosemide and bromobenzene, diquat, *Amanita phalloides* (Death cap mushroom) toxin, and dimethylformamide.

During necrosis one can observe a progression of cellular changes from cellular swelling, dilatation of the endoplasmic reticulum, mitochondrial swelling, nuclear swelling, and rupture of the cell membrane. Fortunately, the liver has significant regenerative potential; however, it can be overloaded by a toxicant, resulting in organ failure as can occur from an acute exposure to certain toxicants (e.g., poisonous mushrooms). The liver has a number of ways to proceed with repair. The principal way repair is accomplished is by the division of mature hepatocytes to restore the structure and functional capacity of the liver. A second way to accomplish repair is through the division and differentiation of a population of stem liver cells known as oval cells that are found along the edges of portal tracts. Failure of these repair mechanisms may result in repair through the recruitment of fiber-producing cells (fibroblasts) and the production of fibrous tissue (scar tissue) to fill the structural gaps where significant hepatocytes have been lost. If significant fibrosis occurs, then the liver is recognized by the disease state known as cirrhosis.

### Lipidosis (Steatosis or Fatty Liver)

Fatty liver, also referred to as steatosis, is a common and often reversible response to acute exposures to toxicants. It is characterized by an increase in hepatic lipid content to greater than 5% of liver weight. In steatosis, the liver enlarges as a result of the accumulation of lipids and triglycerides; sometimes it is associated with necrosis. The lipids appear as vacuoles in the hepatocyte cytoplasm, often displacing the nucleus of the cells. Several factors other than toxicant exposure can cause steatosis, including obesity, alcoholism, and a diet deficient in protein, a common problem in undeveloped countries. Exposure to many chemicals can result in a fatty liver. Carbon tetrachloride is an example of a chemical that can produce lipidosis by interfering with fatty acid oxidation, inhibition of mitochondrial function, and lipoprotein synthesis. Triglycerides accumulate in hepatocytes due to the inability of the cell to balance its rate of synthesis and its extracellular release. Carbon tetrachloride also results in hepatocyte necrosis. Ethanol is another chemical, widely abused, that results in increased production of fatty acids, and chronic exposure can progress to fibrosis and cirrhosis.

### Cholestasis

Cholestasis is the accumulation within the bile canaliculi of bile pigments and other products that restrict the normal flow of bile. The liver retains bile salts and bilirubin, which can lead to their elevation in the blood in the production of jaundice. Cholestasis that is toxicant induced can be reversible or chronic. The general features of canalicular cholestasis include the presence of bile within hepatocytes and canalicular spaces, which can lead to increased blood levels of contents normally excreted in bile, most importantly bile salts and bilirubin. Because bile salts are strong surfactants, their accumulation within hepatocytes can result in cell membrane injury and loss of cellular function. Examples of toxicants that can produce canalicular cholestasis include anabolic steroids, 1,1-dichloroethylene, manganese, organic arsenicals, phalloidin, chlorpromazine, erythromycin, cyclosporin, and oral contraceptives.

## Vascular Injury

The sinusoids of the liver are very delicate structures. Like capillaries, their walls are composed of endothelium. Conditions that result in sinusoid blockage can cause the dilatation of these structures, and consequently the liver can become engorged with blood cells. This is a very serious condition that can lead to shock and death due to the retention of blood cells by the liver. This condition appears to be related to changes in the endothelial cytoskeleton and the collapse of the space of Disse, thereby trapping blood cells in the vascular spaces of the liver. The disruption of hepatic endothelial cells has been shown to be caused by chemicals such as microcystin, beryllium, dimethyl nitrosamines, and some anticancer drugs.

## Cirrhosis

Cirrhosis of the liver is a fibrotic disease that is characterized by the loss of significant hepatic function, which can ultimately result in total organ failure. It is a disease that has been classically associated with the chronic consumption of excessive amounts of ethanol. This inflammatory disease is characterized by a significant accumulation of fibrous tissue and lipids. The normal hepatic extracellular supporting framework of a number of different types of collagens, proteoglycans, and glycoproteins is altered to the extent that it compromises the normal flow of blood within the liver leading to portal hypertension and general cardiovascular compromise. A diet poor in proteins and B vitamins is believed to increase the progression of the disease. In addition to ethanol, chemicals such as carbon tetrachloride, aflatoxins, vinyl chloride, and arsenic have been linked to the disease.

## Tumors of the Liver

Malignant neoplasms have been linked to chemical exposures. Occupational exposures to chemicals such as vinyl chloride and arsenic, for example, have been linked to angiosarcomas. This tumor develops from the cells of the hepatic sinusoids, and although relatively rare in its occurrence, this blood vessel–derived neoplasm rapidly proliferates. Malignant neoplasms also commonly arise from hepatocytes (hepatocellular carcinoma) and from the bile ducts. Cirrhosis of the liver is believed to be one of the important predisposing factors in the development of hepatic cancers. Other examples of hepatic carcinogens include aflatoxin B, safrole, alkylnitrosamines, $CCl_4$, and acetylaminofluorene.

# The Kidneys

### General Considerations

The kidneys perform a number of vital functions in the overall homeostasis of the body (Figure 14.4):

- Regulation of the extracellular milieu
- Elimination of waste products (nitrogen as urea, phosphates, $NH_3$, sulfates, organic acids, and creatinine)
- Regulation of acid–base balance

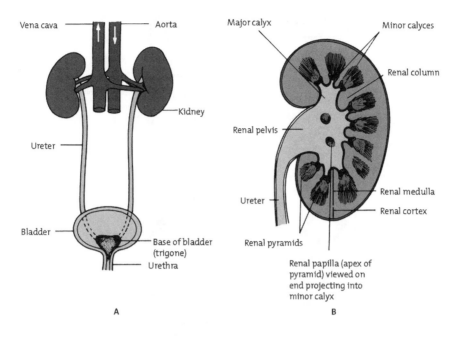

**FIGURE 14.4** The kidneys. *Source:* Courtesy of Leonard V. Crowley, M.D., Century College.

- Erythropoietin production for stimulation of synthesis of red blood cells
- Control of blood pressure and volume by formation of renin and its effect on vascular smooth muscle
- Xenobiotic metabolism (P450 and high glutathione levels)
- Production of glucose and 1,25-diOH vitamin $D_3$

Approximately 25% of the cardiac output is to the kidneys, with about 125 ml/min or 180 l/day of glomerular filtrate produced, most of which is reabsorbed by the tubules of the nephron, the functional units of the kidney (Figure 14.5). The nephron is a complex structure composed of vascular and epithelial tubular components that are specialized for filtration, secretion, and reabsorption. The nephron is divided into the following components:

- Glomerulus: A specialized arrangement of capillaries for high-pressure ultrafiltration into Bowman's capsule. The chemical size limitation for filtration is approximately 60 kDa.
- Bowman's capsule: Where the glomerular filtrate is collected before its modification as it moves along the renal tubules.
- Proximal convoluted tubule: Where approximately 60–80% of glomerular filtrate is reabsorbed (this includes water and $Na^+$, $K^+$, $HCO_3^-$, $Cl^-$, $PO_4^=$, $Ca^{2+}$, $Mg^{2+}$, glucose, amino acids, some small organic acids, peptides, proteins).
- Loop of Henle: Where adjustment of salt content and pH of urine occurs.
- Distal convoluted tubule: Where transport of $K^+$, $H^+$, and $NH_3$ into the lumen occurs.
- Collecting duct: Where reabsorption of water and NaCl occurs.

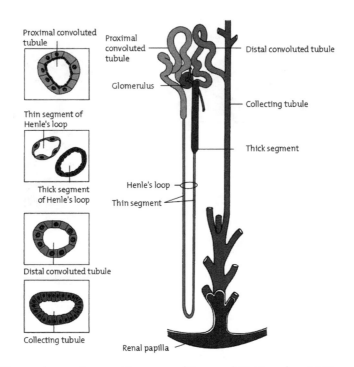

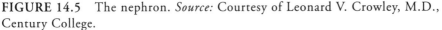

**FIGURE 14.5** The nephron. *Source:* Courtesy of Leonard V. Crowley, M.D., Century College.

## Nephrotoxicants

Many chemicals have been demonstrated to be toxic to the kidneys. Table 14.2 provides examples of several of these nephrotoxicants.

As a group, heavy metals such as chromium, cadmium, lead, and mercury are toxic to the proximal convoluted tubule of the nephron and can lead to acute renal failure. Heavy metals accumulate in the body, leading to the induction of metallothionein by the liver, an important metal binding "detoxification" protein present in most body tissues. Cadmium (Cd) stimulates the production of liver metallothionein, which serves to bind cadmium and thus protects most organs from its toxic effects. The kidney is especially vulnerable to the cadmium–metallothionein complex due to its concentration in the nephron tubules. Beta-2-microglobulin excretion from the kidney is diagnostic of cadmium toxicity. Cadmium's early effects are reversible and repairable. The metal produces damage to the proximal convoluted tubule and over time can result in chronic interstitial nephritis and tubular necrosis, which can result in renal failure. Mercury (Hg) and mercuric compounds such as phenyl mercury and methylmercury affect secretion into the renal tubules by inhibiting important enzyme systems by combining with enzyme –SH groups, thus inhibiting their function. Additionally, mercury and other heavy metals may alter normal $Ca^{2+}$ homeostasis.

Therapeutic agents can also be damaging to the kidney. Long-term use of analgesics (aspirin, ibuprofen, naproxen, and indomethacin), antibiotics, and certain anticancer drugs can result in

**Table 14.2**   Examples of Nephrotoxicants

| Substance | Type of Injury |
| --- | --- |
| Mercury | Proximal tubular necrosis and autoimmune glomerular damage |
| Cadmium | Proximal tubule dysfunction, chronic interstitial nephritis |
| Lead | Chronic tubulointerstitial nephropathy |
| Penicillamine | Glomerular injury |
| Methoxyflurane | Distal tubule injury |
| Tetrachloroethylene | Hyaline droplet nephropathy |
| 1,4-Dichlorobenzene | Hyaline droplet nephropathy |
| Ethylene glycol | Obstructive uropathy |
| Cephaloridine | Cell death |
| Nitric oxide | Cell death |
| Chloroform | Proximal tubule injury |
| Bromobenzene | Proximal tubular cell death |
| Carbon tetrachloride | Acute tubular necrosis |
| Ethylene dichloride | Acute tubular necrosis |

renal toxicity. In addition, polychlorinated biphenyls (PCBs), polybrominated biphenyls (PBBs), tetrachlordibenzodioxin (TCDD), the mycotoxins, ochratoxin A (which has been linked to Balkan nephropathy), and fumonesins from grains such as corn have been associated with renal toxicities.

## Bibliography

Amacher, D. E. (2002). A toxicologist's guide to biomarkers of hepatic response. *Human and Experimental Toxicology, 21,* 253–262.

Batt, A. M., & Ferrari, L. (1995). Manifestations of chemically induced liver damage. *Clinical Chemistry, 41*(12 Pt 2), 1882–1887.

Bock, K. W., Gerok, W., & Matern, S. (Eds) (1991). *Hepatic metabolism and disposition of endo- and xenobiotics.* Dordrecht, The Netherlands: Kluwer.

Crowley, L. V. (2001). *An introduction to human disease: pathology and pathophysiology correlations.* Sudbury, MA: Jones and Bartlett Publishers.

Ganey, P. E., Luyendyk, J. P., Maddox, J. F., & Roth, R. A. (2004). Adverse hepatic drug reactions: inflammatory episodes as consequence and contributor. *Chemico-Biological Interactions, 150,* 35–51.

Hard, G. C., & Khan, K. N. (2004). A contemporary overview of chronic progressive nephropathy in the laboratory rat, and its significance for human risk assessment. *Toxicologic Pathology, 32,* 171–180.

Hook, J. B., Lash, L. H., & Tarloff, J. B. (Eds.) (2005). *Toxicology of the kidney.* Boca Raton, FL: CRC Press.

Klaassen, C. D. (2001). *Casarett & Doull's toxicology. The basic science of poisons.* New York: McGraw-Hill.

Klaassen, C. D., & Watkins, J. B. (2003). *Casarett & Doull's essentials of toxicology.* New York: McGraw-Hill.

Lautt, W. W., & Macedo, M. P. (1997). Hepatic circulation and toxicology. *Drug Metabolism Reviews, 29,* 369–395.

McCuskey, R. S., & Earnest, D. L. (2000). *Comprehensive toxicology: hepatic and gastrointestinal toxicology.* New York: Elsevier Science.

Phillips, S. D., & Waksman, J. C. (2004). Hepatorenal solvent toxicology. *Clin Occup Environ Med, 4,* 731–740.

Plaa, G. L., Hewitt, W. R., & Strauss, S. (1998). *Toxicology of the liver.* Washington, DC: Taylor and Francis.

Prough, R. A., Linder, M. W., Pinaire, J. A., Xiao, G. H., & Falkner, K. C. (1996). Hormonal regulation of hepatic enzymes involved in foreign compound metabolism. *FASEB J, 10,* 1369–1377.

Robinson, P. J. (1992). Physiologically based liver modeling and risk assessment. *Risk Analysis, 12,* 139–148.

Stricker, B. H. (1992). *Drug-induced hepatic injury.* New York: Elsevier Health Sciences.

Ulrich, R. G., Bacon, J. A., Cramer, C. T., Peng, G. W., Petrella, D. K., Stryd, R. P., & Sun, E. L. (1995). Cultured hepatocytes as investigational models for hepatic toxicity: practical applications in drug discovery and development. *Toxicology Letters, 82–83,* 107–115.

U.S. National Library of Medicine, National Institutes of Health, Environmental Health, and Toxicology Specialized Information Services (SIS). (2005). *Toxicology tutorial III.* Retrieved October 2, 2005 from http://www.sis.nlm.nih.gov/enviro/toxtutor.html.

van de Water, B., de Graauw, M., Le Devedec, S., & Alderliesten, M. (2006). Cellular stress responses and molecular mechanisms of nephrotoxicity. *Toxicology Letters, 162,* 83–93.

Williams, G. M., & Iatropoulos, M. J. (2002). Alteration of liver cell function and proliferation: differentiation between adaptation and toxicity. *Toxicologic Pathology, 30,* 41–53.

# CHAPTER 15

# The Cardiovascular System

## General Considerations

The cardiovascular system can be viewed as a muscular pump (the heart) pushing fluid (blood) through a series of tubes (the vasculature, composed of arteries, veins, and capillaries) in an effort to keep tissues supplied with essential nutrients and gases and free of the waste products associated with cellular metabolism (Figure 15.1). Functioning together, the components of the cardiovascular system

- Maintain internal homeostasis
- Regulate body temperature
- Maintain tissue and cellular pH

## Cardiac Physiology

The heart is composed of four pumping chambers and four unidirectional valves. The right and left half of the heart can be considered clinically independent structures because there is no direct communication between the two halves. The right atrium and right ventricle power the pulmonary circulation, pushing blood from the systemic circulation through the pulmonary artery to the lungs for oxygenation. The left atrium and left ventricle receive oxygenated blood by way of the pulmonary veins and pump it into the aorta for systemic distribution.

Valves control the flow of blood into and out of the cardiac chambers. The atrioventricular (AV) valves are flap-like structures controlling blood flow from the atria into the ventricles. The mitral or bicuspid valve separates the left atrium and ventricle, and the tricuspid valve separates the right atrium and ventricle. The outer edges of the valves are connected to the ventricular walls by *chordae tendineae,* which serve to prevent prolapse during ventricular systole. The aortic and pulmonic semilunar valves define the margins between the aorta and pulmonary arteries respectively. The aortic valve opens into the left atrium, and the pulmonic valve into the right atrium. The semilunar and AV valves function sequentially so that the AV valves close as blood opens the semilunar valves. Conversely, closure of the semilunar valves during diastole causes the AV valves to open. This coordinated action is necessary for unidirectional blood flow.

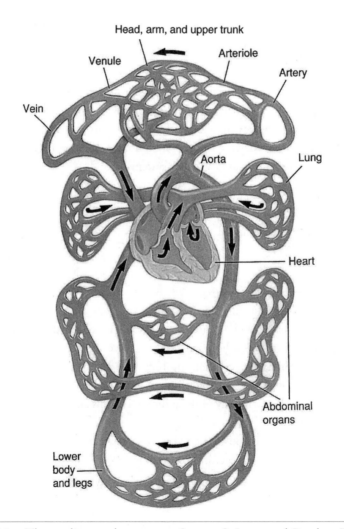

**FIGURE 15.1**    The cardiovascular system. *Source:* © Jones and Bartlett Publishers.

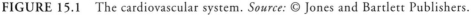

## Cell Types

The heart is composed of

- Cardiac fibroblasts
- Vascular cells
- Purkinje cells
- Connective tissue cells
- Cardiac myocytes

Cardiac myocytes are the primary contractile unit of cardiac tissue; as such they constitute the majority of the tissue mass. That fact, combined with the terminally differentiated nature of cardiac myocytes and the proliferative response of cardiac fibroblasts in the face of injury, highlights the vulnerability of the heart to toxicological insult.

## Cardiac Electrophysiology

### Action Potential

Recall that the cellular action potential is the change in electric potential that causes the membrane potential to go from a negative resting state to a positive state corresponding with the opening of ion channels in the membrane (Figure 15.2). The action potential is necessary for muscular contraction:

- Phase 0: $Na^+$ channels open and membrane rapidly depolarizes.
- Phase 1: $Na^+$ channels close and $K^+$ channels open.
- Phase 2: Plateau as $Na^+$ dissipates and $Ca^{2+}$ enters cell to balance charge.
- Phase 3: Repolarization as $Ca^{2+}$ channels close and $K^+$ leaves cell.
- Phase 4: Continued repolarization and redistribution of Na and K ions by the sodium–potassium pump.

### Signal Conduction

The sinoatrial (SA) node normally determines the heart rate. For this reason it is referred to as the *pacemaker*. Pacemaker cells spontaneously depolarize and pass the current onto adjacent cells. The

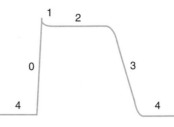

FIGURE 15.2    Phases of a typical cardiac action potential.

SA node is the fastest of sites of spontaneously depolarizing cells, followed by the AV node, the bundle of His, and Purkinje fibers. The latter three are referred to as *latent pacemakers*; they are responsible for setting the cardiac pace should the SA node be damaged by a toxicant or disease process. Excitation begins in the SA node and spreads as a propagating wave along the myocardial sarcolemma from cell to cell. Signal transmission proceeds through the heart as follows:

SA node → AV node → AV bundles (or bundle of His) → Purkinje fibers → cardiomyocytes

These pacemaker cells do not contract; they are responsible for stimulating cardiac myocytes. The depolarization of pacemaker cells differs from traditional cells in that the pacemaker cells lack a constant resting potential. They slowly depolarize to threshold due to "leaky" membranes, allowing the slow influx of $Na^+$ and $Ca^{2+}$ and efflux of $K^+$. Once the threshold is reached, a traditional action potential is triggered. Electrical cardiac activity is controlled by the autonomic nervous system (ANS). Sympathomimetics like norepinephrine can increase both heart rate and myocardial contractility. Parasympathomimetics decrease the rate of depolarization but have very little effect on contractility.

## Contraction of Cardiac Myocytes

Cardiac myocytes are composed of myofibrils. These contractile filaments can be further broken down into thick and thin myofilaments; the thick filaments consist primarily of myosin, whereas the thin filaments are mainly actin. The action potential is conducted to the interior of the cell via the T-tubule system. Calcium is released from the sarcoplasmic reticulum, allowing it to bind troponin in the C subunit of the troponin complex (Figure 15.3). Binding $Ca^{2+}$

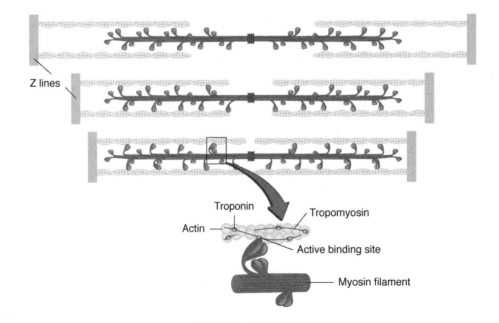

Z lines

Troponin

Actin

Tropomyosin

Active binding site

Myosin filament

**FIGURE 15.3**    Muscle contractile complex.

induces a conformational change in troponin C and tropomyosin, exposing the myosin binding site on actin. Hydrolysis of adenosine triphosphate (ATP) bound to each myosin molecule allows actin to bind myosin and initiate cross-bridge cycling. When $Ca^{2+}$ is present, the cross-bridges attach at 90 degrees. Anything affecting the availability of $Ca^{2+}$ has an impact on the force of the contractions. As the energy of ATP is released, the angle of attachment is decreased forcing the actin filaments to be pulled to the center of the sarcomere.

Detachment results when new ATP is bound to the myosin. Cardiac output has a high metabolic cost; contraction is associated with the hydrolysis of ATP. The ability of the heart to contract is strictly limited by the availability of oxygen.

## Assessing Cardiac Function

The electrocardiogram (ECG) is an important clinical methodology for assessing cardiac function. It takes advantage of propagation of electrical currents generated by depolarization and repolarization throughout the body and its fluids (Figure 15.4). Electrical activity is measured by strategically placed electrodes on the skin surface. Careful examination of the patterns generated can reveal abnormal cardiac activity and damage. The deflections recorded correspond to

- Atrial depolarization (P wave)
- Ventricular depolarization (QRS complex)

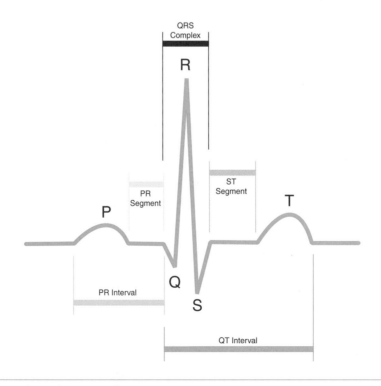

**FIGURE 15.4**    Schematic of ECG

- Ventricular repolarization (T wave)
- PR interval (conduction through the AV node)
- ST interval (ventricular repolarization)

Alterations in the magnitude or duration of the waves can be diagnostically revealing. For example, significant deviations in the ST interval may indicate ischemic damage.

Cardiac output is the primary measure of cardiac function and reflects the ability of the heart to keep up with the demands of the body. It is dependent on volume (ventricular efficiency) and heart rate. Normal cardiac output is approximately 5 L/min for an adult at rest and can be assessed by echocardiography. The Fick principle states that the volume of oxygen taken up by the blood in the lungs, divided by the arteriovenous oxygen content difference, is equal to the cardiac output. Cardiac output is vulnerable to factors that regulate

- Heart rate
- Contractility
- Preload
- Afterload
- Left ventricular size

Toxicants that exert a deleterious effect on cardiac output can have a significant impact on most of the body's systems.

## Effects of Toxicants on the Cardiovascular System

Tissues in the heart and the vasculature are susceptible to toxicant injury (Figure 15.5). Toxicant exposure can alter functionality, inflict structural damage, or cause indirect injury.

A vast array of substances, organisms, and disease states can contribute to cardiomyopathy. There are two basic categories, dilated cardiomyopathy and hypertrophic cardiomyopathy. The former is the result of progressive cardiac hypertrophy that negatively impacts contractility or systolic function. Alcoholic cardiomyopathy caused by chronic alcohol consumption is a form of dilated cardiomyopathy. Hypertrophic cardiomyopathy is characterized by diastolic dysfunction, and most cases are due to inherited diseases.

There are several different injury mechanisms associated with cardiac toxicants:

- Generation of free radicals
- Lipid peroxidation
- Impaired membrane integrity
- Mitochondrial dysfunction
- Sarcoplasmic reticulum dysfunction
- Altered calcium homeostasis

Oxidative stress exerts a wide range of adverse effects through an equally impressive number of mechanisms. Reactive oxygen species can be generated during ischemic events and subsequent reperfusion and are associated with arrhythmias, myocyte injury or death. Reactive oxygen

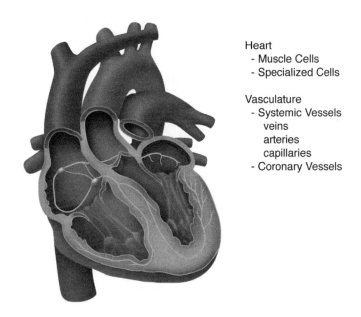

Heart
  - Muscle Cells
  - Specialized Cells

Vasculature
  - Systemic Vessels
      veins
      arteries
      capillaries
  - Coronary Vessels

**FIGURE 15.5**    Susceptible tissues in the cardiovascular system.

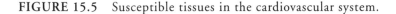

species disturb $Ca^{2+}$ homeostasis, which can impact its uptake, transfer, and exchange. The activities of essential enzymes (ATPases, phospholipase D, and cytochrome oxidase) can be altered by oxidative stress. Exposure to xenobiotics capable of inducing oxidative stress can cause cardiotoxicity. Both ethanol and doxorubicin are considered cardiotoxic because of their ability to generate reactive oxygen species.

Cells derive their energy from the oxidative phosphorylation of ATP during cellular respiration. Cellular respiration occurs in the mitochondria via the electron transport chain. Because cardiac tissues require large amounts of energy to function normally, cardiac myocytes have large numbers of mitochondria. Toxicants like 2,4-dinitrophenol are capable of uncoupling electron transfer from oxidative phosphorylation, which negatively impacts ATP synthesis. Toxicant action can disrupt oxidative phosphorylation at various sites along the mitochondrial membrane.

The sarcoplasmic reticulum in cardiac myocytes is specially adapted to surround the myofibrils and create the T-tubules. The sarcoplasmic reticulum provides the majority of $Ca^{2+}$ required for contraction. Sarcoplasmic reticular function and sarcolemmal membrane integrity are necessary to maintain the large $Ca^{2+}$ concentration gradient. Should either fail, the influx of $Ca^{2+}$ may be enough to trigger apoptosis via signaling pathway activation. Oncocytic cell death may also result. Excessive intracellular $Ca^{2+}$ has been linked to membrane blebbing, DNA fragmentation, and protease activation. $Ca^{2+}$ homeostasis in the cardiac tissues can be adversely impacted by chemicals such as immunosuppressants, ryanodine, and caffeine.

Xenobiotics can affect the intracellular concentration of $Ca^{2+}$ through the inhibition or excitation of $Ca^{2+}$ channels in the cell membranes. The main $Ca^{2+}$ channel in the cells of the human heart is the L-type voltage-gated $Ca^{2+}$ channel. This channel contributes to excitation-contraction coupling; in contrast, the T-type $Ca^{2+}$ channels are associated with the pacemaker potential in the SA node. Blockade of the cardiac $Ca^{2+}$ channels exerts a negative inotropic effect. This is the pharmacological basis of drugs like verapamil and diltiazem, both used to treat tachycardia.

Cardiovascular toxicants can be placed into the basic categories of pharmaceuticals, industrial chemicals, and natural products (Table 15.1). Pharmaceuticals with cardiotoxicant action include antineoplastics, anesthetics, psychotropics, and antibiotics. Some pharmaceutical cardiotoxic effects are seen only when the dose exceeds the therapeutic range. For example, digitalis is used to control ventricular response to fibrillation. It can also induce arrhythmias. Other pharmaceuticals can be cardiotoxic for reasons completely unrelated to their therapeutic use. Antineoplastic drugs are used in chemotherapy for the treatment of malignant tumors. They include anthracyclines such as doxorubicin and daunorubicin. The clinical utility of these drugs is limited by their tendency to induce arrhythmias, left ventricular failure, and cardiomyopathy (long-term usage). Although the mechanisms have not been completely elucidated, it is hypothesized that the toxicity is the result of oxidative stress, defects in mitochondrial integrity, disrupted $Ca^{2+}$ homeostasis, or altered gene expression leading to apoptosis. Centrally acting drugs,

**Table 15.1**    Examples of Cardiotoxicants and the Associated Injuries

| Substance | Type of Injury |
|---|---|
| Ethanol | Cardiomyopathy |
| Isopropyl alcohol | Tachycardia |
| Methanol | Heart rate reduced |
| Amitriptyline | Arrhythmia |
| Toluene | Arrhythmia |
| Chloroform | Decrease cardiac output |
| Doxorubicin | Tachycardia, arrhythmia |
| Methyl chloride | Negative inotropic effect |
| Cobalt | Cardiac hypertrophy |
| Cocaine | Arrhythmias, myocardial infarction, ischemia, congestive heart failure |
| Anabolic steroids | Left ventricular hypertrophy, myocardial infarction, cardiomyopathy |
| Vinyl chloride | Portal hypertension, tumors of hepatic blood vessels |
| Digitalis | Arrhythmia |
| Cobra venom | Ischemia, disturbed ion balance |
| Catecholamines | Tachycardia, cardiac myocyte death |
| Carbon disulfide | Atheroma formation, direct injury to endothelial cells |
| Carbamylhydrazine | Tumors of pulmonary blood vessels |
| Boron | Hemorrhage, edema |
| Paraquat | Vascular damage in the lungs and brain |
| Tetrodotoxin | Blockade of sodium current of myocardial action potential |
| Heavy metals | Alterations in cardiac electromechanical activity |

including tricyclic antidepressants and antipsychotics, can present significant cardiotoxic perils such as ECG abnormalities and sudden cardiac death.

Heavy metals, solvents, and alcohols are some of the industrial chemicals capable of cardiotoxic action. Many industrial solvents rapidly disperse into cells and adversely affect cell membrane properties and signal transduction mechanisms. Halogenated alkanes and many heavy metals exert negative inotropic and chronotropic effects. Heavy metals may also induce myocardial hypertrophy.

Certain natural products, such as certain venoms, cocaine, and mushroom toxins, can produce cardiovascular toxicities. The cardiotoxic effects of drugs like cocaine, alcohol, and anabolic steroids have been fairly well characterized. Cocaine use is associated with cardiac arrhythmias, myocardial ischemia, hypertension, and congestive heart failure. It is used occasionally as a local anesthetic; it produces the numbing effect by inhibiting sodium channels on contact. Cocaine use decreases the rate of action potential depolarization, slows conduction speed, increases the effective refractory period, and inhibits the reuptake of norepinephrine. When cocaine and alcohol are used concurrently, a unique metabolite known as cocaethylene is formed in the liver. Cocaethylene has a significantly lower $LD_{50}$ than cocaine and reaches peak plasma concentrations just as the concentration of cocaine wanes. Adverse cardiovascular effects can be seen with anabolic steroid usage. Steroids can alter plasma lipids, decreasing high density lipoprotein (HDL) and increasing LDL. Consequently, the LDL/HDL ratio rises. Left ventricular hypertrophy, myocardial infarction, and cardiomyopathy have all been associated with anabolic steroids.

## Blood Vessels

The vascular system is a complex array of vessels that carry oxygen and nutrients to tissues while simultaneously ridding them of metabolic wastes. Oxygenated blood leaves the aorta and travels through arteries, arterioles, and continuous capillaries to reach the tissues. Poorly oxygenated blood leaves the tissues via fenestrated capillaries, venules, and veins to be oxygenated anew. Continuous and fenestrated capillaries meet to form a postcapillary or pericytic venule for extravasation in the capillary bed. Water and other exuded plasma components form the interstitial fluid. Interstitial fluid returns to the general circulation through the lymphatic system. Absorbed toxicants encounter the cells of the vascular system irrespective of the initial exposure route. This means the vascular system has an increased risk of toxic insult. Vascular endothelial cells are central in hemostasis, angiogenesis, and the maintenance of vascular tone.

There are similarities in the structure of all blood vessels despite their differences in size and function. Vessel walls are divided into three layers, or tunics. The *tunica intima* is the endothelial lining and associated connective tissue that lines the interior of the vessel. An *internal elastic lamina* separates the *tunica intima* from the middle layer, or *tunica media*. It is composed of smooth muscle and connective tissue cells. Another layer of elastic fibers, the *external elastic lamina,* separates the *tunica media* from the *tunica adventitia*. The *tunica adventitia* consists of a layer of fibroblasts, collagen, elastin, and glycosaminoglycans. In smaller vessels the middle layer is less elastic and contains fewer smooth muscle cells. Arterial vessels tend to be more elastic than their venous counterparts.

Atherosclerosis describes the structural change that occurs in vessel wall after injury or exposure to chemicals like carbon disulfide. After the formation of the initial lesion, extracellular components such as collagen, complex carbohydrates, intra- and extracellular lipids, inflammatory cells, and other blood products adhere to the expanding lesion. The progressively narrowing vessel restricts blood flow to distal tissues. The process may take place over the course of decades, and renal hypertension, stroke, and myocardial infarction are all possible outcomes. Acrolein, heavy metals, carbon disulfide, and homocysteine are all endothelial toxicants capable of injuring the vessel walls and triggering the formation of an atheroma. Diets with excessive cholesterol intake cause an increase in plasma lipoproteins, which has been associated with an enhanced risk of atherosclerosis. There are some indications that the smooth muscle cells in an atheroma may all be the progeny of a single cell, leading some to suggest similarities between the atherosclerotic and neoplastic growth processes.

Changes in blood pressure, especially those occurring over prolonged periods of time, can produce lasting damage to the vasculature. Hypotension can result from heavy metal exposure and central nervous system depressant poisonings. This can lead to circulatory insufficiency that may progress to shock when accompanied by extreme loss of blood or body fluids. Hypertension can be the product of hormonal influence (angiotensin II is a powerful vasoconstrictor) or heavy metal toxicity, a symptom secondary to a disease process, or the result of drug overdose. Sustained hypertension is associated with capillary destruction and is the most important risk factor in the predisposition of coronary and cerebral atherosclerosis. Some substances like the antineoplastic cyclophosphamide are cytotoxic enough to cause hemorrhages in large vessels. Aneurysms can develop if the structural integrity of the vessel wall is compromised. Penicillamine reduces cross-linking of collagen and elastin, and this can lead to decreased tensile strength in vasculature walls. Toxicants can be thrombolytic through several different mechanisms. Fibrinolysis may be inhibited, as with Hg exposure. Oral contraceptives have been linked to thrombosis by disrupting antithrombin III. A portion of the thrombus may detach and travel through the vasculature until it becomes lodged in a vessel of smaller diameter than its own.

Endothelial cells are the first line of defense for the vascular system against toxicants in the blood. Toxicants that disturb ionic regulation impact the vascular reactivity. Nontoxic chemicals may be bioactivated by enzyme systems present in vascular cells. Other tissues can produce angiotoxic chemicals that leave the metabolizing site for the target site. The reactive intermediate may be capable of damaging intracellular and extracellular targets. The oxidation of LDLs is critical to the development of atherosclerosis. The oxidative process produces activated oxygen species capable of directly injuring endothelial tissue. Aromatic hydrocarbons and other common environmental contaminants can be incorporated into the lipid phase of atherosclerotic plaques. The damage caused by such an incorporated toxicant is modulated by cellular, noncellular, and mechanical factors.

Nicotine stimulates sympathetic ganglia with a concomitant increase in heart rate and blood pressure. The cardiovascular effects of cocaine were detailed in earlier sections; hypertension and cerebral strokes are vascular effects that may be seen. Bacterial endotoxicants are an example of natural vasculotoxicants. They can cause vascular damage in hepatic tissues, compromise membrane integrity in pulmonary vasculature, and induce changes in coronary vessels that can result in necrosis. Industrial agents include aromatic hydrocarbons and nitroaromatics. Benzo[a]pyrene and its metabolites have several ways of altering smooth muscle proliferation. They include the formation of DNA adducts, enhanced transcription of growth related genes, and the inactivation of protein kinase C. Dinitrotoluene and carbon disulfide have atherogenic properties.

## Blood

With its ubiquitous distribution and array of proliferative cells, the hematopoietic system is a unique target organ. Erythrocytes, granulocytes, and platelets are produced at a rate approaching 1 to 3 million per second in a healthy adult. Direct and indirect damage to the hematopoietic system may produce hypoxia, hemorrhage, infection, and death (Table 15.2).

Hematotoxicity may be considered primary when blood components are directly damaged. Secondary hematotoxicity occurs when local and systemic effects of a toxicant affect blood cells.

The hematopoietic system generates formed elements of blood; it includes the spleen, liver, and bone marrow. Blood cells include erythrocytes, lymphocytes, monocytes, and granulocytes. The spleen is an active hematopoietic site during fetal development, the liver generates red blood cells during infancy, but the bone marrow is the only blood cell–producing organ at birth. All marrow is involved in hematopoiesis at birth, but the production steadily retreats to the long bones during early childhood. By adulthood, the only active marrow is in the axial skeleton. The marrow of the distal long bones becomes "fatty" but can be reactivated if necessary.

Erythrocytes make up approximately 40% of the blood volume in circulation. They serve as the main vehicle for oxygen transport from the lungs to the tissues. Erythropoietin is produced in the kidneys and stimulates bone marrow stem cells to form proerythroblasts. The proerythroblasts are nucleated cells; nascent erythrocytes shed their nucleus before entering the circulation. Erythrocytes have a life span of 120 days. Expired erythrocytes are removed and catabolized by

**Table 15.2    Examples of Toxicant-Induced Effects on the Blood**

| Chemical | Effect |
| --- | --- |
| Ethanol | Sideroblastic anemia |
| Benzene | Aplastic anemia, leukemia |
| Vinyl chloride | Acquired porphyria |
| Nitrates | Methemoglobinemia |
| Antimony | Neutropenia |
| Arsine | Thrombocytopenia |
| Dichlorodiphenyltrichloroethane | Thrombocytopenia |
| Methylene chloride | Hemolytic anemia |
| Carbon monoxide | Reduced oxygen-carrying capacity of the blood |
| Warfarin | Alterations in blood-clotting mechanism |
| Alkylating agents | Agranulocytopenia |

the spleen. Heme is broken down and excreted in bile. Xenobiotics can interfere with the production, function, and survival of erythrocytes. Agents that decrease the number of erythrocytes in circulation may do so by decreasing their production, increasing their destruction, or interfering with hemoglobin or oxygen-transport function. Carbon monoxide, for example, reduces greatly the oxygen-carrying capacity of hemoglobin with the result that all systems of the body are affected, especially those with the greatest oxygen demands. A hematotoxicant that increases the rate of erythrocyte destruction usually increases the number of reticulocytes in circulation as the body speeds production to compensate for the loss rate.

Erythrocyte production is a continuous process that may be interrupted at several points. The resultant symptoms can pinpoint the trouble. Heme synthesis requires dietary iron; a deficient amount of iron can increase the risk of developing *microcytic anemia.* Defects in the synthesis of heme can occur in several ways. Lead can block the insertion of iron into heme; this leads to an accumulation of protoporphyrin IX in the blood. This is one of the factors behind the central nervous system effects of lead exposure. A defect in the synthesis of heme's porphyrin ring can lead to sideroblastic anemia. Because folate and vitamin $B_{12}$ are required for thymidine synthesis, which is in turn vital to the active DNA synthesis central in marrow proliferation, deficiencies in folate and vitamin $B_{12}$ can induce megaloblastic anemia. Aplastic anemia, characterized by a failure of bone marrow proliferation, can result from exposure to benzene, gold, bismuth, and other chemicals. Aplastic anemia is a life-threatening disorder characterized by bone marrow hypoplasia, reticulocytopenia, and peripheral blood pancytopenia. The mechanism has not been elucidated.

White blood cells and all their precursors include granulocytes, monocytes, lymphocytes, and leukocytes. Granulocytes can be further classified as neutrophils, eosinophils, and basophils; they are named for their characteristic cytoplasmic granules. Granulocytes and monocytes are both phagocytic cells. Lymphocytes are considered immunocytes. White blood cells are synthesized in the bone marrow, and they use the circulatory system to travel to their specified active site. Leukocytes exist to protect the body from foreign materials and organisms.

The granulated leukocytes are important in the mediation of inflammation and phagocytosis of pathogenic microorganisms. Neutrophils, eosinophils, and basophils are associated with inflammation and allergic disorders. Neutrophils and their progenitors have a high proliferation rate. Agranulocytopenia is the most common indicator of chemically induced bone marrow damage due to radiation, alkylating agents, antimetabolites, nonsteroidal antiinflammatory drugs (NSAIDs), and benzene exposures. Granulocytosis is the leukemia caused by benzene exposure.

Monocytes mature to macrophages and reside in the tissues for months. They have an active nitric oxide (NO) synthase that generates NO. When combined with a reactive oxygen species, NO forms peroxynitrite for bactericide.

Lymphocytes mediate the specific immune response. T cells, formed in the thymus, are involved in cell-mediated killing. B cells, formed in the bursa and found in the lymph glands, secrete humoral antibodies and immunoglobulins. The activity of lymphocytes declines with age. It can also be suppressed by corticosteroids. Lymphocytopenia can be caused by chemotherapy and acquired immune deficiency syndrome (AIDS). Acute lymphocytic leukemia (ALL), also referred to as acute lymphoblastic leukemia, is cancer of the white blood cells. It is characterized by a continuous overproduction of malignant and immature white blood cells called lymphoblasts. Left untreated, ALL is fatal. It is also the most common childhood cancer.

Thrombocytes, or platelets, are formed in the bone marrow. Platelets are formed when the cytoplasm of megakaryocytes fragments. They prevent hemorrhage by adhering to exposed collagen fibers on the damaged wall and degranulating. This releases adenosine diphosphate (ADP) and promotes their aggregation. Platelets adhere to one another by adhesion receptors or integrins. The loss of the cell membrane helps form a sticky plug. Blood clotting factor lays down the fibrin network. Fibroblasts complete the process with the formation of a scar.

Thrombocytopenia may develop from decreased production or increased destruction of thrombocytes. It is a common side effect of chemotherapy because of the antiproliferative nature of the drugs used. Antiinflammatory drugs may irreversibly acetylate cyclooxygenases in platelets. This suppresses the formation of thromboxane $A_2$ and blocks platelet aggregation. Platelets cannot synthesize more enzymes to compensate for the loss. Nitric oxide vasodilator drugs like glycerol trinitrate and hydroxylamine trigger the release of NO. This activates guanylate cyclase, stimulating cyclic guanosine monophosphate (cGMP) formation and smooth muscle relaxation.

The disruption of the coagulative process can take place before or after the clot has begun to form. There is a fairly narrow window for the therapeutic use of anticoagulants such as warfarin. Administration must account for a large degree of interindividual variation of response. Too little warfarin can increase the likelihood of thromboembolus formation, and excessive warfarin can lead to hemorrhage. Fibrinolytic agents accomplish the dissolution of a thrombus by converting the inactive zymogen plasminogen to the active proteolytic enzyme plasmin. Use of fibrinolytic agents can generate free plasmin, which can elevate the risk of bleeding. Fibrinolysis can also be inhibited when there is a need to control bleeding. Sufferers of von Willebrand disease have a congenital hemostatic abnormality that leaves them vulnerable to hemorrhage. Fibrinolytic inhibitors like tranexamic acid prevent the binding of plasminogen and plasmin to fibrin.

## Bibliography

Abel, E. D., & Wilkins, M. R. (2004). *Cardiovascular pharmacogenetics*. New York: Taylor & Francis.

Acosta, D. (2001). *Cardiovascular toxicology*. Target Organ Toxicology Series. New York: Taylor & Francis.

Amacher, D. E. (2005). Drug-associated mitochondrial toxicity and its detection. *Current Medicinal Chemistry, 12,* 1829–1839.

American Heart Association. Retrieved December 2005 from http://www.americanheart.org.

Chung, M. K., & Rich, M. W. (1990). Introduction to the cardiovascular system. *Alcohol Health and Research World, 14,* 269–276.

Crowley, L. V. (2001). *An introduction to human disease: pathology and pathophysiology correlations* (5th ed.). Sudbury, MA: Jones and Bartlett Publishers.

Holstege, C. P., & Dobmeier, S. (2005). Cardiovascular challenges in toxicology. *Emergency Medicine Clinics of North America, 23,* 1195–1217.

Jokinen, M. P., Lieuallen, W. G., Johnson, C. L., Dunnick, J., & Nyska, A. (2005). Characterization of spontaneous and chemically induced cardiac lesions in rodent model systems: the national toxicology program experience. *Cardiovascular Toxicology, 5,* 227–244.

Kang, Y. J. (2001). Molecular and cellular mechanisms of cardiotoxicity. *Environmental Health Perspectives, 109*(suppl 1), 27–34.

Klaassen, C. D., & Watkins, J. B. (Eds.) (2003). *Casarett & Doull's essentials of toxicology.* New York: McGraw-Hill.

U.S. National Library of Medicine, National Institutes of Health, Environmental Health, and Toxicology Specialized Information Services (SIS). (2005). *Toxicology tutorial III.* Retrieved December 2005 from http://www.sis.nlm.nih.gov/enviro/toxtutor.html.

Wang, R. (2001). *Carbon monoxide and cardiovascular functions* (1st ed.). Boca Raton, FL: CRC Press.

# CHAPTER 16

# The Respiratory System

## General Considerations

Public health agencies face a number of formidable challenges regarding concerns about diseases and their association with air toxics from the public. The Centers for Disease Control and Prevention (CDC) is working with state and local health departments to establish asthma surveillance activities, for example, that can better clarify previously unrecognized risk factors, including hazardous air pollutants.

The respiratory system, when viewed from a toxicological perspective, is important in that it

- Provides an early warning detection system via olfaction for many airborne toxicants
- Provides an exposure pathway for systemic exposures to many toxicants
- Is a direct target of toxicity from exposures to many airborne chemicals and from some that have been orally consumed
- Is an important organ system for many xenobiotic biotransformations

The respiratory system is subjected to frequent assault by airborne environmental contaminants. The average adult inhales approximately 12 kg of air daily, although this value may increase dramatically with physical activity or exertion. Compared with average daily food (1.5 kg) or water (2 kg) intake, it is obvious that inhaled air is a major source of potential exposures to environmental toxicants. At times, the concentration of airborne chemical contaminants increases to levels immediately dangerous to life and health. Incidents like the accidental release of 40 tons of methyl isocyanate in Bhopal, India in 1984 and the short-term inversion of smoke and sulfur dioxide in London, England in 1952 resulted in thousands of deaths, principally among the sick and elderly. These episodes illustrate the danger that concentrated air pollution may pose. They also offer additional insight into the potential hazards posed by lower concentration chronic exposures and their role in the pathogenesis and exacerbation of respiratory disorders like chronic bronchitis and bronchial asthma. Contaminants do not need to be industrial; those of biological origin can also aggravate existing disease states. Handling and milling grain releases atmospheric dusts that may provoke asthmatic attacks in susceptible individuals.

*Karenia brevis* is a dinoflagellate found in the Gulf of Mexico and the Caribbean, although similar species occur throughout the world. Red tide blooms are associated with massive fish and bird kills. *K. brevis* produces several types of lipid-soluble polyether toxins that are neurotoxic and can be collectively referred to as brevetoxins, including PbTx-2 and PbTx-1. The *K. brevis* organism is fragile, and wave action along beaches results in the organism breaking up and releasing the toxins. During an active red tide outbreak, the aerosol containing the toxins can be carried inland, producing respiratory symptoms in nonasthmatic individuals and bronchoconstriction in asthmatics. The respiratory problems associated with the inhalation of aerosolized toxins are due in part to the opening of sodium channels and the release of neurotransmitters from autonomic nerve endings, particularly acetylcholine, leading to airway smooth muscle depolarizations and contractions.

The respiratory system is responsible for much more than the maintenance of life through gas exchange. It performs many nonrespiratory functions like immune system maintenance, metabolism of endogenous substances like angiotensin, and the metabolism of environmental pollutants. The respiratory system plays an important role in the recognition, metabolism, detoxification, and elimination of xenobiotics. The surface epithelium of the respiratory system is an interface exposed to external contaminants via inhaled breath. Inhaled air contains a variety of nonessential gases, vapors, aerosols, and particulates that may all possess the capacity to induce local injury or systemic injury. The respiratory system can provide a route for systemic toxicants in addition to those that target the system directly. As an example, nitrogen dioxide can cause pulmonary fibrosis upon inhalation without producing systemic toxicity, whereas a volatile organic compound is likely to be absorbed systemically where it can affect the central nervous system.

The respiratory system may also be a target for toxicity from other exposure pathways, such as the ingestion of the pesticide paraquat. The respiratory system is unique in that all xenobiotics present in cardiac output pass through pulmonary circulation before entering systemic circulation. This explains why toxicants can be so rapidly distributed to other organs. One needs only to consider the rapidity of central nervous depression from respiratory exposure to a volatile organic toxicant or clinically to an inhalation anesthetic. The respiratory system is also the principal exposure route for neurotoxicants, carcinogens, and other systemic toxicants (Table 16.1).

**Table 16.1**   Systemic Toxicities Through Respiratory Exposure

| Classification | Examples |
|---|---|
| Irritants | $NH_3$, $NO_2$, $SO_2$, $O_3$, phosgene, halogens, aldehydes |
| Asphyxiants | CO, CN, $N_2$, $H_2$, $CH_4$, $H_2S$, He |
| Central nervous system toxicants | Aliphatic and aromatic hydrocarbons, chlorinated hydrocarbons, acetone, ethyl ether, benzene, $CS_2$, Hg, acrylamide, n-hexane, methyl n-butyl ketone |
| Hepatotoxicants | $CCl_4$, $CCl_3$, ethanol, allyl alcohol, bromobenzene |
| Nephrotoxicants | Heavy metals, $CCl_4$, chloroform, trichloroethylene |
| Hematotoxicants | CO, nitrobenzene, arsine, naphthalene |
| Carcinogens | Polycyclic aromatic hydrocarbons, vinyl chloride, 2-naphthylamine, bis(chloromethyl)ether |

## Nomenclature of Airborne Toxicants

- **Gases:** Of high water solubility where they readily dissolve in the nasal passages, upper airways (e.g., sulfur dioxide); limited water solubility where movement into the deeper airways and alveolar region occurs (e.g., $O_2$, $CO_2$, $O_3$, $NO_2$)
- **Vapor:** Normally a liquid or solid at STP, but due to their high vapor pressure they volatize (e.g., alcohols, ethers, gasoline)
- **Aerosols:** Relatively stable suspensions of solids and/or liquid particles or droplets in the air
- **Dusts:** Small particles of primary material, produced by abrasive processes such as sanding, grinding, or milling (e.g., metals, silica, grains)
- **Fumes:** Produced by combustion, sublimation, or condensation of vaporized material; size tends to be generally <0.3 μm (e.g., zinc vapors and metal fume fever)
- **Smoke:** Particles produced by combustion of organic matter
- **Mists and fogs:** Condensation of moisture on particulate nuclei in air or by the uptake of liquid by hydroscopic particles (e.g., the condensation of $SO_2$ [a water-soluble gas] onto particles of ash that penetrate deeply into the lung)
- **Smog:** Mixture of smoke, particles, and gases (fog) produced by automotive exhaust and other combustion processes and formed by action of sunlight on oxides of nitrogen and volatile organics

## Functional Divisions of the Respiratory System

There are three functional divisions of the respiratory system:

- Nasopharyngeal
- Tracheobronchial
- Pulmonary (alveolar or gas exchange surfaces)

Particulate matter settles in these regions by inertial impaction (nasopharyngeal), sedimentation (trachea to bronchioles), and diffusion (alveoli).

The nasopharyngeal region extends from the nose to the pharynx and is characterized by a well-vascularized mucosa that warms and humidifies the inspired air before it enters into the tracheobronchial region (Figure 16.1).

The nose provides a number of important functions, including the sense of olfaction or smell. Many airborne toxicants can be detected by olfaction, and many potentially injurious toxicants have odor thresholds at levels below which any injury might occur. This is a very important protective mechanism to alert us that the air contains a chemical(s) that normally might not be present in our breathing zone. Olfactory receptors are found in the roof of the nasal cavity along with sustentacular and basal cells; olfactory receptors are modified bipolar neurons whose proximal end contains olfactory cilia thought to be involved in chemoreception and transduction. The nasal mucosa also contains a rich source of xenobiotic metabolizing enzymes; thus it is capable of biotransformation reactions for many airborne toxicants, including those biotransformation reactions that result in bioactivation of precarcinogens.

The tracheobronchial region of the respiratory system is essentially involved in the conduction of air between the nasopharynx and the gas exchange surfaces (alveoli) of the lungs. This portion of the respiratory system contains the trachea, right and left main stem bronchi, and approximately 25 generations of airways whose diameters progressively decrease (as well as air velocity) as the overall surface area increases due to the extent of the branching as we progress distally toward the gas exchange surfaces. Conducting airways contain airway smooth muscle that is regulated by

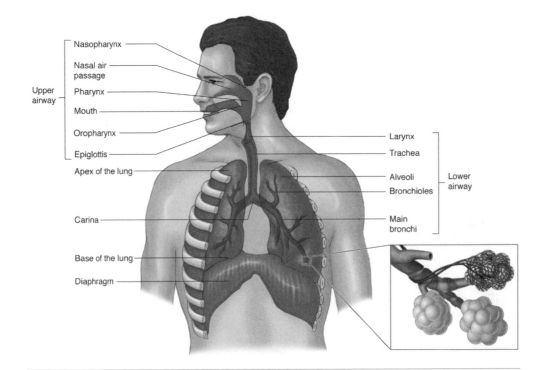

**FIGURE 16.1**    Regions of the respiratory system.

neural and cellular mediators; cholinergic innervation of the airway stimulates contractions of the smooth muscle, and adrenergic stimulation has the opposite effect. The bronchial tubes are complex structures made up of a number of cell types that not only regulate the diameter of the bronchial tube, through contractions of the circularly arranged airway smooth muscle, but are also capable of biotransformation reactions as well. The bronchial mucosa is essentially an environmental interface between the air that we breathe and any chemicals contained therein that may be capable of producing local and/or systemic injury. These airways have mucus-producing ciliated cells and submucosal glands, which form an important clearance mechanism (the mucociliary escalator) that moves the mucus along with trapped particulates at a rate of approximately 3 mm/min from the deep airways toward the pharynx, where it can be swallowed or expectorated.

Clara cells are nonciliated cells found in the epithelial layer of the distal airways. They are primarily found in the central and proximal portion of the transition zone between the conducting airways and the gas exchange region. Clara cells are cuboidal to columnar with long apical microvilli, extensive agranular endoplasmic reticulum, and numerous mitochondria and have high cytochrome P450 activity; thus they are likely to play an important role in xenobiotic metabolism in the airways.

The pulmonary region of the respiratory system is the site of gas exchange; it includes bronchioles, alveolar ducts and sacs, alveoli, and tissues such as capillaries and lymphatics. The basic unit of the pulmonary region is the acinus; there are approximately 200,000 in the human lung. Type I pneumocytes comprise approximately 90% of the surface area of alveoli. These cells are squamous (flattened) and nonciliated to allow for efficient exchange of physiologically important gases (e.g., oxygen, carbon dioxide), nonpolar gases (such as nitric oxide and ozone), volatile organics (generally very lipophilic), and small particulates (<2 μm). Type II pneumocytes secrete surfactant into the alveoli, thus maximizing their surface area. In addition, the pulmonary region contains alveolar macrophages, which are important in the clearance of particulates (e.g., bacteria, silica, asbestos), and interstitial cells, such as fibroblasts and monocytes.

## Respiratory System Injury

Although there may be numerous potentially injurious chemicals in the air, the responses of the respiratory system generally fall into one or more of the following categories:

- Irritative or inflammatory
- Bronchoconstrictive
- Fibrotic
- Oncogenetic
- Necrotic

The type and extent of injury depend on the concentration of the pollutant, dose, duration of exposure, and the physiochemical properties of the chemical. Any part of the respiratory tract might be the target of toxicity. The inhalation of chlorine and ammonia gas, for example, produces airway irritation and bronchoconstriction with a concomitant inability to inhale deeply or rapidly enough to satisfy airway demands. The dyspnea stems from the water solubility of both gases and their removal in the airways. Injury can extend to the gas exchange surfaces in cases of severe exposures.

## Exposures to Air Pollutants

Epidemiological studies have clearly demonstrated a link between air pollutants such as ozone, particulate matter, $SO_2$, and others with acute responses such as the exacerbation of asthma in the general population (Table 16.2). Exposure to ozone (one of the criteria pollutants) is known to induce increases in airway inflammation in nonasthmatics. Low ozone concentrations, even brief exposures, are thought capable of triggering a low grade inflammatory response. In asthmatics the effect of ozone is exaggerated, producing bronchoconstriction, increased neutrophilic inflammation, and increased sensitivity to allergens. Ozone is found naturally in the upper atmosphere and closer to the ground as a component of air pollution. Concentrations typically spike in the summer when oxides of nitrogen and hydrocarbons react to form ozone. There are concurrent increases of other pollutants such as sulfuric and nitric acids that may potentiate the irritant effects of ozone on the respiratory system. It has been demonstrated that ozone is a potent pulmonary irritant, even in healthy individuals. Short-term exposure to low level concentrations can produce symptoms that include chest tightness, increased airway resistance, increased mucociliary transport, and increased respiratory epithelial cell permeability. Ozone is less soluble than many other irritant gases and penetrates into the pulmonary regions more effectively.

Like ozone, nitrogen oxides effectively penetrate deep into the respiratory system. Exposure to nitrogen oxides triggers pathological changes in distal and alveolar regions of the respiratory system; these changes are characterized by proliferation of Clara and Type II cells. Acute exposures to both ozone and nitrogen oxides can result in pulmonary edema, and chronic exposures may be linked to emphysema.

Sulfur dioxide, another major environmental pollutant, is produced by the combustion of sulfur-containing fossil fuels like coal, oil, and kerosene. It is primarily an upper airway irritant due to its high water solubility; as such, asthmatics are especially susceptible to its effects. It is capable of triggering nonimmunological airway smooth muscle contraction that is thought to involve neural and non-neural mechanisms. Prior exposures may result in increased bronchoconstriction in subsequent exposures and increase airways reactivity to challenges from pollutants other than sulfur dioxide.

Photooxidation of hydrocarbons yields a variety of aldehydes such as formaldehyde and acrolein. Formaldehyde represents 50% of total aldehydes. It is a nasal, upper respiratory and ocular irritant. It has an odor threshold of approximately 0.5 ppm and is intolerable to most exposed individuals at exposures greater than 4 ppm. Formaldehyde is used in both industrial and consumer products, thus making exposure difficult to avoid. Acrolein is both more reactive and irritating than formaldehyde, and the damage inflicted by exposure can be irreversible.

Particulate matter is another important pollutant associated with increased disease severity in asthma. Diesel exhaust particles, for example, increase nonspecific airway reactivity in asthmatic

**Table 16.2**    Sources and Effects of Common Air Pollutants

| Pollutant | Description | Sources | Health Effects | Environmental Effects |
|---|---|---|---|---|
| Ozone ($O_3$) | Gaseous pollutant when formed in the troposphere | Primarily vehicle exhaust | Eye and throat and respiratory effects, including the exacerbation of asthma and lung damage | Plant and ecosystem damage |
| Sulfur dioxide ($SO_2$) | Colorless gas that when dissolved in water vapor produces the corresponding acid | Fossil power plants, petroleum industry, manufacture of sulfuric acid, and smelting of ores containing sulfur | Eye and mucous membrane irritation, wheezing, chest tightness, shortness of breath, lung damage | Contributes to acid rain formation, aesthetic damage |
| Nitrogen dioxide ($NO_2$) | Reddish brown highly reactive gas | Motor vehicles, electric utilities, and other industrial, commercial, and residential sources that burn fuels | Lower respiratory irritation and injury, respiratory symptoms (e.g., cough, chest pain, difficulty breathing) | Contributes to smog, acid rain, water quality deterioration, global warming, and visibility impairment |
| Carbon monoxide (CO) | Colorless odorless gas | Motor vehicle exhaust; indoor sources include kerosene or wood-burning stoves | Headaches, reduced mental alertness, heart attack, cardio-vascular diseases, impaired fetal development, death | Contributes to the formation of smog |
| Lead (Pb) | Metallic element | Metal refineries, lead smelters, battery manufacturers, iron and steel producers | Cardiovascular effects, brain and kidney damage, neurological disorders, develop-mental effects | Affects animals, plants, and aquatic ecosystems |
| Particulate matter (PM) | Particles such as aerosols, soot, dust, or other matter | Diesel engines, industries, power plants, windblown dust, wood stoves | Eye irritation, bronchitis, asthma, lung damage, cancer, cardiovascular effects | Visibility impairment, atmospheric deposition, aesthetic damage |

individuals and increase the numbers of airway neutrophils and mast cells. Endotoxin is commonly found in the particulate matter of many grains and has been shown occupationally to produce increased airway symptoms in those workers who encounter it at high concentrations in the workplace. It is capable of producing inflammation in both nonasthmatic and nonallergic individuals and can result in nonspecific airway reactivity in those individuals with asthma.

The pathogenesis of asthma has not been fully elucidated. It is clear that airborne environmental contaminants can be an important contributing factor in both workplace and non-workplace environments. Paradoxically, the incidence of asthma has increased, particularly in urban environments, despite overall improvements in air quality at least with respect to the criteria pollutants. There is no clearcut relationship between respiratory disease and chronic low concentration exposures to environmental pollutants.

Concerns about the effects of toxic air pollutants were legislatively addressed in the Clean Air Act. Inhalation introduces toxicants such as ozone, sulfur dioxide, nitrogen oxides, aldehydes, and a host of other pollutants to the respiratory system. Although the dangers of some compounds have been demonstrated when they are inhaled alone, little is known about the hazards of complex mixtures. More than 180 toxicants were added in the Clear Air Act Amendment of 1990, but the health effects of these substances are virtually unknown. Most information is derived from controlled animal studies, but there are perils associated with the extrapolation of such data and their application to humans. Laboratory studies are conducted under very circumscribed conditions; it may not be defensible to apply findings to real-world systems. Even when the dangers of a chemical seem obvious, underlying health issues can make elucidation of the mechanism more difficult.

## Defense Strategies

The respiratory system has several defense strategies to respond to exposures to inhaled toxicants. These mechanisms attempt to reduce local damage and minimize absorption. Clearance mechanisms are one of the most important of these. Clearance mechanisms refer to the processes involved in the active removal of foreign matter in contact with the epithelial interface. In the respiratory system clearance mechanisms are a nonspecific means of particulate and dissolved chemical removal; they vary with the site of deposition. The two clearance mechanisms are mucociliary transport in the airways and alveolar macrophages in the gas exchange regions. For aerosols, particle size, shape, and physicochemical properties of the particulate are important for determining deposition and distribution. Deposition mechanisms include:

- Impaction of 5 to 30 µm particulates occurring primarily at airway bifurcations
- Interception of particles within the airways that results in their capture
- Sedimentation of 1 to 5 µm particulates in conducting airways involves the settling of particles in insufficiently turbulent air flow
- Diffusion that involves <0.5 µm particulate penetration into the alveoli

Clearance of relatively insoluble inhaled toxicants occurs in the

- Nasal cavity by filtering mechanisms that trap and eliminate larger particles (>10 µm). Sneezing and coughing further eliminate impacted particulates in this region.
- Conducting airways through the process of mucociliary transport
- Alveoli by the action of alveolar macrophages

Submucosal glands and goblet cells in the airways generate a fluid layer of mucus to coat the epithelium, and the ciliated mucosal cells propel the mucus replete with particles and dissolved gases proximally to where they are swallowed or expectorated. Irritants like sulfur oxides and ozone can adversely affect the mucociliary transport system. Clearance in humans is rapid; it generally occurs 1 to 2 days under normal conditions; however, exposures to environmental agents can reduce or increase the clearance rate. Chronic exposure to tobacco smoke can impair the long-term function of the tracheobronchial clearance mechanism and result in bronchitis.

The mucociliary action of the nose performs similar functions to that of the tracheobronchial airways and helps to protect the respiratory system from the toxic effects exerted by inhaled particles. Clearance in the pulmonary region is a two-step process consisting of phagocytosis by alveolar macrophages and subsequent removal of the macrophage from the alveoli via mucociliary transport or through capillary or lymphatic drainage. Alveolar macrophages that originate in the bone marrow circulate as monocytes and migrate into the air spaces of the alveoli where they become alveolar macrophages, now a pulmonary resident capable of cellular division. Pulmonary macrophages are the main clearance mechanism for particulates that have reached the alveoli. Alveolar macrophages, upon encountering a particulate, attach to it and internalize it by the process of endocytosis (phagocytosis), and the now internal and membrane bound particulate fuses with a lysosome in an attempt to digest the particle. The macrophage migrates into the more proximal regions of the respiratory system and is carried by the mucociliary escalator to the nasopharyngeal region for clearance by swallowing or expectoration, thus providing an important nonspecific defense mechanism for particulates that enter into the gas exchange regions.

These particulates are generally less than 1 μm in diameter. Removal is determined by the physiochemical properties of the particle, with soluble particles leaving via pulmonary capillaries and insoluble particles moving from the alveolar air space into the vascular or lymphatic systems or the mucociliary escalator. Macrophages act within minutes of inhalation to engulf inhaled particles, a process that occurs over the course of several hours. Macrophages that progressively accumulate particulates, even those that are relatively inert toxicologically such as carbon, can lead to their reduced phagocytic effectiveness and may result in the release of endogenous chemicals into the surrounding pulmonary tissue. These chemicals include digestive enzymes, fibroblast growth factors, and free radicals, which could lead to secondary toxicity as expressed by lung fibrosis. Alveolar macrophages are therefore an important component of nonspecific pulmonary defense mechanisms; however, when they malfunction, they become a source of chemicals that have the capacity to produce local injury.

Some particulates, especially asbestos and silica, produce macrophage dysfunction and death of the macrophage during the attempt to digest these particles. This is due to the release of lysosomal enzymes into the macrophage, its dissolution, and subsequent release of these enzymes into the surrounding pulmonary tissue. The release of these enzymes into the tissue results in local tissue destruction, inflammation, and fibrosis. Particulate matter and chemicals that can alter macrophage function or numbers have the capacity to either enhance the defense mechanism or reduce its effectiveness and produce local tissue injury. A number of common air pollutants, such as tobacco smoke, carbon monoxide, and many environmental dusts, stimulate increased numbers of macrophages. Some environmental pollutants such as aldehydes and certain heavy metals can reduce the numbers of pulmonary macrophages. Environmental exposures to ozone, heavy metals, and nitrogen dioxide can impair alveolar macrophage function. Alveolar macrophages also phagocytose foreign substances for presentation to lymphocytes and initiate an immune response; thus these cells also represent an important specific pulmonary defense mechanism as well.

Biochemical defense mechanisms in the respiratory system include xenobiotic metabolism, protective proteins, and antioxidant actions, with most activity occurring within the mucosa of the respiratory system. The mucosa is susceptible to direct toxic damage because it is in direct contact with air pollutants. There are enzymes capable of metabolic transformations in all regions of the respiratory system. Nasal mucosa, Clara cells, alveolar macrophages, epithelial cells, and pulmonary endothelial cells are among those active in pulmonary xenobiotic metabolism. Cells in the conducting region are less metabolically active than those cells in the pulmonary and nasal regions. Nasal tissues contain a wide range of enzymes, including cytochrome P450, lipoxygenase, and epoxyhydrolase. The principal phase I enzymes are cytochrome P450 and flavin-containing monooxygenases; these systems modify inhaled organic toxicants through aromatic and aliphatic hydroxylations, epoxidation, deamination, sulfoxidation, dealkylations, and other biochemical transformations. Ideally, metabolic transformations reduce the toxicity of the target compounds; however, it is possible, as previously discussed, to bioactivate substances of relatively low toxicity into more potent metabolites.

The presence of antioxidants in the nasal mucosa is evidence of its role in xenobiotic metabolism. The activity of the nasal mucosa is both protective and adverse. Depletion of glutathione can result in increased covalent binding of formaldehyde to DNA and potentially increased risk for the development of nasal tumors. Alpha-antitrypsin, generated primarily by the liver, is a protective protein in the lung. It functions as an antiprotease and inhibits plasmin, thrombin, and neutrophil elastase. The latter is a broad-spectrum protease capable of digesting many extracellular matrix proteins. When the alveolar surface is exposed to oxidants, the binding of alpha-antitrypsin and elastase may be profoundly altered. Antioxidant systems may help reduce the progression of injury. The respiratory system is subjected to significant oxidative stress. Exposure to ozone, for example, generates free radicals via the glutathione peroxidase enzyme system, despite the assumption that this enzyme is induced to reduce damage.

Other pulmonary defense mechanisms include bronchoconstriction, airway epithelium, olfaction, alveolar macrophages, and immunological defense. Bronchoconstriction can be induced by a variety of means in response to respired particulate matter or chemicals. Bronchoconstriction is considered protective because it reduces air flow to the lungs, thereby limiting pulmonary exposure to inhaled toxicants. Airway epithelial cells are capable of producing inflammatory mediators such as arachidonic acid metabolites, which alter vascular permeability. This recruits inflammatory cells to the injury site. Additionally, because damaged airway epithelial cells produce drastically reduced amounts of the endogenous mediators necessary to maintain airway muscle tone, the airway epithelial cells act as down regulators of airway smooth muscle contractions.

## Types of Injury

Pulmonary responses may be acute in their onset, delayed, or chronic in nature. An irritant gas such as sulfur dioxide may trigger an immediate reflex, producing bronchoconstriction. A delayed response to this insult may involve neutrophil and macrophage accumulation at the injury site and the release of cytokines to trigger an acute inflammatory response, leading to edema, reduced airflow, and bronchitis. Examples of delayed responses are seen from exposures to chemicals such as nitrogen dioxide, ozone, the herbicide paraquat, and aspiration of gasoline into the airways from siphoning. Alveolar injury and pulmonary edema can occur after a delay of approximately 12 hours. The chronic condition, emphysema, is responsible for about 3% of deaths in the United States. Cigarette smoke leads to release of proteases (elastase) from neutrophils and alpha-1-antiprotease in blood, which destroys the partition (septa) between alveoli, leading to the loss of gas exchange surface, inflammation, and fibrosis.

Although the underlying mechanism of sensitization to environmental allergens has not been fully elucidated, it is necessary to consider such exposures and their role in the pathogenesis of environmental asthma. A critical feature of asthma is nonspecific airway hyperresponsiveness; airway epithelial cell damage and mucosal inflammation are important steps in the pathogenesis of this condition. Infiltration of inflammatory cells, evidence of bronchial epithelial damage, airway smooth muscle hyperreactivity, and thickening of subepithelial collagen are examples of some changes to the airways seen in both occupational and nonoccupational environmental bronchial asthma. Avoidance of the aggravating environmental chemical may reverse reticular basement membrane thickening but has little effect on inflammatory cell infiltration, presence of specific airway sensitivity to the chemical allergen, or nonspecific airway hyperresponsiveness.

Several stages may be associated with the clinical airway manifestations associated with the exacerbation of bronchial asthma subsequent to exposure to an environmental chemical. The response may be immediate (within minutes), late (several hours postexposure), or dual, combining both an immediate and late response. The late response appears to be directly associated with airway mucosal inflammation. The late asthmatic response seen in environmental exposures also appears similar to occupational asthma; both are associated with an increase in suppressor-cytotoxic lymphocytes and eosinophils in peripheral blood. Although the pathophysiological manifestations of asthma can be explained, the issue of sensitization cannot. It is not known why specific chemical exposures lead to sensitization whereas others have little to no lasting effect. Some correlations have been drawn between the reactivity of a chemical with proteins and its potential to induce sensitization of the respiratory tract. Recent studies have shown that nonimmunological mechanisms are important in the pathogenesis of bronchial asthma as well. The disastrous release of methyl isocyanate gas in Bhopal, India tragically demonstrated the development of sudden onset asthma accompanied by persistent nonspecific airway hyperreactivity in response to the massive acute exposure. There is more than one type of environmentally induced reactive airways syndrome, but reactive airways dysfunction syndrome (RADS) is an important prototype. RADS is a condition that develops quickly after a brief highly concentrated exposure to generally an irritant gas or vapor in some sort of industrial or environmental accident.

In the alveolar region, alveolar macrophages are linked to the pathogenesis of pulmonary fibrosis. Fibroblast stimulation and fiber deposition depend on a delicate balance between fibroblast proliferation factors and factors that inhibit their proliferation. The promotion of proliferation factor secretion is connected to the chemical–physical interaction between the particle and the surface of the alveolar macrophage. The particulate–cell interaction may be related to the type and spatial arrangement of atoms in the particulate. The physical properties of the particulate (e.g., fiber length) also determine the sort of damage that may be produced. Clearance mechanisms are also influenced by particulate properties. Long fibers, for example, are not readily cleared by alveolar macrophages. These interactions may be aided by serum factors that promote association of the fiber with the cellular surface. Simple activation of the macrophages and initiation of phagocytosis promote an inflammatory response. Other mechanisms are at play in the development of fibrosis. "Activated" macrophages also generate free oxygen radicals when fibers such as chrysotile asbestos open calcium channels on the surface of the macrophage.

Plasminogen activator (PA) is another potent inflammatory mediator secreted by alveolar macrophages after activation. It has been demonstrated that PA activity is increased in certain inflammatory lung disease and theorized that PA secretion is linked to the early stages of asbestos-induced alveolitis.

Pneumoconiosis refers to a disease state such as silicosis or asbestosis characterized by pathophysiological changes in the lungs due to particulate deposition. Small crystalline silica particles from 0.5 to 2 mm that are inhaled can reach the alveoli where they cause lung damage. The particles that reach the alveoli activate the alveolar macrophages, which attempt to engulf them. This often produces injury to the phagocyte, which releases its digestive enzymes into the surrounding tissue, producing inflammation and fibrosis.

The inhalation of quartz ($SiO_2$) results in nodular formations in the upper regions of the lung. The progression of pathological changes in silicosis can occur over the course of several months to years resulting in death or may have a period of latency of a decade or more. Although quartz is not carcinogenetic, the inflammatory changes and fibrosis to the lung (e.g., often seen in the past in sandblasters) can be so extensive that the loss of vital gas exchange surface reduces the lungs to being unable to fulfill their function.

In asbestosis, the size and shape of the fibers influence whether the disease may progress to cancer (Figure 16.2). Fibers that reach the deep lung tend to be <2 μm in diameter and <100 μm in length. The major site of deposition is the bifurcations of the airways. All forms of asbestos are fibrous silicates composed of silicon dioxide with various substituted elements. Examples include chrysotile, which is soluble in acids, has curved fibers containing numerous fibrils, and has a tubular structure, whereas amphiboles are straight fibers, many of which contain iron, a metal associated with oxygen radical formation at their surface, perhaps associated with their greater carcinogenic potential.

Two types of cancer associated with asbestosis are bronchiocarcinoma and malignant mesothelioma. The latter is a cancer of the pleural lining due to penetration into the lymphatic space and was often seen in insulator workers on ships in World War II. Although the shorter fibers are totally digested by macrophages, the longer fibers are not, and this incomplete digestion is associated with the reduced ability of the asbestos-containing macrophage to be cleared from the alveoli where it remains and dies, releasing the fiber to start the process again by another macrophage. The release of destructive tissue chemicals also stimulates proliferation of other cells, and if proliferation is uncontrolled, the stage is set up for lung cancer or mesothelioma to develop.

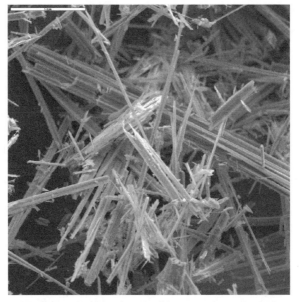

**FIGURE 16.2**    Asbestos fibers. *Source:* Courtesy of the Denver Microbeam Laboratory, USGS.

## Bibliography

Air Pollution Control Orientation Course. Retrieved December 2005 from http://www.epa.gov/apti/course422/ap7a.html.

Bhattacharya, K., Dopp, E., Kakkar, P., Jaffery, F. N., Schiffmann, D., Jaurand, M. C., Rahman, I., & Rahman, Q. (2005). Biomarkers in risk assessment of asbestos exposure. *Mutation Research, 579,* 6–21.

Borm, P. J. (2002). Particle toxicology: from coal mining to nanotechnology. *Inhalation Toxicology, 14,* 311–324.

Brooks, S. M., Fox, R., Lockey, R., Hammad, Y., Richards, I. S., Giovinco-Barbas, J., & Jenkins, K. (1998). The spectrum of irritant-induced asthma: sudden and not-so-sudden onset and the role of allergy. *Chest, 113,* 42–49.

Cashman, T. M., & Murray, P. M. (1995). Respiratory protection in occupational health-update. *Military Medicine, 160*(4), 168–171.

Cohen, M. D., Zelikoff, J. T., & Schlesinger, R. B. (2000). *Pulmonary immunotoxicology.* Boston, MA: Kluwer.

Dietrich, C., Richards, I. S., Bernard, T., & Y. Hammad. (1996). Human stress protein response to formaldehyde exposure. *Experimental and Toxicologic Pathology, 48,* 518.

Dockery, D. W. (2001). Epidemiologic evidence of cardiovascular effects of particulate air pollution. *Environmental Health Perspectives, 109*(suppl 4), 483–486.

Fernandez-Caldas, E., Fox, R. W., Richards, I. S., Varney, T. C., & Brooks, S. M. (1995). Indoor air pollution. In S. M. Brooks (Ed.), *Environmental medicine: concepts and practice* (pp. 419–437). St. Louis, MO: Mosby.

Folinsbee, L. J. (1993). Human health effects of air pollution. *Environmental Health Perspectives, 100,* 45–56.

Gardner, D. E. (2005). *Toxicology of the lung* (4th ed.). Target Organ Toxicology Series Volume 22. Boca Raton, FL: CRC Press Inc.

Genter, M. B. (2006). Molecular biology of the nasal airways: how do we assess cellular and molecular responses in the nose? *Toxicologic Pathology, 34,* 274–280.

Harkema, J. R., Carey, S. A., & Wagner, J. G. (2006). The nose revisited: a brief review of the comparative structure, function, and toxicologic pathology of the nasal epithelium. *Toxicologic Pathology, 34,* 252–269.

IARC monographs on the evaluation of carcinogenic risks to humans. World Health Organization, International Agency for Research on Cancer.

Kimmel, E. C., & Still, K. R. (1999). Acute lung injury, acute respiratory distress syndrome and inhalation injury: an overview. *Drug Chem Toxicol, 22,* 91–128.

Koren, H. S. (1995). Associations between criteria air pollutants and asthma. *Environmental Health Perspectives, 103*(suppl 6), 235–242.

Koren, H. S. (1997). Environmental risk factors in atopic asthma. *Int Arch Allergy Immunol, 113,* 65–68.

Koren, H. S., & Bromberg, P. A. (1995). Respiratory responses of asthmatics to ozone. *Int Arch Allergy Immunol, 107,* 236–238.

Koren, H. S., Devlin, R. B., Graham, D. E., Mann, R., McGee, M. P., Horstman, D. H., Kozumbo, W. J., Becker, S., House, D. E., & McDonnell, W. F. (1989). Ozone-induced inflammation in the lower airways of human subjects. *Am Rev Respir Dis, 139,* 407–415.

Kulkarni, A. P., Cai, Y., & Richards, I. S. (1992). Rat pulmonary lipoxygenase: dioxygenase activity and role in xenobiotic metabolism. *International Journal of Biochemistry, 24,* 255–261.

Kulkarni, A. P., Edwards, J. H., & Richards, I. S. (1992). Metabolism of 1,2-dibromoethane in the human fetal liver. *General Pharmacology, 23,* 1–5.

Kulkarni, A. P., Mitra, A., Chaudhuri, J., Byczkowski, J. Z., & Richards, I. S. (1990). Hydrogen peroxide: a potent activator of dioxygenase activity of soybean lipoxygenase. *Biochemical and Biophysical Research Communications, 166,* 417–423.

Leikauf, G. D., Swiecicowski, A. L., Rosbolt, J. P., & Richards, I. S. (1993). Aldehyde-induced airway hyperreactivity. *Proc. Hung. Biochem. Soc, 3,* 235–240.

Lippmann, M., & Schlesinger, R. B. (2000). Toxicological bases for the setting of health-related air pollution standards. *Annual Review of Public Health, 21,* 309–333.

National Research Council Staff. (1989). Biologic Markers of Pulmonary Toxicology.

Ostro, B., Lipsett, M., Mann, J., Braxton-Owens, H., & White, M. (2001). Air pollution and exacerbation of asthma in African-American children in Los Angeles. *Epidemiology, 12,* 200–208.

Perper, J. A., & Van Thiel, D. H. (1992). Respiratory complications of cocaine abuse. *Recent Developments in Alcoholism, 10,* 363–377.

Peters, A., Dockery, D. W., Muller, J. E., & Mittleman, M. A. (2001). Increased particulate air pollution and the triggering of myocardial infarction. *Circulation, 103,* 2810–2815.

Phalen, P., & Phalen, R. F. (Eds.) (1996). *Methods in inhalation toxicology.* Boca Raton, FL: CRC Press.

Richards, I. S. (1991). Health effects of illicit cocaine use. Pulmonary and critical care update. *American College of Chest Physicians, 7,* 1–7.

Richards, I. S. (1997). Ethanol potentiates the depressant effect of cocaine in human fetal myocardium in vitro. *Journal of Toxicology Clinical Toxicology, 35,* 365–371.

Richards, I. S., & Brooks, S. M. (1995). Respiratory toxicology. In S. M. Brooks (Ed.), *Environmental medicine: concepts and practice* (pp. 166–180). St. Louis, MO: Mosby.

Richards, I. S., & de Hate, R. (2006). Formalin produces depolarizations in human airway smooth muscle in vitro. *Toxicology and Industrial Health, 22,* 1–5.

Richards, I. S., Kulkarni, A., & Bremner, W. F. (1990). Cocaine induced arrhythmias in human fetal myocardium in vitro: potential mechanism for fetal death in utero. *Pharmacology and Toxicology, 66,* 150–154.

Richards, I. S., Kulkarni, A., Brooks, S. M., Lathrop, D. A., Bremner, W. F., & Sperelakis, N. (1989). A moderate concentration of ethanol alters cellular membrane potentials and decreases contractile force of human fetal heart. *Developmental Pharmacology and Therapeutics, 13,* 51–56.

Richards, I. S., Kulkarni, A., Brooks, S., & Pierce, R. (1990). Florida red-tide toxin (brevetoxins) produce depolarization of airway smooth muscle. *Toxicon, 28,* 1105–1111.

Richards, I. S., Miller, L., Solomon, D., Kulkarni, A., Brooks, S., & Sperelakis, N. (1990). Azelastine inhibits acetylcholine-induced contraction and depolarization in human airway smooth muscle. *European Journal of Pharmacology, 186,* 331–334.

Salem, H., & Katz, S. A. (2005). *Inhalation toxicology* (2nd ed.). Boca Raton, FL: CRC Press.

Samet, J. M., & Cheng, P. W. (1994). The role of airway mucus in pulmonary toxicology. *Environmental Health Perspectives, 102*(suppl 2), 89–103.

Samet, J. M., Zeger, S. L., Dominici, F., Curriero, F., Coursac, I., Dockery, D. W., Schwartz, J., & Zanobetti, A. (2000). The National Morbidity, Mortality, and Air Pollution Study. Part II: Morbidity and mortality from air pollution in the United States. *Research report (Health Effects Institute), 94,* 5–70.

Sandstrom, T. (1995). Respiratory effects of air pollutants: experimental studies in humans. *European Respiratory Journal, 8,* 976–995.

U.S. EPA. Retrieved December 2005 from http://www.epa.gov/region09/toxic/noa/clearcreek/index.html.

U.S. National Library of Medicine, National Institutes of Health, Environmental Health, and Toxicology Specialized Information Services (SIS). (2005). *Toxicology tutorial III*. Retrieved October 2, 2005 from http://www.sis.nlm.nih.gov/enviro/toxtutor.html.

# The Nervous System

## General Considerations

Neurotoxicity is the alteration of normal function of the nervous system as the result of exposure to natural or artificial neurotoxicants. The damage may be specific to a particular cell type, a given region, or a particular function. The nervous system is structurally divided into two major anatomical components:

- The central nervous system (CNS), consisting of the brain, cranial nerves, and the spinal cord
- The peripheral nervous system (PNS), consisting of sensory (afferent) neurons, which relay impulses from the receptors to the CNS, and motor (efferent) neurons, which relay impulses from the CNS to effectors such as the glands and muscles of the body.

The efferent division of the PNS can be divided into the voluntary or somatic nervous system, which regulates skeletal muscle activity, and the autonomic or involuntary nervous system, which regulates the glands and cardiac and smooth muscles. The somatic nervous system uses one group of motor neurons to stimulate the effectors, whereas the autonomic nervous system requires both a preganglionic and a postganglionic neuron to stimulate the effector. The autonomic nervous system is composed of both sensory and motor neurons that control the internal environment of the body's internal organs. The somatic nervous system consists of the skeletal and cranial nerves that send sensory information to the CNS and motor nerve fibers that innervate the skeletal muscles. The autonomic nervous system is further divided into the sympathetic and parasympathetic systems (Figure 17.1).

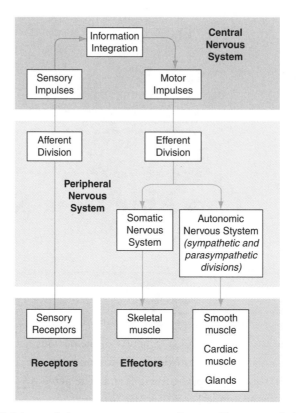

**FIGURE 17.1** Divisions of the nervous system. *Source:* Courtesy of the Toxicology and Environmental Health Information Program of the National Library of Medicine, U.S. Department of Health and Human Services.

The sympathetic division of the autonomic nervous system (the "fight or flight" response system) is responsible for

- Increasing cardiac output
- Elevating blood pressure
- Increasing heart rate
- Bronchodilatation
- Increasing pupil size
- Increasing blood flow from peripheral vessels to skeletal muscle
- Mobilization of glycogen in fat

The parasympathetic division of the autonomic nervous system is generally antagonistic to the sympathetic system and is responsible for

- Decreasing cardiac output
- Decreasing blood pressure
- Decreasing heart rate
- Decreasing pupil size
- Bronchoconstriction

- Increasing digestion and absorption of foods
- Eliminating wastes

The brain can be divided into several regions:

- *Forebrain,* consisting of the cerebrum and the diencephalon (thalamus and the hypothalamus)
- *Midbrain* (mesencephalon), consisting of the tectum and tegmentum
- *Hindbrain,* consisting of the medulla oblongata (myelencephalon) and the metencephalon (pons and cerebellum)

The cerebrum is the largest part of the brain and can be subdivided as follows:

- *Frontal lobe,* which controls such things as creative thought, intellect, problem solving, attention, behavior, abstract thinking, smell, emotions, and coordination of movement
- *Temporal lobe,* which controls such things as language, auditory and visual memory, speech, and hearing
- *Parietal lobe,* which controls such things as tactile perception, responses to internal stimuli, sensory interpretation, and some visual function
- *Occipital lobe,* which processes visual information

The white matter of the CNS is composed of nerve fibers with large amounts of the insulating material called myelin, which facilitates conduction of electrical impulses and is sparse in nerve cell bodies. The gray matter, in contrast, is composed primarily of nerve cell bodies, synapses, and unmyelinated axons, which are all involved in the processing of information. White matter is less vascularized than gray matter and is somewhat more tolerant to lesser levels of oxygen; however, overall the nervous system has little capacity for anaerobic metabolism. The cerebral cortex is most sensitive to hypoxia. The toxicants cyanide and $H_2S$ bind to cytochrome oxidase, thus blocking the mitochondrial transport chain. Carbon monoxide replaces oxygen in hemoglobin and damages neurons and supporting cells in the CNS.

## Cells of the Nervous System

The neuron (single nerve cell) is the functional unit of the nervous system. These are the excitable cells that are capable of generating and propagating an electrical signal, filing and storing information to support basic communication processes and higher functions such as learning, memory, and behavior (Figure 17.2).

The functional classes of neurons are

- Sensory or afferent neurons that carry information to the CNS
- Motor or efferent extrinsic neurons that carry information from the CNS to the tissues and organs

Interneurons in the CNS are "routing" neurons, directing incoming and outgoing signals to other neurons. They provide connections between sensory and motor neurons and are involved in spinal reflexes, coordination of motor impulses, analysis of sensory information, and memory.

A neuron consists of a cell body and two types of extensions, numerous dendrites, and a single axon. The cell body of the neuron is the metabolic center and contains the nucleus, mitochondria,

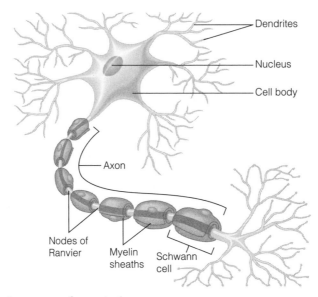

**FIGURE 17.2**    Structure of a typical neuron.

enzymes, and other structures and chemicals that are necessary to support the entire cell. The axon is the main conducting unit that transmits the action potential from one neuron to the next. At the axon hillock, the action potential is initiated, and when a critical membrane potential is reached, an action potential is initiated that travels the entire length of the axon to the axon terminals which communicate with another neuron or effector cell. The axon may extend long distances, over a meter in some cases, to transmit information from one part of the body to another. Some axons are wrapped in a multilayer coating, known as the myelin sheath, which helps insulate the axon from surrounding tissues and fluids and prevents the electrical charge from escaping from the axon. Myelinated neurons have a faster velocity of conduction than nonmyelinated neurons. Motor neurons are typically myelinated, whereas sensory neurons are typically nonmyelinated.

The cellular structure of a "typical" neuron is complex. Generally, neurons can be classified structurally as unipolar, bipolar, or multipolar. Unipolar neurons have dendrite and axon originating from the same process. Bipolar neurons have a single axon and single dendrite opposite one another on the cell body. Multipolar neurons have more than one dendrite.

Because of the length of many axons and their dependence on chemicals produced by the cell body, mechanisms must be in place to provide a system of transport to and from that source. Axonal transport is the process of moving substances from the cell body to the axonal terminal (anterograde) or from the axonal terminal to the cell body (retrograde). Because axons contain no ribosomes, for example, they are dependent on this axoplasmic transport of the necessary proteins required to support its function of conduction. Axonal transport is generally recognized as containing a slow and a fast component. Slow transport is used to carry important chemicals that are not rapidly depleted by the axon, such as enzymes; cytoskeletal elements, such as actin; and other microfilament-associated proteins at a rate of several millimeters per day. Fast axonal transport utilizes proteins such as kinesins and microtubules to actively move such things as old membrane components for recycling, peptides, glycolipids, glycoproteins, acetylcholinesterase (AChE), and serotonin at a rate of several hundred millimeters per day. Axonal transport generally occurs along the microtubules of the axon and requires a number of transport proteins such as kinesin and dynein. Axonal transport is also important for the cell body of the neuron because retrograde transport provides chemicals such as growth factors that are released by effector.

Neuroglial or glial cells are supportive to the nervous system and are represented by several types of cells in the CNS:

- Oligodendrocytes
- Astrocytes
- Ependymal cells
- Microglia

Microglia are macrophages that differ from other glial cells because they are monocyte derived. Astrocytes or astroglia are the most abundant glia; they comprise the largest portion of the blood–brain barrier (BBB). They are located within the CNS and are critical to the maintenance of the BBB and help to regulate concentrations of potassium ($K^+$) and to maintain extracellular pH, glutamate, and water. In addition, they contain enzymes that are important in metabolizing certain chemicals in the brain. 1-Methyl-4-phenyl-1,2,3,6-tetrahydropyridine (MPTP), a contaminant byproduct of synthetic heroin manufacturing, crosses the BBB and is metabolized to $MPP^+$ (the ionized form of MPTP) by monoamine oxygenase by astrocytes, released, and then taken up by dopamine-producing neurons in certain regions of the brain such as the substantia nigra, which is important in feedback control for coordinating muscular activity. Here, the metabolite inhibits oxidative phosphorylation and produces a permanent Parkinson-like effect.

Oligodendrocytes or oligodendroglia are responsible for the production of myelin in the CNS and hence are responsible for normal propagation of action potentials. In the PNS, Schwann cells are responsible for this function. Ependymal cells line the ventricles in the CNS and produce and circulate the cerebrospinal fluid through ciliary activity.

## The Blood-Brain Barrier (BBB)

The BBB is an anatomical and physiological "barrier" between the brain and circulation, which regulates the entry and leaving of both endogenous and exogenous substances into and out of the brain. The key factors that determine this are

- Molecular size
- Lipid solubility
- Molecular charge
- Concentration differences
- Specialized transport mechanisms

The BBB is composed of tight junctions (zonulae occludens) between endothelial cells of brain capillaries and astrocytic cell membrane projections that surround these capillaries. The barrier is relatively ineffective for lipid-soluble molecules, whereas water-soluble substances such as glucose require special mechanisms for transport. Compounds that mimic essential chemicals such as certain ions and nutrients can be actively transported across the BBB as occurs when organic mercury combines with the amino acid cysteine and is transported by amino acid uptake systems. Certain ions such as $Pb^{2+}$ can be transported by normal ion exchange systems. The BBB is not a continuous barrier in that there are places within the CNS where the barrier is relatively ineffective, such as the median eminence, pineal, neurohypophysis, and the hypothalamus. The BBB is not fully developed in children, thus making them much more susceptible to the effects of certain chemicals when compared with the adult brain. Small exposures to lead, for example, are of greater concern in children than in adults due to the more permeable nature of their cerebral capillaries.

## Neuron Action Potential and Synaptic Function

The unequal distribution of ions across a neuron cell membrane, like other excitable cells, is the basis for the nervous action potential. This is brought about by electrical and chemical gradients that are created across the cell membrane by active transport mechanisms and selective membrane permeability. Electrical conduction involves the movement of sodium and potassium ions across the nerve cell membrane through sequential changes in its permeability to sodium ($Na^+$) and potassium ($K^+$) ions. The membrane potential difference can be measured by ascertaining the difference between the electrical charge inside and outside the cell. There are two basic kinds of electrical signals in neurons: graded potentials and action potentials. Graded potentials travel short distances. Action potentials travel over longer distances. They do not lose amplitude as they travel, nor do they vary. When the neuron is not firing, it has a separation of charges across the membrane that creates a resting membrane potential of about −70 to −80 mV, that is, the inside of the cell relative to the outside has a net electronegativity, in part due to an electrogenic Na/K pump (Na/K ATPase), which maintains a higher internal $K^+$ concentration relative to $Na^+$ and exchanges two $K^+$ for every one $Na^+$.

At the terminal end of an axon (i.e., the presynaptic terminal) are synaptic vesicles containing chemicals known as *neurotransmitters* (Figure 17.3). Upon arrival of action potentials at the axon terminals, a neurotransmitter is released that diffuses across the synaptic or neuromuscular junction and activates postsynaptic receptors, thereby initiating another action potential or the response of the effector cell.

Examples of neurotransmitters include

- Acetylcholine
- Catecholamines (dopamine, norepinephrine, epinephrine)
- Serotonin
- Glutamate
- Gamma-aminobutyric acid (GABA -an inhibitory neurotransmitter)
- Peptides

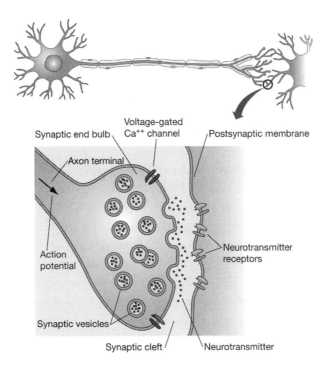

**FIGURE 17.3**   A typical synapse.

Neurotransmitters are mostly stored in synaptic granules and released via membrane fusion between the granule membrane and the plasma membrane. Opening of the $Ca^{2+}$ channels is a voltage-dependent process, requiring depolarization of the synaptic terminal to occur.

## Neurotoxicity

Neuropathic damage can result from exposure to neurotoxicants like carbon monoxide, carbon tetrachloride, mercury, or lead. Lead is a ubiquitously occurring toxicant found naturally in the environment and therefore can be found in water, food, and air, as well as in many manufactured products. Despite the efforts for lead reduction by the U.S. Environmental Protection Agency (EPA) and the U.S. Food and Drug Administration (FDA), lead exposures still remain an important public health concern, especially in children, who are both more likely to be exposed to certain sources and more sensitive to the effects of lead. It is now clear that even relatively low lead exposures during childhood development have neurobehavioral and developmental effects that may persist into adulthood. The problem is still of greatest concern in urban environments where exposures to lead, especially from lead-based paint and plumbing fixtures in old housing, are commonplace.

The idea that certain diseases may be produced or triggered by environmental factors, including exposure to chemical agents, has become widely accepted based on both laboratory studies and human data. An unfortunate and relatively recent event in support of this is the association between the development of Parkinson's disease and exposure to chemicals. A Parkinson-like disease in humans has been linked to exposure to the chemical MPTP, a compound that is the byproduct of synthetic heroin production as previously mentioned. A number of users developed signs and symptoms virtually identical to Parkinson's disease over the course of a week or two after the use of the illicit substance. Normally, the disease generally occurs later in life and develops over the course of many years. MPTP is extremely neurotoxic and produced in these individuals the characteristic lack of muscular control and tremors that are associated with the degeneration of brain cells in the substantia nigra, a region of the brain that produces the neurotransmitter dopamine. Once injected into the blood, MPTP readily crosses the BBB and is metabolized by brain oxygenases, producing charged metabolites that no longer can readily leave the brain. MPTP is today used experimentally in laboratory animals to study neurodegenerative diseases: When injected into laboratory rodents, it produces the signs and symptoms characteristic of the human equivalent.

In the United States during Prohibition, an extract of Jamaican ginger became contaminated with triorthocresyl phosphate (TOCP). The extract from Jamaican ginger had been used in the United States in the 1800s as a medicinal tonic purported to aid in digestion, ward off respiratory infections, and other unsubstantiated claims. The preparation typically contained about 70% alcohol. During Prohibition the ginger extract was legal for sale if it contained 5 g of ginger per milliliter of ethanol. Because of the high content of ginger, the preparation was too spicy to consume in the way one would consume an alcoholic beverage and therefore the government deemed this to be adequate to sell for medicinal purposes. Bootleggers saw this as an opportunity to produce illegal alcohol by distilling the alcohol content, adding a small amount of ginger, and substituting adulterants such as molasses and castor oil to replace the solid content back to 5% in the event that the Department of Agriculture were to test the elixir for quality control. Quality control by the Department of Agriculture was essentially to boil off the alcohol and weigh the solid residue. In 1930, one bootlegger substituted lyndol for castor oil as an adulterant (lyndol was used in varnishes in lacquers). Consumption of this product, which contained the organophosphorus chemical TOCP in the lyndol, resulted in the degeneration of neurons in both the CNS and the PNS in an estimated 20,000 to 100,000 people who consumed the product. Effects were reported as tingling in the extremities, numbness, and various degrees of paralysis. These effects were either temporary or permanent in nature.

Neurons have little capacity for anaerobic metabolism. Respiratory failure, decreased cardiac output, decreased oxygen-carrying capacity, or exposure to carbon monoxide may result in hypoxia. Exposure to carbon monoxide has long been associated with neurological sequelae; it can cause anoxic and cytotoxic toxicity that can affect the integrity of the BBB. Hypoglycemia and metabolic inhibitors interfere with cellular metabolism, and cytotoxic hypoxia can occur despite adequate blood and oxygen supplies. Cyanide, azide, and hydrogen sulfide are all metabolic inhibitors. Cyanide affects the gray and white cortical matter through the inhibition of cytochrome oxidase. Anoxia decreases intracellular pH, increases intracellular lactate, causes nuclear chromatin to clump, destroys mitochondrial granules, increases intracellular sodium, shrinks cytoplasm, induces nuclear pyknosis, and induces cell death. Cerebral edema from anoxia may reflect astrocyte swelling. Some toxicants damage the microtubular substructure necessary for nutrient transport.

Neurotoxicity can be produced in the CNS after exposure to a chemical agent. At the cellular level, injury can occur at

- Motor neurons, producing muscle dysfunction and paralysis
- Interneurons, producing decrements in memory and learning coordination
- Sensory neurons and sensory receptors, producing dysfunction in vision, hearing, and the senses of temperature, pressure, touch, taste, smell, and pain

Injuries to the structure and physiological perturbations in the nervous system include

- Direct cytotoxicity and death of neurons and glia
- Conduction abnormalities and interference with synaptic and neuroeffector transmission

Damage occurs selectively in the tissues of the nervous system, depending on the presence and penetrability of barriers, differences in blood flow, differences in metabolic rates, and differences in metabolic function. Cells of the cerebellum and visual cortex, for example, are preferentially killed by methylmercury.

Toxic responses to the nervous system have been classified as falling into several categories:

- Neuronopathy: damage to neuronal cell body
- Axonopathy: damage to axon or axonal transport
- Myelinopathy: loss of or abnormal formation of myelin
- Conduction/transmission: associated effects where conduction or neurotransmitter functions are altered

Some examples of these types of injury are summarized in Table 17.1.

Toxicants that produce neuromyopathies include lead, methylmercury, and carbon monoxide. Lead can lead to encephalopathy (a degenerative disease in the brain) and learning deficits, especially in children. Methylmercury is incorporated in the CNS by an amino acid uptake system

**Table 17.1    Examples of Neurotoxic Chemicals**

| Chemical | Type of Injury |
| --- | --- |
| Aluminum | Neuropathy: degenerative changes in cortex |
| Arsenic | Neuropathy: axonal degeneration in PNS |
| Methylmercury | Neuropathy: neural degeneration |
| Methanol | Neuropathy: necrosis of putamen, degeneration or retinal ganglion cells |
| Acrylamide | Axonopathy: axonal degeneration |
| Hexachlorophene | Myelinopathy: brain swelling, intramyelinic edema in CNS and PNS |
| Demoic acid | Neurotransmitter-associated injury: neural loss |
| Tellurium | Myelinopathy: demyelinating neuropathy |
| Cuprizone | Myelinopathy: edema, gliosis |
| Lead | Neuropathy: brain swelling, axonal loss |
| Carbon tetrachloride | Neuropathy: enlarged astrocytes in striatum |
| Thallium | Neuropathy: brain swelling, axonal degeneration |

and can cause neural degeneration in the cerebellum and cortex and in children mental retardation and paralysis. Triethyl tin alters normal neuronal energy metabolism, leading to cellular swelling and necrosis.

Axonopathies involve some form of degeneration of the axon and are most often accompanied in myelinated axons by demyelination. In the CNS axons do not normally regenerate, whereas in the PNS regeneration may occur over the course of months or years depending on the extent of the injury. Some of the best-known toxicants that produce axonopathies fall into the broad category of organic solvents, such as carbon disulfide, acrylamide, methyl-*N*-butyl ketone, trichloroethylene, and n-hexane (Table 17.2). Carbon disulfide has been used in the rayon and vulcanized rubber industries for decades and has been linked to chronic peripheral axonopathies by apparently forming cross-linkages with axonal neurofilaments. N-hexane, a common solvent found in such things as adhesives, is metabolized and bioactivated and produces injury to normal axonal transport mechanisms in sensory and motor neurons. N-hexane is metabolized to 2,5-hexanedione (a diketone), which then enters into reactions with the cellular proteins of axonal neurofilaments and tends to accumulate in the distal portion of the axon proximal to a node of Ranvier. There it produces what have been referred to as nodal swellings, which interfere with normal action potential transmission at the node.

**Table 17.2   Common Organic Solvents**

| Compound | Uses |
| --- | --- |
| Acetone | Cleaning solvent |
| Acrylamide | Mining and tunneling, adhesives, waste treatment, ore processing |
| Benzene | Fuel, detergents, paint removers, manufacture of other solvents |
| Carbon disulfide | Viscose rayon, explosives, paints, preservatives, textiles, rubber cement, varnishes, electroplating |
| n-Hexane | Glues and vegetable extraction, components of naphtha, lacquers, metal cleaning compounds |
| Hydrogen sulfide | Sulfur chemical manufacturing, byproduct of petroleum processing, decay of organic matter |
| Methyl-*N*-butyl ketone | Many industrial uses |
| Methylene chloride (dichloromethane) | Solvent, refrigerant, propellant |
| Perchloroethylene | Dry cleaning, degreaser, textile industry |
| Styrene | Fiberglass component, ship building |
| Toluene | Paint, fuel oil, cleaning agents, lacquers, paints and paint thinners |
| 1,1,1-Trichloroethane (methyl chloroform) | Degreaser and propellant |
| Trichloroethylene | Cleaning agent, paint component, decaffeination, rubber solvents, varnish |
| Vinyl chloride | Intermediate for polyvinyl chloride resins for plastics, floor coverings, upholstery, appliances, packaging |
| Xylene | Paint, lacquers, varnishes, inks, dyes, adhesives, cements, fixative for pathologic specimens |

TOCP, an organophosphorus ester and contaminant of illegal alcohols during prohibition in the United States, was responsible for the "Ginger Jake syndrome," discussed above, which produced progressive paralysis about a week or two after consumption of the alcohol. This chemical, similar to an organic phosphorus pesticide, phosphorylated an enzyme referred to as neuropathy-target esterase (NTE), thus deactivating it. The progressive effects, seen experimentally with some organophosphate pesticides, have been referred to as organophosphate-induced delayed neuropathy (OPIDN). Some chemicals that have been used in the treatment of certain malignancies such as colchicine, vincristine, and Taxol (from the yew tree) have been shown to affect axonal microtubules polymerization, thus blocking normal axonal transport mechanisms.

A myelinopathy is characterized by degeneration or unwrapping of the myelin sheath from neuronal axons. The term *demyelination* refers to the degeneration of axonal myelin. Chemicals that produce injury to the myelin produce decrements in impulse conduction velocity. Chemicals that have been associated with demyelination include diphtheria toxin, triethyl tin, hexachlorophene, tellurium, and lead. Triethyl tin has been used in a number of applications as a stabilizing agent, preservative, and biocide. It primarily results in the demyelination of peripheral motor axons as a result of myelin accumulation of water. The demyelination of axons of the retina has been demonstrated. The chlorinated aromatic hydrocarbon hexachlorophene has been used in the past as an antimicrobial agent against *Staphylococcus*. The chemical can readily pass through the skin to affect both the PNS and the CNS. In the CNS it is associated with brain swelling due to an accumulation of fluids (intramyelinic edema) as a result of alterations in normal electrochemical gradients. Lead has been associated with segmental demyelination due to the decreased synthesis of myelin lipids.

The term *synapse* refers to the space between the axon terminal of a neuron and a postsynaptic cell. The average neuron receives thousands of signals per second. Synaptic integration allows neurons to prioritize stimuli using summation and facilitation. The postsynaptic cell may be another neuron or it may be a muscle or gland cell. Technically, a synapse refers to nerve-to-nerve information transfer, whereas the neuromuscular junction is a term reserved for nerve-to-muscle information transfer. Synapses and neuromuscular junctions are the sites of chemical neurotransmission. The presynaptic bouton releases the chemical signal. Its effect is determined by the receptor on the postsynaptic membrane. The same neurotransmitter can induce excitatory or inhibitory responses, depending on the receptor. Neurotransmitter receptors are classified metabotropic or ionotropic based on their functional and physical characteristics. Ionotropic receptors form an ion channel pore and generate faster action than their metabotropic counterparts. Metabotropic receptors are linked through second messenger cascades. Specific receptors are defined by their pharmacological affinities; for example, all acetylcholine receptors respond to acetylcholine but respond to other molecules as well. Nicotinic acetylcholine receptors are especially responsive to nicotine, whereas muscarinic acetylcholine receptors are sensitive to muscarine.

Signal transmission can be disrupted in a variety of ways. The neuromuscular junction can be blocked; botulinus toxin irreversibly binds to the axon terminal and prevents the release of acetylcholine, whereas tetrodotoxin selectively blocks sodium channels. Compounds like dichlorodiphenyltrichloroethane (DDT), lindanes, and organochlorines depolarize the presynaptic nerve

terminal, which causes repetitive firing and seizures. Stimulants, depressants, receptor antago-
nists, and anticholinesterases can all disrupt signal transmission. Neurotransmission-associated
toxicities represent a category of toxicities that refer to any chemical that

- Affects the function of synaptic vesicles
- Blocks or activates synaptic or effector receptors
- Blocks the release of neurotransmitter
- Blocks the reuptake or degradation of neurotransmitter
- Produces uncontrolled release of neurotransmitter
- Interferes with action potential conduction

Chemicals that can produce neurotransmission-associated toxicities include those that

- Block impulse conduction along axons (e.g., local anesthetic and tetrodotoxin blockade of
  $Na^+$ channel function)
- Block synaptic function by interfering with the normal calcium channel activity, which
  triggers the release of synaptic vesicles (e.g., metals such as cadmium, lead, nickel, and
  cobalt; toxins such as curare, alpha-bungarotoxin)
- Activate synaptic function (e.g., nicotine)
- Block reuptake or breakdown of neurotransmitter resulting in receptor overstimulation
  (e.g., organophosphates, carbamates, which competitively bind acetylcholinesterase, thus
  blocking breakdown of acetylcholinesterase; cocaine, which blocks catecholamine reuptake)
- Produce massive release of neurotransmitter (e.g., black widow spider venom increases
  acetylcholine and amphetamine increases norepinephrine releases)
- Block the release of neurotransmitter (e.g., botulinum toxin blockage of acetylcholine release)

# Bibliography

Bajgar, J. (2004). Organophosphates/nerve agent poisoning: mechanism of action, diagnosis,
    prophylaxis, and treatment. *Advances in Clinical Chemistry, 38,* 151–216.

Bellinger, D. C. (2006). *Human developmental neurotoxicology.* Boca Raton, FL: CRC Press.

Blum, K., Manzo, L., & Blum, B. (2001). *Neurotoxicology* (Vol. 3). New York: Marcel Dekkar.

Bondy, S. C., & Campbell, A. (2005). Developmental neurotoxicology. *Journal of Neuroscience
    Research, 81,* 605–612.

Cory-Slechta, D. A. (2005). Studying toxicants as single chemicals: does this strategy adequately
    identify neurotoxic risk? *Neurotoxicology, 26,* 491–510.

Crofton, K. M., Makris, S. L., Sette, W. F., Mendez, E. , & Raffaele, K. C. (2004). A qualitative
    retrospective analysis of positive control data in developmental neurotoxicity studies.
    *Neurotoxicology and Teratology, 26,* 345–352.

Deng, W., & Poretz, R. D. (2003). Oligodendroglia in developmental neurotoxicity. *Neuro-
    toxicology, 24,* 161–178.

Gobba, F. (2003). Occupational exposure to chemicals and sensory organs: a neglected research
    field. *Neurotoxicology, 24,* 675–691.

Harry, G. J., & Tilson, H. A. (1999). *Neurotoxicology series: target organ toxicology series.* Boca
    Raton, FL: CRC Press.

Kaufmann, W. (2003). Current status of developmental neurotoxicity: an industry perspective. *Toxicology Letters, 140–141,* 161–169.

Klaassen, C. D. (2001). *Casarett & Doull's toxicology. The basic science of poisons.* New York: McGraw-Hill.

Klaassen, C. D., & Watkins, J. B. (2003). *Casarett & Doull's essentials of toxicology.* New York: McGraw-Hill.

LoPachin, R. M. (2004). The changing view of acrylamide neurotoxicity. *Neurotoxicology, 25,* 617–630.

LoPachin, R. M., Jones, R. C., Patterson, T. A., Slikker, W., Jr., & Barber, D. S. (2003). Application of proteomics to the study of molecular mechanisms in neurotoxicology. *Neurotoxicology, 24,* 761–775.

Massaro, E. J. (Ed.) (2002). *Handbook of neurotoxicology* (Vol. 1). Boca Raton, FL: Humana Press.

Massaro, E. J. (Ed.) (2002). *Handbook of neurotoxicology* (Vol. 2). Boca Raton, FL: Humana Press.

Schmid, C., & Rotenberg, J. S. (2005). Neurodevelopmental toxicology. *Neurologic Clinics, 23,* 321–336.

Shafer, T. J., Meyer, D. A., & Crofton, K. M. (2005). Developmental neurotoxicity of pyrethroid insecticides: critical review and future research needs. *Environmental Health Perspectives, 113,* 123–136.

Slikker, W., Xu, Z., & Wang, C. (2005). Application of a systems biology approach to developmental neurotoxicology. *Reproductive Toxicology, 19,* 305–319.

Spencer, P. S., Schamburg, H. H., & Ludolph, A. C. (2000). *Experimental and clinical neurotoxicology.* New York: Oxford University Press.

U.S. National Library of Medicine, National Institutes of Health, Environmental Health, and Toxicology Specialized Information Services (SIS). (2005). *Toxicology tutorial III: cellular toxicology, neurotoxicity.* Retrieved October 2, 2005 from http://www.sis.nlm.nih.gov/enviro/toxtutor.html.

Valciukas, J. A. (2002). *Foundations of environmental and occupational neurotoxicology.* New York: Transaction Publishers.

Wallace, D. R. (2005). Overview of molecular, cellular, and genetic neurotoxicology. *Neurologic Clinics, 23,* 307–320.

# The Practice of Toxicology

Toxicological information is important in making rational decisions with respect to protecting the public health from the chemical agents we are exposed to, by identifying those chemicals that pose the greatest risk for toxicity and by enabling safer chemicals to be developed. Toxicologists commonly work in industry, government, and academia. An important role of toxicologists is to develop safer pharmaceuticals, household products, industrial and agricultural chemicals, and food additives. Emphasis must always be placed on the protection of workers, consumers, and the environment, and thus products need to be tested under controlled laboratory conditions to assess for any toxic potential. The extent of toxicological testing depends on the potential use of the product. A new pharmaceutical or food additive, for example, is tested much more extensively than a chemical used by a few scientists under highly controlled conditions in a university research laboratory. Industrial toxicologists often work closely with regulatory agencies to ensure that a product and the processes used to make that product conform to established rules and regulations.

Toxicologists also work in academic institutions as instructors of toxicology and as researchers in their own areas of interest. Toxicologists who work in academia often work closely with industry and government as both consultant (e.g., serving on advisory committees) and scientific investigator (e.g., principal investigator on a research grant or testing contract).

Clinical toxicologists most often have medical degrees, typically in emergency medicine and pediatrics, with knowledge and clinical training in toxicology, requisite for the rational management of individuals who have been poisoned. Common situations include adverse effects of clinically relevant drugs; consumption of or exposure to chemicals while at home or on the job; ingestion of plants; and exposure to toxins from insects, spiders, snakes, or other animals. Clinical toxicologists provide advice not only on the management of poisoned patients, but also on issues related to environmental and occupational hazards associated with chemical exposure. Most clinical toxicologists work in hospitals, often with clinical pharmacologists, and may supervise the overall operations of a regional poison control center as well.

Probably most people have observed some aspect of toxicology practice through the media on issues related to the medicolegal aspects of drugs and poisonings, ranging from simple assessments concerning driving under the influence of alcohol to cases where accidental or intentional poisonings are suspected.

The forensic toxicologist may be called on as an "expert witness" to establish, determine, or justify the following:

- The methodology used to identify, isolate, and quantify a toxic substance in a biological sample
- The amount or concentration of chemical present in the sample analyzed
- When the exposure occurred and by what route
- If metabolism can affect the concentration and effect of the chemical on the body
- If the presence or absence of a specific chemical could account for a specific clinical behavior or condition
- Whether a therapeutic chemical was correctly taken, or if an accidental or intentional overdose resulted
- Whether other factors such as drug interactions, age-related differences in response, tolerance, and individual or genetic differences are involved

Environmental toxicologists, sometimes referred to as ecotoxicologists, study the effects on the environment of chemicals that have been discharged into the air, water, and soil. These effects include both the interactions of chemical agents with their physical surroundings and the immediate and long-term responses of organisms in the environment. Although environmental toxicologists may focus their immediate efforts on individual organisms for study, the ultimate concern is the effect of chemicals on populations and ecosystems. The environmental toxicologist tracks the movement of pollutants through aquatic and terrestrial food chains and assesses the potential for bioaccumulation. Although DDT (dichlorodiphenyltrichloroethane), was used for decades without serious incident in humans, evidence of bioaccumulation in plants and animals resulted in it being banned in the United States in 1972. Rachel Carson is credited by environmental advocates for first noting the egg shell thinning that later became the impetus for banning the insecticide in much of the world. The environmental impact of chemicals is now a major concern in regulating their use and disposal. The identification of changes in exposed populations from pollutants is of special concern, because lessons learned in the past have clearly shown that a particular species may lose its ability to compete for resources or suffer irreversible reproductive and genetic effects. An ultimate aim of environmental toxicology is to develop models that have the ability to predict the transport and fate of chemicals within an ecosystem.

Regulatory toxicologists need to consider what the standards for toxicological testing should be and the nature and limitations of toxicity testing. The objective of testing must be to produce and quantify the adverse effects of chemicals with respect to exposure and dose and to define, in a mechanistic fashion, the nature and scope of the harmful effect(s) produced. The regulatory toxicologist recognizes that sufficient information to fully assess a hazard may often be lacking, but in the absence of all the information needed to fully assess any hazard, they can still make rational decisions to predict the level of risk to public health in a given situation. Regulatory toxicologists are typically employed by governmental organizations and industry.

Based on toxicological data in laboratory animals, regulatory toxicologists often need to assess whether or not the data provided in support of a new drug, for example, satisfies the legal requirements needed to further test the drug clinically. Working with toxicologists and health professionals in various disciplines, regulatory toxicologists review current standards for acceptable exposures in both occupational and environmental settings or review and determine whether or not a chemical (e.g., pharmaceutical, food additive, pesticide) should be withdrawn from the market. Thalidomide is a classic example of the limitation of animal models to predict adverse human effects. Although some studies were done with rabbits that suggested birth defect (teratogenic) potential of the drug, the vast majority of animal studies gave thalidomide the proverbial "clean bill of health." In the 1950s thalidomide was considered safe enough by physicians in Europe and Canada for use during pregnancy; however, the U.S. Food and Drug Administration refused to grant it approval for use in the United States because of some troubling evidence of irreversible peripheral neuropathy. Despite this, it was imported from Canada and prescribed as a sleep aid and antinausea drug by American physicians under the name "Kevadon." By 1962 there were 8,000 reports of birth defects in 46 countries. Thalidomide was a danger to the developing fetus during the organogenic phase of development, resulting in limb abnormalities, organ dysfunction, and sometimes fetal death. The March of Dimes estimated that more than 10,000 infants were born with some sort of defect causally related to maternal use of thalidomide. Interestingly, it has been considered for limited use for Hansen's disease (leprosy), acquired immune deficiency syndrome, and for mitigating some of the symptoms of lupus, macular degeneration, some cancers, and rheumatoid arthritis. Those who take the drug must follow very precise instructions; women of childbearing age agree to use two forms of birth control and take monthly pregnancy tests, and men using thalidomide must agree to use condoms or undergo a vasectomy.

Many toxicologists have very specialized interests in toxicology. The Society of Toxicology Membership Directory, as an example, further illustrates the diversity of interests and specialties in toxicology. Specialty sections include biological modeling, carcinogenesis, comparative and veterinary toxicology, dermal toxicology, food safety, immunotoxicology, *in vitro* toxicology, inhalation toxicology, mechanistic toxicology, metals toxicology, molecular toxicology, neurotoxicology, epidemiology, occupational health, regulatory and safety evaluation, reproductive and developmental toxicology, risk assessment, and toxicological and exploratory pathology. This is by no means a comprehensive list; however, it serves to identify some of the major specialized interests within the very broad discipline of toxicology.

# Expectations and Requirements for Toxicologists: An Example Using a State Toxicologist

Practicing toxicologists hold a Masters or Doctoral degree and their experience is varied, as are the requirements for positions. The following job descriptions serve as examples of positions for State Toxicologists at different levels of responsibility.

## ASSOCIATE TOXICOLOGIST

Description:
Advises on the toxicological properties of chemicals for the purpose of advising on health and/or environmental problems; interprets and evaluates the less specialized experimental study results in terms of toxicological properties and hazards; evaluates, advises, and consults on the adequacy of toxicological data submitted by other organizations; advises on precautionary labeling for hazardous chemicals and products; may testify as an expert witness in hearings and court procedures; may serve in a lead capacity over other scientific and technical staff; and prepares reports and scientific papers for publication.

Education/Experience:
Possession of a Doctoral Degree in Toxicology, Biochemistry, Environmental Health, or a closely related specialty or a Master's Degree and 3 years of experience in designing and managing toxicological studies, interpreting results, and conducting hazard assessment or safety evaluations.

Knowledge of:
General principles of toxicology, with emphasis in environmental and occupational health concerns; laboratory and testing procedures for toxicological investigations; principles and procedures of risk assessment; and provisions of laws, rules, and regulations pertaining to the use, processing, and handling of toxic substances.

Must be able to:
Evaluate research studies in the fields of toxicology and pharmacology for application to issues of public health; work cooperatively with outside agencies and departmental staff; interpret and apply environmental and public health standards; communicate effectively; and analyze situations accurately and take effective action.

## SENIOR TOXICOLOGIST

Description:
Under general direction, originates, designs, and carries out toxicological studies and investigations; in a specific area of expertise, acts as statewide expert on the toxicological properties of chemicals for the purpose of advising on health and environmental problems; interprets and evaluates experimental study results in terms of toxicological properties and hazards, especially in the

area of expertise; evaluates, advises, and consults on the adequacy of toxicological data submitted by other organizations; advises on precautionary labeling for hazardous chemicals and products; provides technical consultation in areas such as legislation, rule, and regulation promulgation and policy development; testifies as an expert witness in hearings and court procedures; prepares reports and scientific papers for publication; and may serve in a lead capacity over other scientific and technical staff.

Education/experience qualifications:
Possession of a Doctoral Degree in Toxicology, Biochemistry, Pharmacology, or a closely related field and 4 years of experience in designing and managing toxicological studies, interpreting results, and conducting hazard assessment or safety evaluations.

Knowledge of:
All of the above and principles of toxicology and public health applicable to the recognition, identification, and quantification of relative hazards from exposure to chemicals in the environment; and one or more specialized areas in toxicology or a closely related field.

Must be able to:
All of the above and provide leadership in the evaluation and development of programs to implement toxicological practices and procedures on a statewide basis; and function as a specialist in one or several areas of toxicology.

## SUPERVISING TOXICOLOGIST (MANAGERIAL)

Description:
Under general direction, incumbents are responsible for providing significant input into departmental policy as it relates to toxicologic issues, monitoring those policies to ensure compliance, and possessing the authority to provide for the interpretation of those policies beyond the standard operating procedures. Incumbents also act as supervisor through subordinate supervisors over a moderate to large group of scientific and technical staff (10–20). Incumbents are responsible for the design and management of major projects addressing toxicological issues, participate in budget preparation and operational planning, and act as liaison with other managerial and administrative staff. The greatest portion of time is spent performing administrative and managerial duties.

Education/experience qualifications:
Two years of experience in the state service performing the duties of a Senior Toxicologist and Possession of a Doctoral Degree in Toxicology, Biochemistry, Pharmacology, or a closely related specialty.

Or

Five years of postdoctoral experience in toxicology or closely related field in positions of increasing responsibility. This experience must have included the interpretation of toxicological findings relative to probable human health hazards, 1 year of experience in the development and design of toxicological research and investigative studies, and two years of experience in supervisory or management positions.

Must possess knowledge of:
Principles and techniques of effective supervision and program budget management; and the ability to supervise the work of others; develop program policies, standards and procedures; organize the work of others effectively.

Based on the above discussion, you can see that our toxicologists may wear many hats and may be involved in

- Developing policy and regulations
- Research and development
- Scientific writing
- Public relations
- Legal proceedings as an expert witness
- Product safety and labeling
- Evaluation of test results
- Risk analysis

## Websites

Agency for Toxic Substances and Disease Registry (ATSDR):
http://www.atsdr.cdc.gov/

American Association of Poison Control Centers:
http://www.aapcc.org

American College of Medical Toxicology:
http://www.acmt.net/main/

Centers for Disease Control and Prevention (CDC):
http://www.cdc.gov/

ChemFinder:
http://chemfinder.cambridgesoft.com/

Environmental Protection Agency (EPA):
http://www.epa.gov/

EXTOXNET:
http://extoxnet.orst.edu/

Extremely Hazardous Substances (EHS):
http://yosemite.epa.gov/oswer/ceppoehs.nsf/EHS_Profile?openform

Food and Drug Administration (FDA):
http://www.fda.gov/

Hazardous Materials:
http://www.usfa.fema.gov/subjects/hazmat/

HSDB Hazardous Substances Data Bank:
http://toxnet.nlm.nih.gov/cgi-bin/sis/htmlgen?HSDB

IRIS Integrated Risk Information System:
http://toxnet.nlm.nih.gov/cgi-bin/sis/htmlgen?IRIS

IUPAC:
http://www.iupac.org/dhtml_home.html

ITER International Toxicity Estimates for Risk:
http://toxnet.nlm.nih.gov/cgi-bin/sis/htmlgen?iter

Material Safety Data Sheets Online:
http://www.ilpi.com/msds/index.html

Medwatch Homepage:
http://www.fda.gov/medwatch/report/hcp.htm

National Institute of Environmental Health Sciences (NIEHS):
http://www.niehs.nih.gov/

National Institutes of Health (NIH):
http://www.nih.gov/

National Institute for Occupational Safety and Health (NIOSH):
http://www.cdc.gov/niosh/homepage.html

National Report on Human Exposure to Environmental Chemicals:
http://www.cdc.gov/exposurereport/

National Toxicology Program:
http://ntp-server.niehs.nih.gov/

Occupational Safety and Health Administration (OSHA):
http://www.osha.gov/

Poisonous Plants Informational Database:
http://www.ansci.cornell.edu/plants/

Recognition and Management of Pesticide Poisonings:
http://npic.orst.edu/rmpp.htm

Registry of Toxic Effects of Chemical Substances:
http://www.cdc.gov/niosh/97-119.html

Right to Know Hazardous Substance Fact Sheets:
http://www.state.nj.us/health/eoh/rtkweb/rtkhsfs.htm

Toxicon Multimedia Project:
http://www.uic.edu/com/er/toxikon/

TOXLINE:
http://toxnet.nlm.nih.gov/cgi-bin/sis/htmlgen?TOXLINE

TRI Toxics Release Inventory:
http://toxnet.nlm.nih.gov/cgi-bin/sis/htmlgen?TRI

United States Department of Agriculture:
http://www.usda.gov/

World Health Organization:
http://www.who.int

## Bibliography

Hayes, W. A. (Ed.) (2001). *Principles and methods of toxicology* (4th ed.). New York: Taylor & Francis.

Klaassen, C. D. (2001). *Casarett & Doull's toxicology. The basic science of poisons*. New York: McGraw-Hill.

Klaassen, C. D., & Watkins, J. B. (2003). *Casarett & Doull's essentials of toxicology*. New York: McGraw-Hill.

U.S. National Library of Medicine, National Institutes of Health, Environmental Health, and Toxicology Specialized Information Services (SIS). (2005). *Toxicology tutorial III*. Retrieved October 2, 2005, from http://www.sis.nlm.nih.gov/enviro/toxtutor.html.

# CHAPTER 19

# Regulatory Considerations

## Standards, Guidelines, and Regulatory Agencies

The purpose of exposure guidelines and standards is to protect the public from the potentially harmful effects from certain chemical agents. They represent what are believed to be (at the time they were written) both achievable and reasonable exposure levels, that is, levels deemed to be safe under defined conditions (exposure time, temperature, level of personal protective equipment, etc.). There are differences between guidelines and standards. Guidelines are recommended levels of exposure, not to exceed a certain maximum level. They are not legally enforceable but are rather voluntary levels developed by both regulatory and nonregulatory bodies. In contrast, a standard results from formal governmental rule-making and is legal and enforceable to the extent that violators may be subject to fines and/or imprisonment.

Federal, state, and local regulatory agencies have the authority to establish environmental and occupational standards and guidelines. Federal regulatory agencies establish standards for consumer products, drugs, and foods. In the United States there are numerous federal laws and agencies in place to protect the public's health from exposures to potentially toxic chemicals. Examples of federal agencies that oversee this activity include the following:

- Food and Drug Administration (FDA)
- Consumer Product Safety Commission (CPSC)
- Department of Agriculture (USDA)
- Environmental Protection Agency (EPA)
- Occupational Safety and Health Administration (OSHA)

- National Institute for Occupational Safety and Health (NIOSH)
- Department of Transportation (DOT)
- Drug Enforcement Agency (DEA)

Examples of federal laws that have been enacted to define and regulate exposures to potentially hazardous chemicals are numerous and diverse:

- Federal Food, Drug, and Cosmetics Act (FFDCA): regulated by the FDA and covers food, drugs, medical devices, cosmetics, food and color additives, and so on
- Food Quality Protection Act (FQPA): under the Federal Food, Drug, and Cosmetic Act (FDCA), the EPA establishes tolerances (maximum legally permissible levels) for pesticide residues in food
- Federal Hazardous Substance Act (FHSA): regulated by CPSC for toxic household products
- Consumer Product Safety Act (CPSA): regulated by CPSC to oversee hazardous consumer products
- Occupational Safety and Health Act: OSHA and NIOSH regulation of hazardous chemicals in the workplace
- Federal Insecticide, Fungicide and Rodenticide Act (FIFRA): EPA regulation of pesticides
- Clean Air Act (CAA): EPA regulation of air pollutants
- Clean Water Act (CWA): EPA regulation of water pollutants
- Safe Drinking Water Act (SDWA): EPA regulation of contaminants in drinking water
- Toxic Substance Control Act (TSCA): EPA regulation of toxic chemicals not covered by other laws

Many of the federal regulatory agencies listed carry out numerous activities and deal with multiple laws that are often complex in nature. This can be reflected in a considerably wide organizational "division of labor." The FDA, for example, has a number of centers involved in evaluating the safety and effectiveness of chemicals that are presently being used and those that may in the future be used by American consumers (both human and nonhuman). These centers are as follows:

- Center for Drug Evaluation and Research (CDER): regulates human drugs and biological drug products
- Center for Food Safety and Applied Nutrition (CFSAN): monitors food products, dietary supplements, and cosmetics
- Center for Veterinary Medicine (CVM): regulates products used by animals like medicine and feed.
- National Center for Toxicological Research (NCTR): conducts research to elucidate the mechanisms of action underlying the toxicity of products regulated by the FDA. NCTR also develops methods to improve assessment of human exposure and risk. FDA's research activities provide the scientific basis for regulatory actions and guiding the setting of regulatory standards.

## Public Awareness and Public Outrage

The history and growth of these agencies and the enactment of protective laws (acts) has frequently been sparked by the public's awareness of problems or incidents that have affected or potentially could adversely affect the environment, the individual's health, the general quality of life, or the health of a community or susceptible group within a community (e.g., children, the elderly, or individuals with a preexisting medical condition).

The practice of adulteration of foods and medications with untested preservatives or other chemicals was commonplace when there were no regulatory controls in place to define and enforce standards for food and drug purity and safety. Some of the early history of governmental attempts to address these issues is interesting but shocking by today's standards. Consider the dozen men who beginning in 1903 knowingly sat down to dine on food containing suspected toxic chemicals:

> O, they may get over it but they'll never look the same, that kind of bill of fare would drive most men insane. Next week he'll give them mothballs, a la Newburgh or else plain; O, they may get over it but they'll never look the same.
>
> (Chorus from "Song of the Poison Squad," Lew Dockstader's Minstrels, October 1903)

This human experiment took place over a period of approximately 5 years in the basement (complete with kitchen, dining room, and laboratory) of the USDA's former Bureau of Chemistry (now the FDA) in Washington, DC. The project was largely spearheaded by chief chemist Harvey W. Wiley, MD, often considered the founding father of the FDA. One of his concerns was the common practice of using borax as a food preservative and the fraudulent use of the term "pure" for many items of food. Wiley and other scientists recruited healthy young male volunteers who worked within the USDA to dine on wholesome meals to which substances suspected as being harmful were added. The volunteers agreed not to hold the government responsible for any injury or illness that might result from the consumption of these meals. Congress had even appropriated funds to carry out the proposed "hygienic table trials." This activity, of course, also fed the news media, who described these individuals as the "The Poison Squad" (Figure 19.1). Several preservatives, including borax, sodium benzoate, sulfuric acid, salicylic acid, and formaldehyde, were tested over a period of 5 years and at a dose range from 0.5 g to 4 g daily. Early in the experiments the volunteers developed a distaste for some of the additives and began to eat less and less of the foods that were distasteful to them, until they eventually avoided that food altogether. It was therefore decided that the preservatives would no longer be hidden in the food but rather they would be administered inside of a gelatin capsule to be consumed some time during the middle of the meal. This remained the protocol over the 5-year period of study.

Dr. Wiley stopped the testing only when the chemicals had made several of the volunteers so ill with stomachaches, nausea, and vomiting that they could not function at work. Stories of this ran so rampant in the media throughout the United States that it helped Dr. Wiley gain a congressional hearing, thus helping to pave the way for federal regulation of foods and drugs in the United States by enactment of the Pure Food and Drug Act of 1906, also called the "Wiley Act."

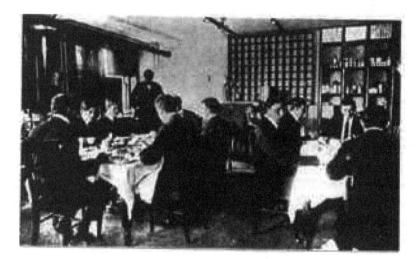

**FIGURE 19.1**   The "Poison Squad." *Source:* Courtesy of U.S. Food and Drug Administration.

Although the Food and Drug Act of 1906 prohibited interstate transportation of adulterated drugs and foods, it did little to ensure safety and quality for the consumer from potentially dangerous chemicals present in "therapeutic" preparations and in foods. As is often the case, it would take a tragic incident to rethink better ways to protect the health of the public. One such incident occurred in 1937, when approximately 100 people died from ingesting an elixir of sulfanilamide produced by the S.E. Massengill Company. Sulfanilamide had long been used in solid form to treat certain bacterial infections. An elixir was developed by Harold Watkins with the intent to make the product easier to swallow, especially by children. Unfortunately, diethyl glycol was used as a solvent, and whereas a small amount of it on the tip of the tongue may have passed Watkins's taste test, he did not realize that this chemical, commonly known as antifreeze, would be toxic in larger doses. Children being treated for bacterial infections of the throat were among those affected by the elixir. Over the course of several weeks, individuals experienced nausea and vomiting, severe abdominal pain, and cessation of urine production. Once notified of the problem, the FDA sent their investigators into the field. The investigators eventually tracked down the remaining supply of elixir and took it off of the shelf. Ironically, S.E. Massengill Company did not violate existing laws despite producing an unsafe product. Simple toxicity tests on animals or even a review of the currently existing scientific literature would have revealed diethyl glycol to be toxic to the kidneys, possibly resulting in renal failure. Unfortunately, in 1937 the existing laws did not prohibit the sale of untested or dangerous drugs. Dr. Samuel Evans Massengill, the firm's owner, said, "My chemists and I deeply regret the fatal results, but there was no error in the manufacture of the product. We have been supplying a legitimate professional demand and not once could have foreseen the unlooked-for results. I do not feel that there was any responsibility on our part." Harold Watkins did not share this sentiment and committed suicide after learning of the effects of his formulation.

The only charge against the company was of mislabeling. The FDA indicated that the term *elixir* implied that the product was an alcoholic solution, whereas in fact it did not contain alcohol but rather the toxic diethylene glycol solution. If the product had been labeled a "solution" instead of an "elixir," there would have been no violation of existing laws and the FDA would have had no legal authority to even recover any remaining product still on the shelf.

FDA Commissioner Walter Campbell, who was then pressing for better federal regulation of drugs, said, "These unfortunate occurrences may be expected to continue because new and relatively untried drug preparations are being manufactured almost daily at the whim of the individual manufacturer, and the damage to public health cannot accurately be estimated. The only remedy for such a situation is the enactment by Congress of an adequate and comprehensive national Food and Drugs Act which will require that all medicines placed upon the market shall be safe to use under the directions for use. . . ."

The year after the incident resulted in the replacement of the Pure Food and Drug Act of 1906 by the Federal Food, Drug, and Cosmetic Act of 1938. This new law required that proof of safety be provided to the FDA before any drug was sold to the public. The definition of a drug, as it is written in the FDCA in 1938, is any product used to diagnose, cure, mitigate, treat, or prevent a disease. Safety was the key issue here, not whether the drug in fact provided any benefit at all. It took almost 25 additional years for Congress to pass, in 1962, the Kefauver-Harris Drug Amendments, which added the requirement that drugs must also be effective.

## Regulatory and Nonregulatory Agencies: Their Role in Protecting Public Health from Chemical Exposures

### FDA

Protecting the public health from chemical-induced injury can involve extensive safety testing and the expenditure of significant financial resources, especially for any chemical that would be intentionally consumed by the public (e.g., a food preservative or a drug). As an example, let's look briefly at the process by which chemicals can receive the FDA approval requisite for their use by the American public. Our chemical is a food preservative developed by the Kracklin Good Cereal Company.

Our hypothetical food preservative was developed approximately 5 years ago and is present in several hundred boxes of bran wheat flakes at a final formulated concentration of 0.50 ppm. These boxes have remained on storage shelves within the company. Inspection of the cereal after 5 years has shown no apparent deterioration of the product. The cereal maintained the typical flavor and crunchiness that one would expect from that which was freshly produced, even boxes that were opened a year or more ago, "resealed," and replaced back on the shelf. Indeed, the food chemist (also the company owner) who developed this patented preservative has consumed a sizable bowl of this well-preserved cereal each morning over the past 2 years.

Realizing the marketing potential of this chemical, the owner consults with the FDA (Center for Food Safety and Applied Nutrition) to see what is required to get his product on the market. It becomes clear to him that compliance with the Federal Food, Drug, and Cosmetic Act (FDCA) of 1938 is required. This Act gives the FDA authority over food and food ingredients and defines the requirements for truth in labeling for ingredients. In addition, the Food Additives Amendment to the Food Drug and Cosmetic Act (1958) requires FDA approval for the use of an additive's inclusion in food.

The Food Additives Amendment exempts two groups of substances from this regulation process. All substances that the FDA or the USDA had deemed safe for use in specific foods before the 1958 amendment are designated as prior-sanctioned substances (e.g., sodium nitrite and potassium nitrite used to preserve processed meats). The other excluded category from the food additive regulation process is the Generally Recognized As Safe (GRAS) chemicals (e.g., salt, sugar, spices, vitamins, and monosodium glutamate). This category includes chemicals whose use is generally recognized by experts as safe, based on published scientific evidence or their extensive history of use in food before 1958. An additive may not receive approval or may lose its approval if it is found to cause cancer in humans or animals. This clause is often referred to by the name of its congressional sponsor, Rep. James Delaney (D-N.Y.).

To market the new preservative, the Kracklin Good Cereal Company must provide convincing evidence to the FDA that

- There are no comparable preservatives in current use that have the same preservation capability as the new chemical.
- The new preservative indeed performs as is claimed by the manufacturer.
- The new preservative is safe to humans at both the highest level of short-term or long-term consumption that any individual could realistically achieve (consumption of 2 pounds of cereal per day for 365 days per year is possible but not likely; consumption of 20 pounds of cereal per day for 365 days per year is not a realistic exposure scenario).

Convincing evidence to the FDA about safety goes well beyond the incidental information that the owner has, over the past several years, himself consumed cereal formulated with the preservative without any apparent adverse effects. For the FDA, animal studies using very large doses of the additive over a long period of time may be necessary to show that it would not be harmful at the expected levels of human consumption, and indeed at levels far greater than could possibly be achieved by humans.

Information for FDA consideration is typically as follows:

- Proposal for its use as a food preservative (technical effect)
- Amount to be added to food
- Identity and chemical composition of the preservative
- Chemical quantitation methods for its detection in food
- Laboratory toxicology studies
- Environmental information (for EPA compliance)

Safety information must be provided to the FDA so they can determine whether the additive is safe to use as intended, in what types of foods it can be used, the maximum amounts to be used, and how it should best be identified on food labels. Although the owner can provide the FDA with a great deal of the technical information that is required, his company is not qualified to provide any toxicological assessments. To establish no harmful effects at the highest expected levels of human consumption for the new preservative requires toxicity studies using large doses of the preservative over both short and long periods of time. Because absolute safety can never be proven, the FDA must base safety on the best information and tests available.

The company in this case would need to contract for these toxicity tests using a certified contract laboratory. The type of toxicity tests that the FDA may require are as follows:

- Acute oral study with rodent
- Metabolism studies
- Feeding study (at least 28 days) with rodent
- Subchronic feeding study (90-day) using rodent with *in utero* exposure
- Subchronic feeding study (90-day) with rodent
- Subchronic feeding study (90-day) with nonrodent species
- Lifetime feeding study (~2-year) using rodent with *in utero* exposure for carcinogenesis and chronic toxicity
- Lifetime feeding study (~2-year) with rodent for carcinogenesis
- Feeding study (at least 1 year) with nonrodent species
- Multigenerational reproduction feeding study (minimum of two generations) with teratology phase using rodent
- Teratology study

Because the preservative would be present in the formulated cereal at a maximum concentration of 0.50 ppm (=500 parts per billion), the FDA expressed a "significant level of concern" requiring both short- and long-term tests to be performed, including multigenerational reproductive and carcinogenic studies. It became apparent to the owner that conducting these types of tests would be very costly.

The rationale and appropriate forms for specific toxicological tests can be located on FDA websites (e.g., FDA "Redbook" website Toxicological Principles for the Safety Assessment of Food Ingredients: http://www.cfsan.fda.gov/~redbook/). If you view the online templates, you can directly see the amount of detail required in support of an application for our hypothetical food preservative. Short-term, long-term, and even multigenerational studies would likely be required by the FDA, and this is understandable in light of a no current requirement for premarketing studies in humans. So although the consumption of cereal over the past several years by the owner of the company is of interest to the FDA, animal toxicity tests serve as the basis for either accepting or rejecting the application to market the food preservative. In deciding whether the additive should be approved, the FDA considers all the factors that bear on safety; however, absolute safety for any substance can never be proven, and thus a determination must be made under the proposed conditions of use and based on the best information available at the time.

If our hypothetical additive is approved, the FDA would issue regulations that may include the types of foods where it may be used, the maximum allowable amounts to be present, and how it should be identified on the appropriate food labels. Regulations known as Good Manufacturing Practices (GMP) limit the amount of the preservative to that which is necessary to achieve the desired effect. If approval is granted, the FDA monitors the extent of consumer consumption as well as any new research concerning its safety; generally, there is a period of time where the scientific community will jump on an opportunity to test a new chemical for its biological effects. The FDA operates an Adverse Reaction Monitoring System (ARMS), which is a computerized database to assist officials in determining whether any reported adverse reactions may represent a true public health hazard.

As we have seen, there is no current FDA premarketing requirement for human safety testing of our hypothetical new food preservative, despite the fact that it may be consumed by millions of people on a daily basis. For any new chemical whose use is intended as a drug, the premarketing process requires *both* safety test results from animals and test results from humans.

The process of drug discovery and screening is one where, ideally, a new chemical is produced that has the desired benefits to the body and is without significant toxicity. Today, the principal sponsors of drug discovery, the pharmaceutical companies and universities, facilitate the process of discovery by using very sophisticated computer modeling to identify, "manufacture," and manipulate compounds that, at least in theory, should produce the desired effect on the body ("structure–activity" relationships). From the theoretical to the actual involves the synthesis and purification of the new chemical and its testing for safety and efficacy in living systems. Before this chemical can be given to humans, first its safety must be clearly established through the use of appropriate surrogate models that are acceptable to the FDA. Laboratory animal testing needs to include sufficient information to assess safety, because a new drug candidate has the potential, like any chemical, to produce toxicity at either a high enough single dose or through multiple lower doses. As such, extensive testing may be required to predict by inference the chemical's physiological and pathological effects in humans. During this preclinical period, short-term animal studies provide toxicokinetic information concerning the absorption, distribution, metabolism, storage, elimination, and acute toxicity of the chemical. Longer term animal studies may concentrate on issues related to reproduction, teratogenicity, or carcinogenicity.

With the appropriate animal test results, the sponsor would apply to the FDA by filing an Investigational New Drug (IND) application. This is not a marketing application but rather a request for an exemption from a federal statute under the Food and Drug Act of 1906 that prohibits the transport of unapproved drugs in interstate commerce. Sufficient information must be contained within the IND (e.g., preclinical safety information from toxicity tests in laboratory animals, *in vitro* assays, chemical information and manufacturing processes, quality control information, a proposal for initial testing in humans) to allow the FDA to evaluate the likelihood of proceeding to limited testing in humans (clinical trials, Phase I). Pharmaceutical companies "outside" of the United States and FDA regulatory authority may provide evidence about the safety and efficacy of a new compound from human studies, thus providing additional support to proceed with clinical testing in the United States. Once the

FDA approves the IND, clinical trials may begin in the United States. The FDA has 30 days by law to review the IND and provide notification to the sponsor as to the acceptability of the application. The CDER monitors clinical trials to ensure the test subjects are not exposed to any unnecessary risks.

The objective of a clinical trial is to provide information about human safety and efficacy. Clinical trials are typically conducted in three distinct phases:

- Phase I: The sponsor tests the new chemical for safety, usually in a small volunteer group of 20–80 healthy individuals. The goals at this stage of clinical study include the elucidation of the toxicokinetics of the chemical, any manifestations of toxicity or side effects, a dose range that is suitable for later clinical testing, and the determination of the maximum tolerated dose (MTD). The MTD may be defined as a dose that results in either an unexpected toxicity or a predictable toxicity in a certain percentage of the subjects being studied (toxicity may be manifested as an objective sign, e.g., change in blood pressure or changes in blood chemistry, or a subjective symptom, e.g., a feeling of nausea or dizziness).

- Phase II: Based on the information from Phase I, the sponsor further tests the product's safety and effectiveness and establishes the most likely range of doses for a larger group of individuals; however, at this point they are *patient* volunteers. The objective of this phase is to establish the effectiveness of the chemical in individuals who have the appropriate medical condition for which the drug was developed (e.g., high blood pressure, high cholesterol, asthma), that is, to establish the efficacy of the drug candidate in a larger group of subjects (often several hundred).

- Phase III: By evaluating the results from large-scale, multicenter, clinical trials, the sponsor can provide the support that the drug candidate is both safe and effective and thus marketed in the United States.

With the completion of the above-referenced studies, the sponsor of the new drug candidate can apply to the FDA for marketing approval. The application, called a New Drug Application (NDA), contains preclinical and clinical data as well as other relevant information required by the FDA (Figure 19.2). The development of new drugs is extremely costly and time consuming, and most new chemicals are abandoned early in the process if they do not appear to be promising for continued development. It is not uncommon for a new chemical to take a decade of development and testing before it receives approval for marketing.

Recognizing that this is a long process, the FDA has made approval possible outside of the traditional

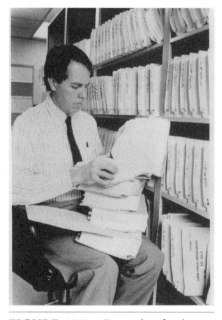

**FIGURE 19.2** Example of volume of information required to market new drug. *Source:* Courtesy of U.S. Food and Drug Administration.

pathways through the "accelerated development" and "parallel track" (Figure 19.3). Accelerated development is reserved for drug candidates that would be used for very serious and life-threatening illness and where other available therapies have been shown to be ineffective or minimally effective as treatments. A surrogate end-point and restricted use are FDA requirements. A "surrogate end-point," as defined by the FDA, is a laboratory finding or physical sign likely to predict benefit to the patient. As an example, the shrinkage of a tumor (which was unresponsive to other available treatments) could be the surrogate for increased patient survival. This pathway of drug development requires that the sponsor continues to test the drug for benefit and safety after approval of clinical testing. The parallel track allows greater use of experimental chemicals for the treatment of certain disease states. It was developed in response to the acquired immune deficiency syndrome (AIDS) epidemic by the U.S. Public Health Service as a policy that permits these individuals, whose compromised immune status would otherwise prohibit inclusion in controlled studies, to receive treatment with promising investigational drugs.

A third nontraditional pathway is via the "treatment investigational new drugs" alternative. This pathway may be used for desperately ill patients to receive investigational new drugs as early in the clinical stage of the drug development process as possible. There must be acceptable preliminary evidence of drug efficacy and no comparable alternative drug or therapy available to treat that stage of the disease.

Although the FDA can approve the use of a chemical as a drug, it does not establish a standard for exposure to it. What it does is provide guidance for usage and ensures that appropriate warnings concerning adverse effects are in place. The pharmaceutical manufacturer must provide this information to both the medical personnel who can prescribe the drug and to the con-

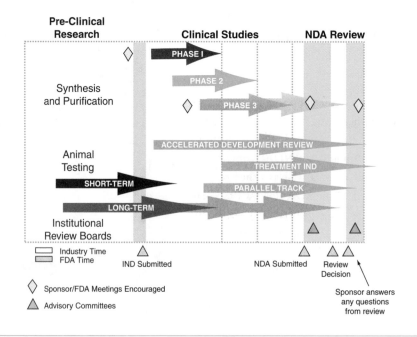

**FIGURE 19.3**    Procedure for new drug development source. *Source:* Courtesy of U.S. Food and Drug Administration.

sumer (patient) who uses it. Information is generally provided through several means, including labeling and package inserts that accompany a drug, the *Physicians Desk Reference (PDR)*, and publications in journals. Clearly, early in the history of any new drug, information concerning its effects, both positive and negative, largely comes from the manufacturer who provides information about

- Chemical description
- Available forms
- Pharmacology
- Indications and usage
- Dosage and administration
- Warnings
- Precautions
- Contraindications
- Adverse reactions
- Overdosage
- Drug interactions

Another consideration is who is responsible for ensuring the safety of cosmetics. Despite the enormous usage by the American population of items that we typically lump into the category of cosmetics, these products and the ingredients contained therein are not subject to any pre-marketing approval by the FDA, with the exception of color additives. The FDA can, however, inspect cosmetic manufacturing facilities for issues related to product adulteration and mislabeling. But it is the cosmetic firms who are solely responsible for ensuring the safety of their product and the ingredients that are used in its production before marketing. Failure to do so could result in a misbranded product unless a warning statement is conspicuously displayed on the product label, such as "Warning—The safety of this product has not been determined." As found in "21 CFR 740.10."

The Code of Federal Regulations (CFR) is the codification of the general and permanent rules published in the *Federal Register* by the executive departments and agencies of the federal government. It is essentially a compilation of the administrative laws that govern federal regulatory agency practice and procedure. It is divided into 50 titles that represent broad areas subject to federal regulation. It is revised annually and contains the whole of the daily *Federal Register* along with previously issued but still current regulations. The number preceding CFR indicates the title number (e.g., 21, Cosmetics) and the number following is that of the rule number. These regulations can be purchased in book/hardcopy form or they can now be viewed online at www.access.gpo.gov.

A number of ingredients are specifically prohibited or have restricted use as cosmetic ingredients. These include bithionol (an antibacterial agent that can cause skin phototoxicity), mercury, vinyl chloride, methylene chloride, chloroform, and aerosols containing zirconium.

The FDA does not have the authorization to require the recall of cosmetics; however, it does monitor company product recalls and may request a company to remove a product from the market that is deemed to be "dangerous" should the company not voluntarily do so. In addition, any cosmetic that is mislabeled or adulterated may be subject to FDA regulatory action through the Department of Justice and the federal court system, including restraint against further man-ufacture and distribution, seizure of product, and criminal action against an individual or com-pany violating the law.

Cosmetic manufacturers are neither required by law to register their establishment with the FDA nor are they required to file information concerning the composition of their product or report cosmetic-related injuries. The FDA, however, encourages manufacturers of cosmetics to register and file a Cosmetic Product Ingredient Statement with them as part of the FDA's Voluntary Cosmetic Registration Program.

## EPA

The EPA, established in 1970, is charged with ensuring the protection of the environment and overseeing our nation's environmental health through the activities of environmental standards setting, environmental monitoring, enforcement, and research. The agency developed out of the National Environmental Policy Act of 1969. Before its inception, industry was often able to sidestep local regulations; however, with the creation of a federal entity, nationwide enforcement of legislation was possible. For over 30 years the EPA has been working to provide the American public with a cleaner and healthier environment.

The EPA is an extremely large and complex federal agency (Figure 19.4). The responsibilities of the EPA are enormous and include the development and enforcement of environmental reg-ulations, publication of information on environmental issues for public awareness, research sup-port to educational and other institutions outside of their own in-house research efforts, techni-cal publications, advancing educational efforts for environmental awareness and protection, sponsorship of programs for industry and nonprofit organizations, research and educational institutions, and state and local governments.

The following environmental acts of Congress are examples through which the EPA carries out its activities:

- 1947 Federal Insecticide, Fungicide, and Rodenticide Act
- 1948 Federal Water Pollution Control Act (also known as the Clean Water Act)
- 1955 Clean Air Act
- 1965 Shoreline Erosion Protection Act
- 1965 Solid Waste Disposal Act
- 1970 National Environmental Policy Act
- 1970 Pollution Prevention Packaging Act
- 1970 Resource Recovery Act
- 1971 Lead-Based Paint Poisoning Prevention Act
- 1972 Coastal Zone Management Act
- 1972 Marine Protection, Research, and Sanctuaries Act
- 1972 Ocean Dumping Act
- 1973 Endangered Species Act
- 1974 Safe Drinking Water Act
- 1974 Shoreline Erosion Control Demonstration Act
- 1975 Hazardous Materials Transportation Act

- 1976 Resource Conservation and Recovery Act (RCRA)
- 1976 Toxic Substances Control Act (TSCA)
- 1977 Surface Mining Control and Reclamation Act
- 1978 Uranium Mill-Tailings Radiation Control Act
- 1980 Asbestos School Hazard Detection and Control Act
- 1980 Comprehensive Environmental Response, Compensation, and Liability Act (CERCLA)
- 1982 Nuclear Waste Policy Act
- 1984 Asbestos School Hazard Abatement Act
- 1986 The Superfund Amendments and Reauthorization Act (SARA)
- 1986 Asbestos Hazard Emergency Response Act
- 1986 Emergency Planning and Community Right to Know Act
- 1988 Indoor Radon Abatement Act
- 1988 Lead Contamination Control Act

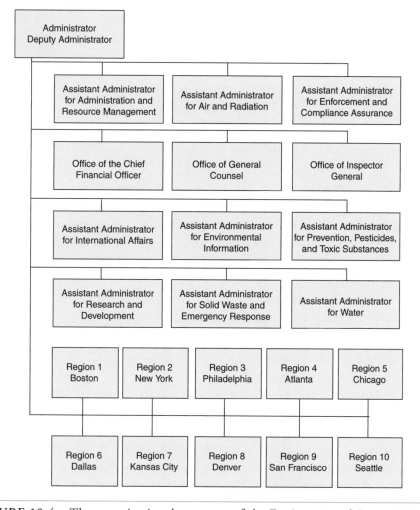

**FIGURE 19.4**  The organizational structure of the Environmental Protection Agency. *Source:* Courtesy of the EPA.

- 1988 Medical Waste Tracking Act
- 1988 Ocean Dumping Ban Act
- 1988 Shore Protection Act
- 1990 National Environmental Education Act

An early goal of the EPA was to establish baseline standards for healthy air and water by amending those earlier acts dealing with air and water, thus resulting in what are commonly referred to today as the Clean Air Act (CAA) and the Clean Water Act (CWA). Air quality standards are issued by the EPA under CAA, including air emissions standards for industry and national ambient air quality standards (NAAQS). When air emissions exceed the levels established for industry, additional control measures by industry are acquired to reduce the discharge of pollutants to an acceptable level. The primary NAAQS pertain to human health, whereas secondary standards exist to protect nonhumans (e.g., animals, crops, physical structures, visibility). Air quality standards have been established for what are referred to as the criteria pollutants: oxides of sulfur and nitrogen, carbon monoxide, ozone, lead, particulates, and hydrocarbons (Table 19.1).

Amending existing laws is an ongoing activity of EPA as well as other agencies; the purpose is to better reflect the best available data and changing views concerning protecting the environment and the health of the public. As an example, recent amendments to the Clean Air Act include considerations to the ozone layer and the effects of acid rain to the environment. Supplemental legislation, like the Toxic Substances Control Act (TSCA), addresses areas not explicitly covered by the CAA and the CWA . The realization that some species are at risk for extinction from environmental exposure to pesticides led to the Endangered Species Act. Pesticides cannot be marketed until they have been registered by the EPA in accordance with the FIFRA. To register a new pesticide or to re-register a currently used one with the EPA requires extensive toxicity testing, chemical analyses, and environmental fate and transport analysis. The EPA has also established standards for the amount of pesticide permissible on foods, referred to as pesticide tolerances. As an example, you may have a tolerance for the organophosphate pesticide malathion at 0.0001 ppm (= 0.1 ppb) for cucumbers.

The EPA is also charged with regulating standards for water through the CWA and the SDWA. The maximum contaminant level (MCL) is a standard that if exceeded requires immediate attention to reduce the level of contaminant. The MCL is different depending on the particular chemical. For example, for the pesticide chlordane it is 0.002 mg/l, for lead it is 0.05 mg/l, and for TCE it is 0.005 mg/l of water. In addition, the EPA can also propose recommended guidelines for chemicals in drinking water where a standard may not be available or if that standard is currently under review. For example, a maximum contaminant level goal (MCLG) may be recommended for long-term exposures to contaminants in drinking water, or health advisories (voluntary exposure guidelines) may be issued for short- and long-term exposures to chemicals that are noncarcinogenic.

The EPA also issues exposure guidance in ambient water quality criteria for groundwater not intended for drinking purposes but rather for recreational purposes (e.g., swimming, fishing). The regulation of hazardous wastes by EPA comes under the guidance of the Resource Conservation and Recovery Act (RCRA) and the Comprehensive Environmental Response,

**Table 19.1**    National Ambient Air Quality Standards

| Pollutant | Primary Standard (Public Health) | | | Secondary Standard (Public Welfare) | | |
|---|---|---|---|---|---|---|
| | Level | Averaging Time | Form | Level | Averaging Time | Form |
| Ozone | 0.12 ppm | 1 hour | More than 3 days over 3 years | Same as primary standard | | |
| | 0.08 ppm | 8 hours | 3-year average of annual fourth highest daily minimum | Same as primary standard | | |
| Particulate matter 10 μm or smaller ($PM_{10}$) | 150 μg/m$^3$ | 24 hours | 3-year average of annual 99 percentiles | Same as primary standard | | |
| | 50 μg/m$^3$ | Annual | Not to be exceeded | | | |
| Particulate matter 2.5 μm or smaller ($PM_{2.5}$) | 65 μg/m$^3$ | 24 hours | 3-year average of annual averages | Same as primary standard | | |
| | 15 μg/m$^3$ | Annual | 3-year average of 98 percentiles | | | |
| Carbon monoxide | 35 ppm | 1 hour | More than once per year | No secondary standard | | |
| | 9 ppm | 8 hours | | | | |
| Sulfur dioxide | 0.14 ppm | 24 hours | More than once per year | 0.50 ppm | 3 hours | More than once per year |
| | 0.03 ppm | Annual | | | | |
| Nitrogen dioxide | 0.053 ppm | Annual | Not to be exceeded | Same as primary standard | | |
| Lead | 1.5 μg/m$^3$ | Quarterly | Not to be exceeded | Same as primary standard | | |

ppm = parts per million.

*Source:* Data from: http://www.epa.gov/air/index.html.

Compensation and Liability Act (CERCLA), commonly known as Superfund. CERCLA was enacted by Congress in 1980 for the purpose of creating a pool of funds dedicated to the cleanup of hazardous chemicals from highly contaminated and generally abandoned sites (Figure 19.5); it was funded by a tax on petroleum and chemical industries.

The Superfund Amendments and Reauthorization Act (SARA) amended CERCLA in 1986. It took lessons learned from the enforcement of CERCLA and attempted to close loopholes and simplify some of the complexities. Additionally considered was the importance of providing more permanent solutions for dealing with hazardous waste sites, the increasing role that states should play in dealing with Superfund issues, new ways to enforce regulation and settle disputes, and an emphasis on potential health problems associated with contaminated sites to both

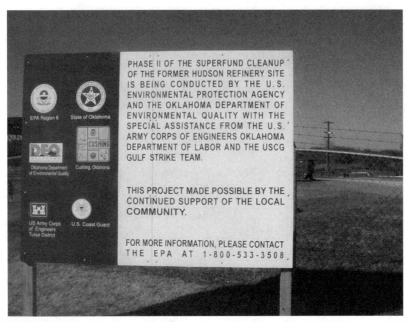

**FIGURE 19.5**    Posting notice for a Superfund site. *Source:* Courtesy of EPA.

surrounding community and Superfund workers. The EPA has developed a list of sites, dubbed the National Priorities List (NPL). The identification of a site for the NPL serves several purposes for the EPA, including:

- Determining which sites should be further investigated
- Determining the extent of contamination and human health and environmental risks associated with the site
- Identifying what if any CERCLA-financed remediation may be necessary
- Notifying the public concerning those sites that the EPA believes warrant further investigation
- Notifying the responsible parties about a potential EPA-initiated CERCLA remedial action

The EPA has developed web-based tools designed to make it easier for citizens to research their own communities and locate NPL sites in their cities and states. The NPL should be viewed as informational. Its purpose is to identify those sites that *may* require some remediation. Inclusion of a site on the NPL in and of itself is neither a judgment against the activities of any owner or operator of a property nor does it assign any liability or requirement for them to take any action.

## Occupational Agencies

In 1970 OSHA and NIOSH were established by the enactment of the Williams-Steiger Act by President Richard M. Nixon. At that time, OSHA was within the Department of Labor and NIOSH was within the Department of Health, Education, and Welfare. OSHA was established in response to a growing concern for work-related injuries and deaths. One of the first actions taken by OSHA was to consolidate standards of existing agencies like the American National Standards Institute (ANSI) and the American Conference of Governmental Industrial Hygienists (ACGIH) into the CFR.

Today, for industries that do not comply with OSHA standards, fines and other sanctions may be imposed. One of the tasks of OSHA related to the mission of reducing workplace injuries is to set reasonable standards for worker exposures to chemicals. OSHA promulgates permissible exposure levels (PELs) to specific chemicals in the workplace. These levels represent standards for the safe exposure (generally via breathing) for nearly all workers to a number of specific chemicals over the course of an 8-hour workday in a 40-hour workweek. This is known as the time-weighted-average (TWA) PEL. Adverse effects should not be encountered with repeated exposures at the TWA PEL. Safe is taken to mean 30 years of exposure without adverse effects.

OSHA also sets short-term exposure limits (STELs) PELs, ceiling limit PELs, and PELs that carry a skin designation. The STELs are concentration limits for substances in air that a worker may be exposed to for a maximum period of 15 minutes. The 15-minute STEL is generally considerably higher than the 8-hour TWA exposure level. For example, for trichloroethylene the TWA PEL is 50 ppm, whereas the STEL PEL is 200 ppm. Ceiling limit PELs are airborne concentration limits that should never be exceeded. Skin and eye exposures, in addition to respiratory exposure, are possible for many occupational chemicals, thus contributing to the overall dose that a worker may receive.

Another OSHA designation is *IDLH* (*immediately dangerous to life and health*). This represents a maximum level of exposure (airborne concentration) for any given chemical over a 30-minute period from which one could escape without personal protective equipment and without sustaining a serious health effect.

The ACGIH (a nongovernmental organization) promulgates guidelines for worker exposures to occupational chemicals. These guidelines are referred to as the threshold limit values (TLVs) and are generally more restrictive (lower concentrations for exposure) than OSHA PELs. In addition, there are more chemicals covered by the TLVs than by the OSHA PELs. The TLVs are exposure limits for airborne concentrations of chemicals and are believed to represent values that nearly all workers may be repeatedly exposed to, day after day, over a working lifetime without adverse health effects. The TLVs are published yearly, and this may imply that they are updated on a yearly basis. This is somewhat misleading because only a small percentage of the chemicals listed may have been under current review, whereas others may have not been considered for several years. Indeed, stricter limits are often adopted internally by some companies to better ensure worker safety.

NIOSH is the nonenforcement governmental arm for issues related to workplace safety. This agency is technically a part of the Centers for Disease Control and Prevention (CDC), which in turn is a division of the Department of Health and Human Services (DHHS). It is charged with conducting research and making recommendations for the prevention of workplace injuries in general, including those that can be produced from exposure to chemicals. NIOSH also has established guidelines called recommended exposure limits (RELs). These concentration limits are considered as being protective to worker health over a working lifetime and are frequently expressed as a TWA exposure to a chemical for up to a 10-hour work day, 40-hour workweek.

NIOSH maintains a health hazard evaluation (HHE) program whereby employees, their representatives, or employers can request an on-site evaluation to identify workplace hazards, including exposures to chemical agents that may pose health risks to employees. Where worker exposures and the development of chemical-induced illness are of real or potential concern to NIOSH during their assessments, recommendations can be made to help reduce the level of exposure by methods that are within the financial resources of the company, including engineering modifications to reduce airborne chemical concentrations, the adoption of personal protective equipment, or both.

Recommended occupational exposure limits (OELs) should not be viewed as absolute levels above which adverse health effects occur and below which they do not. An OEL should rather be viewed as a level above which the probability *begins* to increase that an adverse health effect may occur. If worker protection were the only consideration for setting exposure limits, then they would be much more stringent. The World Health Organization's (WHO) "Recommended Health-Based Occupational Exposure Limits" are generally stricter and more protective than our national safety standards because they are based entirely on health considerations as "the ultimate goal" for standard setting of chemical agents, without considerations of other factors, such as technology and socioeconomic constraints.

## Industrial versus Environmental Standards

From the preceding discussion we see there are several types of OELs based on which governmental agency was responsible for developing it. The goal of an OEL is to protect workers for their entire working lifetime, approximately 40 years. Another important aspect of OEL is that they are meant to apply to a work force, not the general public.

Let's consider some airborne contaminant standards environmentally and occupationally. The EPA has regulatory control for air pollution as stipulated in the 1970 CAA Amendments (CAAA). The CAAA established the NAAQS for six criteria pollutants and then added a seventh one in 1990. There are two types of national air quality standards: Primary standards set limits to protect public health, including the health of "sensitive" populations such as asthmatics, children, and the elderly, and secondary standards set limits to protect public welfare, including protection against decreased visibility and damage to animals, crops, vegetation, and buildings. The criteria pollutants are carbon monoxide, hydrocarbons, nitrogen dioxide, sulfur dioxide, particulates ($PM_{10}$ and $PM_{2.5}$), ozone, and lead. The purpose of the NAAQS was to define the allowable airborne concentrations of the criteria pollutants that may exist but would be anticipated to have no adverse health effect.

The ozone that we breathe is a major active product of photochemical smog and affects almost exclusively the respiratory system by acting as a potent oxidant and irritant. Ozone has low water solubility, exerting its principal effects on the lower respiratory tract. Sulfur dioxide is a concern both because of its health effects and because it contributes to acid rain and the formation of sulfates. Sulfur dioxide is an irritant gas and can trigger bronchial constriction and asthma attacks. The sulfates, also called acid aerosols, can cause adverse respiratory effects. Nitrogen dioxide, like ozone, can stimulate free radical production and local oxidative injury, mostly involving lipid peroxidation. Carbon monoxide, a byproduct of incomplete combustion of carbon-based fossil fuels, is the major air pollutant generated by industry. Carbon monoxide is one of the few inhalable pollutants that does not cause local effects in the lungs but exerts its effects systemically. Airborne lead levels continue to be a concern even decades after leaded gasoline is no longer available in the United States. Exposure to lead has various health effects, from fatigue and headaches to infertility, encephalopathy, seizures, and renal failure.

A comparison between the environmental limit standards (NAAQS) and occupational limit standards (OSHA) for several of the criteria pollutants is shown in Table 19.2.

The standards for environmental exposures are lower than those set for occupational exposures. Environmental exposures are calculated taking into account the general population, including children, adults, and elderly people, both healthy and ill. Therefore a considerable portion of the general population has a higher susceptibility to pollutants even if they are in small concentrations. The occupational standards are designed for an adult healthy population that is exposed to certain agents only for the duration of the workday; this drives the OELs at levels above the environmental ones. In the case of the workers who are spending most or all of their work time outside, the applicable standard limits are still those set and enforced by OSHA. Employers must comply with the OSHA exposure limits for the duration of the workday, regardless of where their employees are working. In the case of workers doing outdoor activities, their exposure to airborne contaminants is usually at a lower level. If, on the other hand, they are working on a day where the pollution is so bad that it even exceeds the occupational standards, then in principle the employer is out of compliance. When they go "off the clock," then they go "off the occupational standard" as well, and EPA standards for environmental exposure limits apply.

**Table 19.2**    Environment and Occupation Standards for Air Pollutants

| Chemical | NAAQs | OSHA TWA PELs | ACGIH TWA TLVs |
|----------|-------|---------------|----------------|
| Carbon monoxide | 9 ppm (10 mg/m$^3$)/8 hours | 50 ppm | 25 ppm |
| Lead | 1.5 µg/m$^3$/3 months | 50 µg/m$^3$ | 0.5 µg/m$^3$ |
| Nitrogen dioxide | 0.053 ppm (100 mg/m$^3$)/yearly | 5 ppm | 3 ppm |
| Ozone | 0.08 ppm/8-hour average | 0.1 ppm | 0.05 ppm |
| Sulfur dioxide | 0.03 ppm/yearly average | 5 ppm | No TLV |

ACGIH values are guidelines, *not* standards.

# The Agency for Toxic Substances and Disease Registry

Another agency responsible for assessing health hazards and contributing to the development of standards and guidelines for exposures to chemical agents is the Agency for Toxic Substances and Disease Registry (ATSDR). The ATSDR is an agency of the DHHS and is charged with serving the public "by using the best science, taking responsive public health actions, and providing trusted health information to prevent harmful exposures and disease related to toxic substances." The ATSDR under congressional mandate is empowered to

- perform public health assessments of hazardous waste sites
- respond to emergency releases of hazardous materials
- perform health consultations
- maintain a health surveillance and registry for toxic substance exposures
- conduct applied research
- produce both technical and lay documents about hazardous substances
- support education and training

One of the most comprehensive reviews of selected hazardous substances comes from the ATSDR Toxicological Profiles. These publications represent a comprehensive review of information about the potential health risks to humans and other species from exposure to a particular chemical. Other informative publications in the ATSDR include "Medical Management Guidelines," "Chemical Fact Sheets" (ToxFax's), "Case Studies in Environmental Medicine," and "State Fact Sheets" (ATSDR activities within a state).

The ATSDR works with its sister agency, the CDC, and other agencies, including the EPA, Congress, industry, national organizations, health care providers, state and local governments, and communities.

The ATSDR collected information that indicates significant risks associated with exposure to hazardous substances released from Superfund sites to communities residing nearby. Some of these health-related effects considered include

- Cancer
- Kidney dysfunction
- Lung and respiratory diseases
- Birth defects and reproductive disorders
- Immune function disorders
- Liver dysfunction
- Neurotoxic disorders

Additionally, the ATSDR has been concerned with the increase of asthma, particularly in inner-city children under the age of 5 years. Their research has been helpful in further advancing scientific knowledge and identifying areas for additional epidemiological investigations. They have been able to identify children with asthma by evaluating hospital discharge data and school health records in an attempt to establish a better link between asthma and specific air pollutants.

## The National Toxicology Program

Although there are many interdisciplinary agencies that contribute greatly to the decision-making considerations regarding exposures to chemical agents, the National Toxicology Program (NTP) clearly stands out as a leader. The NTP was established on November 15, 1978 by Joseph Califano, Jr., Secretary of Health, Education and Welfare (today known as the DHHS). The program had the broad goal of strengthening the department's activities in the testing of chemicals of public health concern as well as the development and validation of new and better integrated test methods. Currently, three federal agencies form the core of the NTP: the NIEHS at the National Institutes of Health , the CDER at the FDA, and NIOSH at the CDC. These agencies work together to form the core of the NTP, which is not a regulatory agency *per se* but rather a coordinated interagency effort to provide information and experience to regulatory decision-making processes in response to concerns about potential chemical hazards.

Some highlights of the NTP include studies that underpin many of the important regulatory and private sector decisions about protecting human health. In 1997, for example, NTP studies as well as others on the agent phenolphthalein produced a response in the FDA and private sector to ban all over-the-counter laxatives containing this agent. The proposal to reclassify phenolphthalein as unsafe was based on a review of animal carcinogenicity studies carried out under the NTP and presented during a recent FDA meeting. It was decided by the FDA to recall the three versions of the over-the-counter laxative Ex-Lax, which contained the chemical. The manufacturer subsequently removed this chemical from any newly manufactured product. Although the decision to do this was based entirely on laboratory studies with rodents that were exposed to large amounts of the chemical, the FDA concluded that the long-term use of phenolphthalein in humans could potentially cause cancer. Probably a more rational basis for the decision was that the American consumer had access to more than two-dozen effective laxative products without this ingredient; thus the benefits of using phenolphthalein did not outweigh the risks.

Another example where the NTP had an effect on policy was the occupational use of the chemical 1,3-butadiene. Studies from NTP showed lung tumors at exposures that were as low as 6.25 ppm in laboratory mice. In 1996 OSHA reduced the occupational exposure limit from 1,000 ppm to 1 ppm in response to this research.

Over 2,500 agents have been tested in cancer bioassays and in noncancer end-points by the NTP, and over 580 technical reports have been produced over the past 25 years. The agents under assessment by the NTP are quite broad and extend from hazardous pollutants, particulates, herbal supplements, medicines, to safe drinking water.

An important publication of the NTP is the "Report on Carcinogens"; the 11th report was released in 2005. It has a listing of approximately 250 agents that are identified as "reasonably known" to be human carcinogens. Another activity of the NTP, initiated in 1998, was the creation of The Center for Evaluation of Risk to Human Reproduction (CERHR). This center has analyzed over a dozen chemical agents of concern to date and has produced documents to inform the public and regulatory agencies on their safety with respect to reproductive health.

In the area of methods development, the NTP is evaluating the application of genomics and proteomics, immunotoxicity screens, and new transgenic models for toxicity and hazard assessment. The NTP has formed partnerships with other international agencies resulting in the formation of The Interagency Center for the Evaluation of Alternative Toxicological Methods. In 2005 six alternative methods have been validated for regulatory use in partnerships with international agencies and another 10 are under review.

## Consumer Product Safety Commission

An agency does not need to be large to serve an important purpose. The CPSC has the task of "protecting the public from unreasonable risks of serious injury or death from more than 15,000 types of consumer products under the agency's jurisdiction." It was created in 1972 to ensure product safety in the consumer products not covered by other agencies. Consumer exposure standards have been developed for hazardous substances and articles by this agency. Their authority under the Federal Hazardous Substance Act (FHSA) pertains to things other than foods, drugs, cosmetics, fuels, pesticides, and radioactive materials.

The responsibilities of the CPSC are as follows:

- To develop voluntary standards for industry
- To issue mandatory standards for some products
- To ban products that cannot be made safe
- To arrange for the recall and repair of defective products
- To conduct research on new products
- To inform and educate the public

Although only a small portion of their effort deals with chemicals, the CPSC has played an important role in ensuring adequate labeling for many commonly used household chemicals, including very dangerous ones such as drain openers. The CPSC requires a warning label on any consumer product that is toxic, corrosive, irritating, or sensitizing.

Identification of the words *dangerous, poison, warning,* and *caution* are today commonplace on consumer household products. Reading product labels is important for those products to work as they are intended to, but more importantly it is to prevent any injury to ourselves and others. Reading labels, such as to ensure that we do not mix together any household products that contain bleach and ammonia, is always preferable to an unfortunate lesson learned.

# Websites

Agency for Toxic Substances and Disease Registry (ATSDR):
http://www.atsdr.cdc.gov/

American Association of Poison Control Centers:
http://www.aapcc.org

Centers for Disease Control and Prevention:
http://www.cdc.gov/

ChemFinder:
http://chemfinder.cambridgesoft.com/

Clinical Trials:
http://www.clinicaltrials.gov/

Environmental Protection Agency:
http://www.epa.gov/

Extremely Hazardous Substances:
http://yosemite.epa.gov/oswer/ceppoehs.nsf/EHS_Profile?openform

Food and Drug Administration:
http://www.fda.gov/

GENE-TOX Genetic Toxicology (Mutagenicity):
http://toxnet.nlm.nih.gov/cgi-bin/sis/htmlgen?GENETOX

Hazardous Materials:
http://www.usfa.fema.gov/subjects/hazmat/

Hazardous Substances Data Bank (HSDB):
http://toxnet.nlm.nih.gov/cgi-bin/sis/htmlgen?HSDB

Integrated Risk Information System (IRIS):
http://toxnet.nlm.nih.gov/cgi-bin/sis/htmlgen?IRIS

IUPAC:
http://www.iupac.org/dhtml_home.html

Healthy People 2010:
http://www.healthypeople.gov/

International Toxicity Estimates for Risk (ITER):
http://toxnet.nlm.nih.gov/cgi-bin/sis/htmlgen?iter

Material Safety Data Sheets Online:
http://www.ilpi.com/msds/index.html

MEDLINEplus:
http://medlineplus.gov/

Medwatch Homepage:
http://www.fda.gov/medwatch/report/hcp.htm

National Institute of Environmental Health Sciences:
http://www.niehs.nih.gov/

National Institutes of Health:
http://www.nih.gov/

National Institute for Occupational Safety and Health:
http://www.cdc.gov/niosh/homepage.html

National Report on Human Exposure to Environmental Chemicals:
http://www.cdc.gov/exposurereport/

National Toxicology Program:
http://ntp-server.niehs.nih.gov/

Occupational Safety and Health Administration:
http://www.osha.gov/

Poisonous Plants Informational Database:
http://www.ansci.cornell.edu/plants/

Recognition and Management of Pesticide Poisonings:
http://npic.orst.edu/rmpp.htm

Registry of Toxic Effects of Chemical Substances:
http://www.cdc.gov/niosh/97-119.html

Right to Know Hazardous Substance Fact Sheets:
http://www.state.nj.us/health/eoh/rtkweb/rtkhsfs.htm

TRI Toxics Release Inventory:
http://toxnet.nlm.nih.gov/cgi-bin/sis/htmlgen?TRI

U.S. Department of Agriculture:
http://www.usda.gov/

World Health Organization:
http://www.who.int

# Bibliography

Chan, V. S., & Theilade, M. D. (2005). The use of toxicogenomic data in risk assessment: a regulatory perspective. *Clinical Toxicology, 43,* 121–126.

Klaassen, C. D. (2001). *Casarett & Doull's toxicology. The basic science of poisons.* New York: McGraw-Hill.

Klaassen, C. D., & Watkins, J. B. (2003). *Casarett & Doull's essentials of toxicology.* New York: McGraw-Hill.

Travis, K. Z., Pate, I., & Welsh, Z. K. (2005). The role of the benchmark dose in a regulatory context. *Regulatory toxicology and pharmacology: RTP, 43,* 280–291.

U.S. National Library of Medicine, National Institutes of Health, Environmental Health, and Toxicology Specialized Information Services (SIS). (2005). *Toxicology tutorial III.* Retrieved October 2, 2005 from http://www.sis.nlm.nih.gov/enviro/toxtutor.html.

Wu, K. M., Farrelly, J., Birnkrant, D., Chen, S., Dou, J., Atrakchi, A., Bigger, A., Chen, C., Chen, Z., Freed, L., Ghantous, H., Goheer, A., Hausner, E., Osterberg, R., Rhee, H., & Zhang, K. (2004). Regulatory toxicology perspectives on the development of botanical drug products in the United States. *American Journal of Therapeutics, 11,* 213–217.

# CHAPTER 20

# Toxicity Testing

## The Nature and Scope of Toxicity Testing

Responsible safeguarding of the public's health must include the identification of potential health risks from exposures to chemicals. There are over 100,000 chemicals that are in regular use in the United States, and several thousand new chemicals are synthesized annually worldwide for both personal and industrial use. There is no instrument that can directly assess toxicity; therefore a number of testing methodologies have been devised to overcome this difficulty. There are two purposes of toxicity testing. There is a quantitative effort to elucidate a dose–effect relationship, and there is a qualitative determination of the toxicity of the agent relative to other known chemicals. Both are accomplished using laboratory animals and *in vitro* methods. There are ethical concerns associated with whole animal studies as the intent of toxicity testing is to produce harm to the animal and then extrapolate the results to humans. Extrapolation magnifies error, so standards have been developed using uncertainty factors and modifying factors. Application of the results from animal testing can improve safety and help prevent injury.

The toxic effects of chemicals are determined by the nature of the chemical hazard, the dose or quantity to which the individual is exposed, the pathway(s) of exposure, and the pattern and duration of the exposure. In toxicity testing the importance of the dose or concentration and the hazardous nature of the chemical may vary considerably depending on the route of exposure. A chemical may be poorly absorbed through the skin but well absorbed orally. Because of such route-specific differences in absorption, toxicants are often ranked for hazard in accordance with the route of exposure. For example, a chemical may be relatively nontoxic by one route of exposure and highly toxic via another route of exposure. Accordingly, toxicity testing should be conducted using the most likely routes for human exposure.

The importance of toxicity testing is to provide safety evaluations of these chemicals, ideally by first discovering any adverse effect(s) from exposures in test animals and not in humans. It is therefore important that we establish conditions, at least initially, for the safe use of chemicals through acceptable nonhuman surrogate testing methodologies. Safety testing, as required by appropriate enactments of legislation, may help avoid repeating incidents of death and injury (e.g., death from elixir of sulfanilamide, eye injury by the eyebrow/eyelash dye Lash-Lure) that we have seen in the past. Similarly, concerns about environmental and occupational exposures to chemicals have resulted in legislation for the control and toxicity testing of chemicals that place workers at risk or may produce adverse effects to plant and animal communities.

Toxicity information is obtained primarily by

- Use of laboratory animals (*in vivo* studies)
- Surrogate animal models such as cell culture systems *(in vitro* studies)
- Human data obtained from intentional or accidental exposures to chemical agents
- Nonbiological models (computers, structure–activity relationships [SARs])

A great deal of information is available on the toxicity of chemicals from whole animal studies, *in vitro* studies, and epidemiological studies. There are advantages and disadvantages for each of these types of studies (Table 20.1).

## Toxicity Test Objectives and Considerations

One of the most important considerations in toxicology is the duration and frequency of exposure to a chemical. This is also an important consideration in developing toxicity tests. There are basically four types of exposure durations:

1. Acute: Generally refers to an exposure lasting less than 24 hours, and in most cases it is a single or "continuous" exposure over a period of time within a 24-hour period. For example, a single oral exposure to 10 ml of an organophosphate pesticide or the inhalation of toluene in the air that we are breathing at 150 ppm over a period of 3 hours would constitute examples of acute exposures.
2. Subacute: Generally refers to repeated exposure to a chemical for a period of 1 month or less.
3. Subchronic: Generally refers to repeated exposure for 1–3 months.
4. Chronic exposure: Generally refers to repeated exposure for more than 3 months.

**Table 20.1** Advantages and Disadvantages of *In Vivo, In Vitro,* and Epidemiological Studies

| Advantages of *In Vivo* Studies | Advantages of *In Vitro* Studies | Advantages of Epidemiological Studies |
|---|---|---|
| Can study effects of toxicants under well-controlled conditions in a "complete" mammalian system. | May help reduce the number of animals used for *in vivo* tests. | Direct inferences without extrapolation from animal data. |
| Mammals share many similar aspects of anatomy, physiology, and biochemistry, thus making extrapolations to humans reasonably valid scientifically. | Pure chemicals and/or mixtures of chemicals can be tested in a relatively simple system in the absence of their biochemical modifications by other body cells and tissues. | Greater level of confidence for medicolegal purposes. |
| Most regulatory approvals cannot take place without *in vivo* testing. | Most *in vitro* tests are relatively simple to perform and quantify. | A great number of individuals can be studied over long periods of time. |
| Longest established testing procedures with a greater abundance of studies. | Screening of new chemicals using human cells is possible and less expensive than animal *in vivo* tests. | Human health outcomes and or changes in human physiology are measured in populations. |
| **Disadvantages of *In Vivo* Studies** | **Disadvantages of *In Vitro* Studies** | **Disadvantages of Epidemiological Studies** |
| Time consuming and expensive. | May not satisfy regulatory demands and/or provide scientifically adequate information as evidence. | Relatively few in number. |
| Variation in structure and function from one species to another. | Difficult to relate *in vitro* dosages to those that produced toxicity to whole animals. | Unrecognized factors may contribute to bias because humans are not a relatively "homogeneous" group such as that which can be produced using genetically "uniform" laboratory animals. |
| Extrapolating information from extremely high doses in animals may not be predictive for a target human population that will be exposed to much lower doses. | Results may be highly variable between laboratories or cannot be repeated (issues related to test validation). | Epidemiology cannot prove causation, only association or high probability. |
| Institutional and other concerns about animal use: Pressure to explore alternative testing methods. | The route of exposure for an *in vitro* test (e.g., introduction of chemical directly to cells in culture through their culture medium) is not comparable with an *in vivo* exposure. | Results may depend on self-reporting of evidence. |

Potential outcomes from chemical exposures include the severity of effects and whether those effects are reversible or irreversible, immediate or delayed. Tissue repair in response to chemical insult may vary significantly depending on which tissue or tissues are affected and their ability to repair the damage that was produced. Those tissues with good regenerative capacity such as epithelia are more likely to keep pace with the insult when compared with one that lacks such reserve capacity (e.g., brain cells). Exposure to a toxicant may result in a local effect, a systemic effect, or both. Local effects occur at the exposure site (e.g., an irritant response). Systemic effects require the absorption and distribution of the toxicant into the body. The tissue or organ that is the most sensitive to the chemical under the conditions of exposure that have been either established experimentally or observed in the case of human exposures represents the "target."

Toxicity studies are conducted for chemicals that have the potential for public exposure; however, the extent of the toxicity testing and therefore the complexity of the study depend on several considerations:

- The specific type of chemical hazard
- How it is to be used
- The projected levels of human exposure
- The extent of its release into the environment

As you might anticipate, any study involving chemicals such as food additives, agricultural chemicals, pharmaceuticals, and veterinary drugs would undergo more extensive toxicity testing than chemicals that have limited use, perhaps in a specific industrial or research application. Toxicity testing using laboratory animals is often the only initial means by which human toxicity can be predicted and is often the only acceptable means for safety testing that satisfies certain regulatory requirements.

The National Toxicology Program (NTP) has been at the forefront of evaluating chemical agents of public health concern. It has been on the cutting edge of scientific research and has developed and applied modern biological and toxicological methodologies to address these concerns. Toxicity testing using laboratory animals is important to provide information necessary to make rational inferences concerning human health effects, despite its limitations.

The objective of toxicity testing, for any chemical, is to produce and quantify the *adverse effects* of that chemical with respect to the route(s) of exposure and dose. In addition, elucidating in a mechanistic fashion the nature and scope of the harmful effects that are produced from a chemical is important to understand and develop rational treatments for individuals or populations that may become ill from exposure to that chemical. Toxicity testing also provides a rational basis, and often the only basis, for making regulatory decisions concerning the use and conditions of use for any particular chemical. It is therefore reasonable that the types of studies required for regulatory compliance for any particular chemical depend on its proposed use and the likely extent and levels of exposures to humans or to plant and animal communities.

To be meaningful, any test for toxicity must include:

- An appropriate biological model
- An end-point that can be qualitatively and quantitatively assessed
- A well-developed test protocol

The model represents the system that is used for evaluation. This may involve the use of whole animals (*in vivo* testing) or an appropriate *in vitro* test system. When *in vitro* models are used, one should be selected that best represents what is believed to be occurring in the whole animal.

The measurement end-point is an appropriate parameter that can be used to predict toxicity. Toxicological end-points are the biological responses to chemical insult. They represent a measure of interaction between toxicant and living system. The term *toxicodynamics* is sometimes used to refer to this dynamic interaction. This end-point can be as crude a measure as lethality or as subtle as a nonclinically detectable change in cellular DNA, that is, one that may be detectable only by using molecular biological methods (Table 20.2). The test protocol is the schedule that defines the conditions related to dosing and time, and provides *all* experimental details, including statistical methodology.

## Animal Use and Extrapolation to Humans

Safety testing using laboratory animals has become routine and standardized. Because a goal of toxicity testing is to establish safe levels of exposure to chemicals, it should be clear that this could not be accomplished without also establishing hazardous levels and conditions of exposure as well. The exposure of experimental animals to often very high doses of chemicals is a form of substitution to using thousands of animals in testing. High doses in small groups can be used for mathematical low-dose extrapolation to estimate human risk.

**Table 20.2    Examples of Toxicological End-Points**

| End-Point of Toxicity | Measurement |
|---|---|
| Inflammation | Indicators of a local or systemic response |
| Enzyme inhibition and biochemical uncoupling | Interruption of a specific biochemical pathway or interference with synthesis |
| Lethal synthesis | Incorporation of a toxic substance into a biochemical pathway that results in changes leading to cytotoxicity and cell death |
| Necrosis | Tissue death that results from toxicant exposure, either acutely or chronically |
| Neoplasia | Aberrant cell division and growth |
| Covalent binding | Electrophilic reactive metabolites binding to a nucleophilic macromolecules as for example a genotoxic mutagen would bind to DNA |
| Lipid peroxidation | Perturbation of cellular phospholipids resulting from the free radical oxidation of cellular fatty acids |
| Receptor interaction | Normal biological responses that are mediated by receptor function are modified |
| Immunosuppression | Decreased immune function in response to a chemical exposure (e.g., chemotherapy treatments) |
| Immune-mediated hypersensitivity | An allergic response triggered by a chemical |
| Developmental and reproductive toxicity | Adverse effects on conception and the structure and function of the conceptus |

The use of laboratory animals provides important information on the toxicity of chemicals for both acute and chronic exposures. Acute studies, along with the physicochemical properties of a chemical, can be used as a basis to propose warning statements, safety precautions, and first aid instructions on product labels and in material safety data sheets. We are familiar with how the degree of toxicity is reflected in the labeling of the hazards: *poison* and *danger* denoting a substance of high toxicity, *warning* meaning the substance is moderately toxic, and *caution* indicating that the hazard possesses relatively low toxicity. Long-term toxicity studies can provide important information on safety as it relates to reproductive and developmental effects. Animal toxicity data can also assist in determining safe levels (acceptable daily intake [ADI]) from exposure to a chemical over the course of an individual's lifetime, as might be obtained from exposures to food additives or pesticide residues in food. The ADI refers to an intake level for a chemical that is believed to be safe for humans over the course of a lifetime as based on current information. The ADI for a chemical is derived experimentally from the no observed adverse effect level (NOAEL) of the most sensitive laboratory species that has been studied with that chemical. In addition, this value is adjusted downward by a factor of 100 times or more (safety factor) based on the uncertainty of extrapolating toxicity data from animals to humans, individual variation of responses, and other factors that may come to bear on uncertainties between humans and animals (Table 20.3).

Toxicity studies using laboratory animals thus provide a basis for

- Understanding how a chemical may potentially produce an adverse response in humans
- Demonstrating a range of exposure levels and gradation of toxicity from no observable effects to severe toxicity
- Justification for public health risk assessments

It must be recognized, however, that although the intent of such studies is to provide information that would be predictive of effects in humans, responses vary between animal species because of anatomical, physiological, and biochemical differences, and this limits to some extent our confidence as to human applicability.

## Animal Use Concerns

The laboratory animals that are used for toxicity studies are primarily rats and mice and to a lesser extent guinea pigs and rabbits. Occasionally, dogs and primates may be used for certain tests as well. Although there has been an increased use of *in vitro* toxicity tests worldwide, con-

**Table 20.3**   Extrapolation of Animal Results to Humans

| Body Weight Assumptions | Uncertainty Factors | Modifying Factors |
|---|---|---|
| "Average" male, 70 kg | 10 for human variability | 0.1–10 if LOAEL used |
| "Average" female, 60 kg | 10 for species variability | (accounts for study methodology) |
| | 10 for less than a chronic exposure | |
| | 10 if LOAEL used instead of NOAEL | |

cern about making inferences from a relatively simple *in vitro* system to a highly complex *in vivo* mammalian system is still a major concern and limitation for their use. The use of laboratory animals *in vivo* will likely continue to provide the main line of information about the toxic properties of chemicals.

The Society of Toxicology (SOT) adopted in 1999 a Public Policy Statement concerning the use of animals for toxicological studies:

- Research involving laboratory animals is necessary to ensure and enhance human and animal health and protection of the environment.
- In the absence of human data, research with experimental animals is the most reliable means of detecting important toxic properties of chemical substances and for estimating risks to human and environmental health.
- Research animals must be used in a responsible manner.
- Scientifically valid research designed to reduce, refine, or replace the need for laboratory animals is encouraged.

The NTP had used rodents, *in vivo*, for evaluating the safety of chemical agents. Published results of short-term toxicity tests for selected chemicals can be found in the NTP toxicity reports (prechronic toxicity studies) available online (http://ntp.niehs.nih). The results of 2-year toxicology and carcinogenesis studies are published in the scientific literature and in the NTP technical reports. Toxicity studies carried out as grant or contract research at universities and other testing facilities use protocols that are consistent with those developed by the NTP or in collaboration with the NTP. The NTP has also developed requirements for contract testing laboratories that are in compliance with the Laboratory Animal Welfare Act of 1966 and adhere to the principles of animal welfare in the "Guide for the Care and Use of Laboratory Animals" (NRC, 1996) and other animal care documents such as the "Institutional Animal Care and Use Committee Guidebook, 2002" (http://grants.nih.gov/grants/olaw/GuideBook.pdf).

### Species Considerations

Traditional toxicological testing using laboratory animals is based on the assumption that mammalian physiology is similar, whether rodent or human. The idea that a human is essentially a 70-kg rat and that toxicity or safety can be reasonably extrapolated from laboratory animal studies by simply adjusting the total dose received in humans, that is, by standardizing the dose to kilogram of body weight, is still a methodology for assessing risk to humans, at least from a regulatory perspective (Table 20.4).

## Practical Aspects in Measuring Toxicity Experimentally

In developing a meaningful toxicity testing protocol, a number of considerations must be met. First, a selection of at least three dose levels should be selected to establish a threshold dose and a dose–response relationship. Second, the route of exposure should represent one that best fits

**Table 20.4** Equivalent Dose Levels in Several Species

| Species | Body Weight (kg) | Oral Dosage (mg/kg) | Total Oral Dose (mg/animal) | Body Surface Area (cm$^2$) | Dosage (mg/cm$^2$) |
|---|---|---|---|---|---|
| Human | 70 | 10 | 700 | 18,000 | 0.7000 |
| Rat | 0.2 | 10 | 2 | 325 | 0.0061 |
| Mouse | 0.02 | 10 | 0.2 | 46 | 0.0043 |
| Dog | 12 | 10 | 120 | 5,770 | 0.0207 |

the anticipated human exposure route(s). Third, although toxicity testing is normally conducted with young adult animals, consideration as to age, sex differences, and pregnancy outcome may be required in certain instances, which may require testing of, for example, newborn or pregnant animals or older animals.

To "measure toxicity" in response to a chemical exposure, we need to establish what the actual measurement of toxicity should be. To have meaning, any measure of toxicity must be objective, quantifiable, and repeatable. These "toxicological end-points" can be as crude as death or as subtle as a small alteration in the DNA. There are a number of standardized test procedures. This means that the procedure has gained scientific acceptance as a methodology that would yield the most meaningful data and by inference would predict human toxicity.

There are standardized tests to determine experimentally

- Acute toxicity
- Dermal toxicity
- Ocular toxicity
- Subacute toxicity
- Chronic toxicity
- Reproductive toxicity
- Developmental toxicity
- Cancer development
- Genetic toxicity
- Neurotoxicity

As examples, neurotoxicity tests are available using laboratory animals to assess for chemical toxicity to the nervous system. Both sensory and motor tests are available as well as neuro-histopathology. A delayed neurotoxicity test using hens has been developed to assess injury from exposure to anticholinergic substances such as organic phosphate pesticides. Genetic toxicity (genotoxicity) can be assessed using laboratory animals such as mice in gene mutation tests that expose mice, breed them, and look for chromosomal changes in offspring. Chromosomal effects from exposure to chemicals can be determined by a number of different tests using both whole animals and *in vitro* methods. Common whole animal tests include, for example, the use of male rats or mice that are first exposed to chemicals suspected of being genotoxic and then mated with nontreated females. Death of the embryo or fetus is taken as an indication of a chemical-induced genetic defect in the DNA of the male sperm. This test is sometimes referred to as the dominant lethal mutation assay. Another toxicity test, the rodent chromosomal assay, uses whole animals to determine whether a chemical can produce any chromosomal injury. Rats or mice may be exposed to a single dose of a chemical, followed by an examination of the bone marrow or peripheral blood cells for chromosomal aberrations. Chromosomal damage, in the form of broken chromosomes, which may become encased within a nuclear membrane (micronucleus test) or by fragments joining their sister chromatid (sister chromatid exchange assay), may be observed.

## Acute Local Toxicity: Tests for Irritancy and Corrosiveness

Irritation and corrosion tests are examples of local tissue responses. The chemical being tested is applied, for example, to the skin of the test animal and over a period of time, generally hours to a few days, the skin is examined for signs of inflammation. When these types of tests are performed on the eyes, it is referred to as the Draize test. Some chemicals have the potential to produce a direct irritating/inflammatory skin response while others may need to first be processed by immunological sensitization. In the latter process, skin injury is not the direct effect of the chemical on the skin, but rather an indirect response from the release of mediators of inflammation upon reexposure in the sensitized individual. Rabbits are generally used for these types of studies. To determine whether the chemical produces a primary irritant response (contact dermatitis), the substance is applied to the skin and any changes are observed over the course of several days. To assess for an immunological response, guinea pigs are first treated with the chemical by its topical application to the skin for several hours (sensitization phase). There should be no inflammatory changes to the skin over the course of a week or two. The substance is then reapplied to the skin (skin challenge) and observations are made over a period of one to several days.

The ocular toxicity of irritants is determined by the brief application of the substance to the eyes of several test animals, which are usually rabbits. Examination of the eyes is conducted over a period of 3 days to assess for any injuries that may have been produced to the conjunctiva, cornea, or iris. Substances have been demonstrated to produce a range of effects from no observable reaction or simple reversible irritation to severe irritation and corrosion. The Draize test, which was developed in the 1940s in response to human injuries produced by cosmetics has been the subject of a good deal of controversy regarding its use. The test has been a reliable indicator for the responses in humans, and the test allows for the use of an anesthetic in the eye of the test animal in the event of distress. Other *in vitro* tests have been developed as surrogates for animal *in vivo* testing, and other alternative procedures that do not use live animals are being developed. Despite the controversy over the use of animals in these types of tests, both regulatory officials and toxicologists agree on the usefulness of this testing to provide a basis for the quantification and standardization for a products potential to produce irritation or serious injury to the eye.

## Acute Systemic Toxicity: Use and Limitations of $LD_{50}$

Typically, toxicological prechronic tests involve the use of rodents of both sexes, over a period of either 24 hours (acute), 14 days (the subacute or 2-week study), or 90 days (the subchronic or 13-week study). A simple end-point measure used for many years is the $LD_{50}$. This is a dose (generally orally administered) that is statistically derived from laboratory animals and represents the dose at which 50% of the test animals would be expected to die. In the late 1920s the $LD_{50}$ test was developed as a measure of the toxicological potency of chemicals intended for human use such as insulin and digitalis. The use of the test was expanded to one that was generally recognized as an acceptable *in vivo* animal surrogate to rank chemical toxicity and became accepted for regulatory purposes as an important source of safety information for new chemicals, including drugs, household products, pesticides, industrial chemicals, cosmetics, and food additives.

As an example, consider the results of a study conducted for regulatory purposes that determined the acute effects of a new food preservative using laboratory rodents and lethality as the end-point for toxicity. Based on this experimentally derived curve, you can observe that the dose anticipated to produce death in 50% of the test animals would be between 15 and 20 mg/kg of body weight (Figure 20.1).

It must be recognized that the $LD_{50}$ acute toxicity test is a poor indicator of human health effects because death is the least desirable measure of toxicity. Additionally, the test provides virtually no information concerning long-term or chronic effects, and information about the mechanisms of toxicity is absent or very limited.

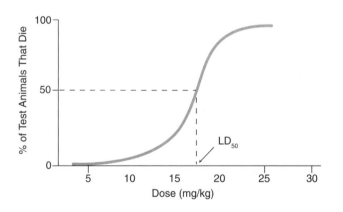

**FIGURE 20.1**    $LD_{50}$ curve. *Source:* Courtesy of the Toxicology and Environmental Health Information Program of the National Library of Medicine, US Department of Health and Human Services.

Because of the large number of animals killed or injured as toxicological end-points, there's been much criticism about the use of animals for these and other types of biomedical studies.

## Alternative In Vivo Tests to Predict LD$_{50}$

Several alternative animal toxicity tests to the classical LD$_{50}$ have been developed as methodologies for acute toxicity testing based on a reduction in the number of animals used, lower maximum dose limits, and, for some tests, end-points other than death. These include the fixed dose procedure, the up and down procedure, and the acute toxic class method. In 1984 the British Toxicology Society proposed an acute oral toxicity test that avoided the use of death as the end point and rather relied on clear signs of toxicity produced in response to a fixed dose level. The method that became known as the fixed dose procedure (FDP) allows for the toxicity testing of chemicals broadly compatible with the traditional LD$_{50}$ acute oral toxicity test while using fewer animals and causing less mortality and distress. The idea is to examine how a series of fixed dose levels affects animals by observation for any objective sign of toxicity at any dose level. The acute toxic class (ATC) method uses fixed dose levels and retains mortality as a main end-point for toxicity. In the up and down procedure, (UDP) animals are dosed in a sequential manner, with the dose for each animal being either increased or decreased as determined from the responses of previously tested animals. In this procedure, single animals are sequentially dosed generally at 24- or 48-hour intervals. The dose that the first animal receives is either a level that is below the toxicologist's best estimate of the LD$_{50}$, or a starting dose of 175 mg/kg if no estimate of lethality for that chemical can be made. A second animal is dosed at a higher level if the first animal survives. If the first animal dies or appears to be ill, then the second animal receives a lower dose. Generally, dosing does not exceed 2,000 mg/kg of body weight, although higher levels may be required for specific regulatory purposes.

Although these three alternative acute toxicity tests have been used more extensively in Europe, especially for the testing of new industrial chemicals, they have not gained wide acceptance in the United States. The United States, for regulatory purposes, requires a point estimate and slope to satisfy the requirements for most types of acute toxicity testing and thus relies more heavily on the classical LD$_{50}$ test.

When referring to lethal toxicity from chemical exposures via inhalation, we would refer to a concentration and accordingly an LC$_{50}$ value would represent the concentration at which 50% of the test animals would die from exposure (Table 20.5).

**Table 20.5**   Comparison of Lethality by Route of Exposure

|  | Oral LD$_{50}$ (mg/kg) | Dermal LD$_{50}$ (mg/kg) | Inhalation LC$_{50}$ (mg/m$^3$/4 hr) |
|---|---|---|---|
| Harmful | 200–2,000 | 400–2,000 | 2,000–20,000 |
| Toxic | 25–200 | 50–400 | 500–2,000 |
| Very toxic | <25 | <50 | <500 |

## Efficacy, Toxicity, and Lethality

For many chemicals that we intentionally use, some benefit is derived from their use. For example, a prescribed medication is anticipated to produce a beneficial effect if properly taken. The level of benefit (efficacy) can also be quantitatively measured; thus an $ED_{50}$ would represent the lowest dose that is beneficial (efficacious) in 50% of the test population. It should be apparent that for a chemical intended to produce some benefit to the body at a certain dose, the likelihood of some toxicity may also result from the same chemical at some dose beyond therapeutic. Any dose that results in a toxic end-point (nonlethal) can be abbreviated TD. Thus, a $TD_{50}$ would represent the dose of a chemical toxic to 50% of the population (Table 20.6).

For chemicals that produce a beneficial effect (e.g., a drug), a comparison of the doses that produce efficacy and those that produce toxicity can yield important information regarding its safety. Compare the doses that produce efficacy and toxicity in Figure 20.2. As you can observe, at the $ED_{50}$ level there is no apparent toxicity, whereas at the $ED_{90}$ level a small amount of toxicity is observed (Figure 20.2).

If the toxicity curve is shifted slightly to the right, it would be more apparent that there would be less toxicity when compared with the dose that produces 90% efficacy and that the doses required to produce toxicity become greater as the curve shifts further and further to the right of the efficacy curve. The further apart that the efficacy and toxicity curves are, the safer the drug; the closer together they are, the less the "margin of safety." For pharmaceutical agents, a therapeutic index (TI) is a comparison of the effective dose of the drug with its toxic dose at the 50% dose response levels, that is, the $ED_{50}/LD_{50}$. If the $LD_{50}$ of a drug is 100 mg/kg and the $ED_{50}$ is 10, then the therapeutic index would be 10. The higher the TI, the greater the safety of the drug, particularly when the efficacy and toxicity slopes of the curves are similar (Figure 20.3).

Perhaps a better designation to describe the safety of a drug is that of the margin of safety (MOS), which overcomes the problem of any significant differences in the response slopes between toxicity and efficacy curves (Figure 20.4). The MOS represents the ratio of lethality at

**Table 20.6**    Common Abbreviations of Beneficial, Toxic, and Lethal Doses

|  | Efficacy | Toxicity | Lethality |
|---|---|---|---|
| $ED_{10}$ | Effect Dose to 10% of the Population | | |
| $ED_{50}$ | Effect Dose to 50% of the Population | | |
| $ED_{90}$ | Effect Dose to 90% of the Population | | |
| $TD_{10}$ | | Toxic Dose to 10% of the Population | |
| $TD_{50}$ | | Toxic Dose to 50% of the Population | |
| $TD_{90}$ | | Toxic Dose to 90% of the Population | |
| $LD_{10}$ | | | Lethal Dose to 10% of the Population |
| $LD_{50}$ | | | Lethal Dose to 50% of the Population |
| $LD_{90}$ | | | Lethal Dose to 90% of the Population |

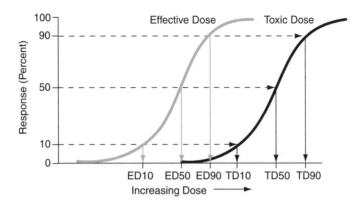

**FIGURE 20.2**    Two curves showing efficacy and toxicity for the same chemical.
*Source:* Courtesy of National Library of Medicine.

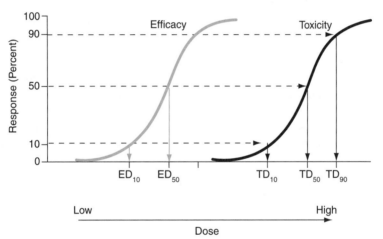

**FIGURE 20.3**    Two curves showing efficacy and toxicity for the same chemical with no measurable toxicity at the higher dose levels for efficacy.

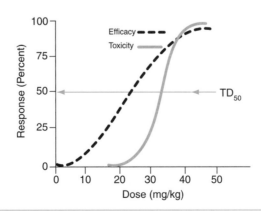

**FIGURE 20.4**    Two curves showing efficacy and toxicity for the same chemical with measurable toxicity at the lower dose levels for efficacy.

a very low level (e.g., 1%) compared with efficacy at the 99% level (MOS= $LD_1/ED_{99}$). Again, the higher the value, the safer the drug.

## A Hypothetical Acute Oral Toxicity Study

Let us consider the acute toxicity of a hypothetical chemical "X" (Table 20.7). Our empirically derived data table does not precisely tell us what the $LD_{50}$ is, other than it rests somewhere between 20 and 30 mg/kg and can be better approximated by drawing a horizontal line from the 50% lethality point on the curve and then a perpendicular line to the dose intercept (Figure 20.5). Because the dose–response curve is not a straight line, caution must be used in making an $LD_{50}$ estimate.

There are a number of methodologies to more precisely calculate the $LD_{50}$. In a population that is normally distributed, the mean ± 1 standard deviation represents 68.3% of the population, the mean ± 2 standard deviations represents 95.5% of the population, and the mean ± 3 standard deviations represents 99.7% of the population. Because dose–response characteristics are usually normally distributed, the percent of response can be converted to units of deviation from the mean, or what is referred to as normal equivalent deviations. The probit (from *proba*bility un*it*) is by convention the normal equivalent deviation + 5. A 50% response is a probit of 5, a + 1 deviation becomes a probit of 6, and a – 1 deviation is a probit of 4 (Table 20.8). A pro-

**Table 20.7    Acute Lethality from Oral Doses of Chemical "X" in Laboratory Rats**

| Dose (mg/kg) | No. of Rats Tested | No. of Rats Killed | % Killed |
|---|---|---|---|
| 10 | 50 | 9 | 18 |
| 15 | 49 | 13 | 26.5 |
| 20 | 48 | 21 | 43.8 |
| 30 | 50 | 31 | 62.0 |
| 50 | 49 | 41 | 83.6 |
| 70 | 50 | 46 | 92.0 |

**Table 20.8    Probit Referenced to % Response and Normal Equivalent Deviations**

| % Response | NED | Probit |
|---|---|---|
| 0.1 | –3 | 2 |
| 2.3 | –2 | 3 |
| 15.9 | –1 | 4 |
| 50 | 0 | 5 |
| 84.1 | +1 | 6 |
| 97.7 | +2 | 7 |
| 99.9 | +3 | 8 |

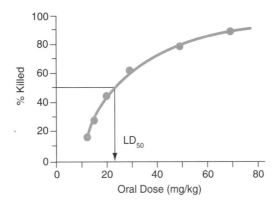

**FIGURE 20.5**    Acute lethality from oral doses of chemical "X" in laboratory rats.

bit transform of our data would produce a graph with a straight line (Figure 20.6). Dose is expressed in both mg/kg and log of dose.

The slope of the probit plot may change depending on the chemical and the end-point measured. In the case of the $LD_{50}$, for example, the doses of two chemicals may be the same but the slopes may be different (Figure 20.7).

There are limitations to the use of $LD_{50}$ values. Importantly, values obtained in one species are not directly applicable in another species. Consider, for example, $LD_{50}$ values of dioxin in mammals. On the basis of $LD_{50}$, dioxin is 1,000 times more potent in guinea pigs than hamsters (Table 20.9).

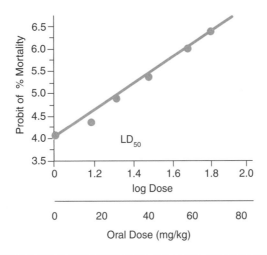

**FIGURE 20.6**    Acute lethality from oral doses of chemical "X" in laboratory rats: probit graph.

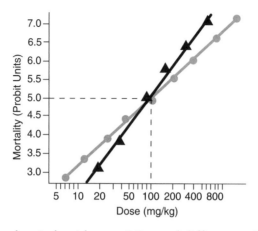

**FIGURE 20.7**    Two chemicals with same $LD_{50}$ and different toxicity slopes.

**Table 20.9**    Oral $LD_{50}$ Values of 2,3,7,8-TCDD in Several Vertebrates

| Species | Sex | Oral $LD_{50}$ ($\mu$g/kg) |
|---|---|---|
| Guinea pig | Male | 1 |
| Guinea Pig | Female | 2 |
| Rat | Male | 22 |
| Rat | Female | 50–500 |
| Rabbit | | 115 |
| Hamster | | 1,000–5,000 |
| Frog | | 1,000 |

# Other Examples of Prechronic Toxicity Testing in Laboratory Animals

To assess toxic effects that do not result in lethality as an end-point for the acute toxicity test, toxicologists can expose rodents to much lower doses than those used in determining the $LD_{50}$. The purpose of the 2-week toxicity protocol is to provide a range of toxicities and potential target organs to help establish the setting of doses for subchronic (13-week) exposure studies. Prechronic tests also determine the no observed adverse effect level (NOAEL) for the test chemical. Subacute or repeated-dose studies examine the effects of *multiple dose exposures* over the course of 14 days. Test animals are monitored for changes in their appearance, behavior, appetite, thirst, growth rate, and body chemistries. Subchronic toxicity tests typically last 90 days. The lowest observed adverse effect level (LOAEL) and the NOAEL are determined in this phase. Additionally, the subchronic tests reveal the target organ or organs affected by repeated exposures, the nature of the tissue damage sustained, and differences in interspecific response. Researchers typically use two different species for the subchronic testing, and all animals are sacrificed and neropsied at the end of the 90-day period. In these subchronic tests lower doses are given to groups of test animals over this more extended period which represents about 10% of their life span (approximately 3 months for rats).

For any toxicity study using laboratory rodents, there is a period of quarantine for approximately 2 weeks before assigning treatment groups. In a subacute test, for example, animals are randomly assigned to one of five treatment groups. The animals of each treatment group are administered a different concentration of the chemical under consideration for each gender and species (Table 20.10). The doses that are studied would typically encompass several levels (e.g., one low, two medium, two high), with toxicity ranging from none to death. Usually, a single dose of the chemical (generally contained in corn oil) is administered and the animals are observed over a 2-week period.

For all animals that either die from exposure to the chemical or are sacrificed at the end of the study, a comprehensive pathological examination of the external body and the internal organs is conducted. Internal organs are examined and may be prepared for microscopic examination (histopathological examination) on those organs/tissues showing gross visible evidence of treatment-related injury and compared with nontreated control animals.

Subchronic (13-week) toxicity testing is important because the data are used to detect any adverse response that may not have been readily apparent from acute single exposure toxicity tests and to determine a range of doses for each species of animals that will be used in 2-year toxicology/carcinogenesis protocols. Subchronic toxicity testing is generally performed by ingestion or inhalation as the exposure routes using dose levels less than those used for acute toxicity testing.

## Chronic Toxicity Testing in Laboratory Animals

Chronic studies represent an important way to identify those chemicals that have the potential to produce adverse health effects, including reproductive and developmental effects and cancer, at levels of exposure that would be reasonably anticipated to occur in humans. The purpose of reproductive toxicity testing is to assess the potential of a chemical to alter in any way normal reproductive function and structure. This testing may include hormonal effects and gonadal

**Table 20.10**  Animal Use in a 2-Week Toxicity Study

| Group | Number of Animals | | Sexes | | Number of Species Per Dose Tested | | Dose Groups | | Total Number Tested |
|---|---|---|---|---|---|---|---|---|---|
| Treatment | 5 | x | 2 | x | 2 | x | 5 | = | 100 |
| Controls | 5 | x | 2 | x | 2 | x | 1* | = | 20 |
| | | | | | | | | | 120 |

* Control animals would be subjected to the same dosing procedure as treatment animals (i.e., would receive corn oil but without the chemical present).

function; changes in mating, birth, or conception; and the growth and development of the off-spring. Generally, the route of exposure for reproductive toxicity testing is oral, and the period of observation includes both male and female parent rodents, their offspring ($F_1$), and the offspring of the next generation ($F_2$) until a generation achieves young adult status.

Developmental toxicity testing of chemicals is conducted to assess the potential of any chemical to produce birth defects, including teratogenic effects, and/or any injury to the developing embryo or fetus. These tests are typically conducted in at least two species of laboratory animals using young adult pregnant animals. Three or more dose levels are used before breeding and during the entire pregnancy. Offspring are observed for any signs of growth retardation and abnormal function during infancy.

Carcinogenicity tests are a specialized chronic toxicity test using two species of rodents over a period of approximately 2 years. Young adult animals are used, and several dose levels are selected based on subchronic toxicity testing. At the least three dose levels are selected, with the highest dose level producing minimal toxicity over an exposure period of 18 to 24 months.

These chronic studies typically involve the use of both sexes of mice (B6C3F1 hybrid) and rats (Fischer 344/N) at several dose levels of exposure, five times per week, in addition to untreated controls in groups of 50 animals, and may extend over a period of 2 years (Table 20.11). This information is important in making rational regulatory decisions concerning reasonable exposures to human populations from chemicals to which humans are either likely to be intentionally or unintentionally exposed.

## Human Studies

Toxicity information from human studies may come from a number of sources:

- Case reports from individuals that have been accidentally or intentionally poisoned
- Reported adverse reactions to drugs
- Clinical studies from various sized groups of individuals that have been intentionally exposed to an investigational chemical, such as a new pharmaceutical
- Epidemiological studies that attempt to determine whether a causal relationship exists in a study population that has been exposed to a substance that may produce adverse health effects when compared with an unexposed population that has been matched for such fac-

**Table 20.11**   Animal Use in a 2-Year Toxicity Study

| Group | Number of Animals | | Sexes | | Number of Species Per Dose Tested | | Dose Groups | | Total Number Tested |
|---|---|---|---|---|---|---|---|---|---|
| Treatment | 50 | x | 2 | x | 2 | x | 3 | = | 600 |
| Controls | 50 | x | 2 | x | 2 | x | 1 | = | 200 |
| | | | | | | | | | 800 |

tors as age, gender, race, and economic status. An example of such a study might be to determine whether a greater incidence of a specific disease (e.g., asthma) in a community is associated with the discharge of pollutants from a specific geographical area.

Case reports represent accounts of illness in one or a small number of individuals and are generally written by occupational health physicians who attribute a particular illness to workplace exposure to chemicals. Any isolated case reports are essentially anecdotal and need to be corroborated by other similar reports before any causality can be established between the chemical agent and a particular illness or adverse effect.

Epidemiological studies, in contrast to case reports, study groups of individuals with particular illnesses in an attempt to establish whether an illness was produced or exacerbated from chemical exposures either environmentally or at work. To establish a causal link between a specific chemical agent and a particular disease requires a study design that adequately compares the individuals with the disease or illness with those not exposed, as far as can be determined. There are several commonly developed methodologies to accomplish this. Common methods are case-control studies, cross-sectional studies, and cohort studies. Case-control studies are relatively easy to conduct and investigate causality by essentially comparing people with an illness or disease and a control group that is without the disease. In cross-sectional studies the occurrence of a specific disease or clinical sign (e.g., blood pressure, cholesterol level) is examined in individuals who have been exposed to the chemical agent(s) of concern and an appropriate control group.

The more complex cohort studies, also referred to as incidence studies or follow-up studies, examine groups of individuals (cohorts) classified according to disease or outcome. Cohort studies are essentially of two types. The retrospective study is of a relatively simple design and attempts to identify cohorts that have had a previous chemical exposure and have been followed up over a period of time. Many retrospective studies come from occupational exposures where specific industrial processes and chemicals are used by workers who would typically be receiving levels of exposure far greater than that received for the same chemical in the general population. Prospective studies attempt to identify those cohorts who are presently being exposed to a specific chemical(s) and monitoring them over time to identify any clinically relevant outcomes.

Epidemiological studies are often either difficult to design or difficult to interpret. Fundamental to a well-designed epidemiological study is a control population as similar as possible to the population with the specific disease(s). Factors that must be equalized include age, race, sex, social status, and lifestyle and environmental influences. Additionally, an adequate period of time to detect statistically significant effects is critical. As an example, consider epidemiological studies that might focus on the relationship between a specific cancer(s) and exposure to a specific chemical substance(s). The development of many cancers requires a relatively long period of time before they are clinically apparent, and thus an epidemiological study might require a period of several decades of data collection before making any definitive assessments with regard to causality. The possibility that conclusions may be drawn based on factors that were not adequately controlled for may introduce serious bias to the study. Examples may include confounding factors due to a poorly matched control population, information that is based on the recall of individuals, or the misclassification of a disease.

The entire cohort is followed to assess if there are any health differences between the exposed and the unexposed groups. Although epidemiological studies offer obvious advantages over laboratory studies, there are nonetheless a number of disadvantages:

- The tests are often expensive to conduct.
- Good quantification of exposures is frequently difficult.
- Large numbers of individuals are acquired for meaningful statistical evaluation.
- Exposure quantification in humans is frequently difficult because of simultaneous exposures to multiple chemical, physical, and biological agents.
- Epidemiological studies generally require long periods of time before information is made available through the appropriate published resources.

## Alternative Toxicity Testing Methods

In the United States and other countries, there has been a growing concern about the use and ethical treatment of laboratory animals for toxicological studies and biomedical research. Advances in *in vitro* technology and computer modeling have fueled the growth of internet databases to provide guidance and information on alternatives to traditional animal toxicity testing. Numerous websites have consolidated much available information so that toxicologists can avoid needless experimental duplication of studies that may have already been conducted. In addition, these sites provide a way to easily investigate techniques that may be applicable to their own work. Often, such websites represent the combined efforts of academia, industry, government, and advocacy groups. Examples of these websites include:

- Altweb: Alternatives to Animal Testing on the Web. Altweb unites academic, government, industry, and activists in a comprehensive resource: http://altweb.jhsph.edu
- Alternatives to Laboratory Animals (ATLA): http://altweb.jhsph.edu/publications/journals/atla/atla-index.htm
- National Agricultural Library's Animal Welfare Information Center (AWIC), U.S. Department of Agriculture. Mandated by Congress to aggregate and share information on alternatives to animal and to improve procedures for humane treatment of research animals: http://www.nal.usda.gov/awic/
- European Centre for the Validation of Alternative Methods (ECVAM), Scientific Information Service. International reference center for the development, scientific, and regulatory acceptance for alternative testing: http://ecvam-sis.jrc.it/index.html
- Fund for the Replacement of Animals in Medical Experiments (FRAME). Attempting to integrate computer modeling and *in vitro* techniques to assess human risk without using animals: http://www.frame.org.uk
- The (U.S.) Interagency Coordinating Committee on the Validation of Alternative Methods (ICCVAM) and NTP Interagency Center for the Evaluation of Alternative Toxicological Methods (NICEATM): http://iccvam.niehs.nih.gov
- INVITTOX. An online database of *in vitro* techniques in toxicology: http://embryo.ib.amwaw.edu.pl/invittox

- Johns Hopkins Center for Alternatives to Animal Testing (CAAT). Promotes the use of alternatives to animal testing: http://caat.jhsph.edu/
- Netherlands Centre for Alternatives to Animal Use (NCA). Supports the alternatives to animal experiments platform, a collaborative effort between the Dutch government, industry, and animal protection organizations: http://www.nca-nl.org/
- Society of Toxicology (SOT): http://www.toxicology.org
- Society for *In Vitro* Biology (SIVB): http://www.sivb.org
- Alternatives Research & Development Foundation (ARDF): http://www.aavs.org/home.html
- The Humane Society of the United States (HSUS): http://www.hsus.org

Toxicologists as well as other scientists who use animals for research and testing purposes have been encouraged to explore the "3R's" of animal alternatives:

- **Replace** the animal with another appropriate test.
- **Reduce** the total number of animals used.
- **Refine** the study to reduce the distress of laboratory animals.

The replacement of laboratory animals with an appropriate *in vitro* test is often not a viable option. Accepting an *in vitro* methodology as a suitable surrogate for an *in vivo* test requires its validation. The *in vitro* methodology must be implementable by multiple laboratories, and consistent results must be produced, that is, the new methodology must be validated. Validation may be defined as a process by which the credibility of a new test is established for a specific purpose and its reliability and reproducibility have been verified by independent sources. Although a large number of *in vitro* tests are available, most of them have not been validated and are unacceptable for regulatory purposes.

However, a great deal of effort has and will continue to be spent on the development of alternative methods for toxicological research. These include state-of-the-art technologies such as the use of *in vitro* methodologies, including cell culture models from both mammalian (including human) and nonmammalian species; microchip array technology; and computer-based predictive toxicology models. As an example, ICCVAM evaluated and recommended four validated test methods for assessing the dermal corrosivity hazard potential of chemicals: Corrositex(r), EPISKIN(tm), EpiDerm(tm) (EPI-200), and the rat skin transcutaneous electrical resistance assay. At the request of the U.S. Environmental Protection Agency, ICCVAM established performance standards for the three proprietary dermal corrosivity test methods (Corrositex(r), EPISKIN(tm), EpiDerm(tm) [EPI-200]) and the nonproprietary rat skin transcutaneous electrical resistance test method and in May 2004 published the *Recommended Performance Standards for In Vitro Test Methods for Skin Corrosion* (http://iccvam.niehs.nih.gov/methods/ps/ps044510.htm).

ICCVAM was established in 1997 by the Director of the National Institute of Environmental Health Sciences to implement Public Law 103–43. This law attempts to establish wherever possible guidelines, recommendations, and regulations that "promote the regulatory acceptance of new or revised scientifically valid toxicological tests that protect human and animal health and the environment while reducing, refining, or replacing animal tests and ensuring human safety and product effectiveness." This committee is represented by 15 federal research and regulatory agencies:

- Agency for Toxic Substances and Disease Registry
- Environmental Protection Agency
- Consumer Product Safety Commission
- Food and Drug Administration
- Department of Agriculture
- National Institutes of Health
- Department of Defense
- National Cancer Institute
- Department of Energy
- National Institute of Environmental Health Sciences
- Department of the Interior
- National Institute for Occupational Safety and Health
- Department of Transportation
- National Library of Medicine
- Occupational Safety and Health Administration

The use of computers for structure–activity relationships (SARs) has provided another methodology for the toxicologist. It is based on the concept that the structure of a chemical may possess significant information upon which predictions concerning toxicity can be made, for both the parent compound and any metabolites that could theoretically be produced from cellular metabolism. SARs can be useful because they may allow us to predict the toxicological properties of uninvestigated substances, based on the known properties of chemically related substances (e.g., the N–N=O functional group tends to confer the property of carcinogenicity for a chemical). In addition, it hypothesizes the mechanisms by which the chemicals may interact with the biological system. This information is expressed in quantitative terms, through the formulation of equations that can make predictions about toxicity under a variety of conditions.

## Examples of *In Vitro* Tests for Several Toxicological End-Points

Numerous *in vitro* methodologies are available to study various aspects of biological responses to chemical insult. Several tests have been organized into a limited number of toxicological end-points, as examples, and are briefly discussed.

### Mutagenicity and Chromosome Damage

Bacteria and animal cells in culture provide a rapid and relatively inexpensive way to screen chemicals for their potential effects on the genetic material. These effects can include mutagenic effects, carcinogenic effects, or damage to the chromosomes. The best-known and most widely used of these tests is the *Salmonella* mutagenicity test (commonly known as the Ames test). This involves growing special bacteria in the laboratory and exposing them to the chemical in question. The procedure evaluates the mutagenic potential of test chemicals by their effect on strains of the bacterium *Salmonella typhimurium,* which cannot produce their own histidine. The amino acid histidine is required by the bacteria to survive and grow in culture and must be supplied to the culture medium. A test chemical that is either first metabolized by an *in vitro* rat liver metabolizing enzyme or the unmetabolized chemical is added to the culture medium of the bacteria to assess if some of the bacteria will mutate back to the form that can produce their own histidine and thus survive and multiply in media that has not been supplemented with this amino acid.

DNA damage is a prerequisite for mutagenesis. A commonly used test to assess for DNA damage is the unscheduled DNA synthesis (UDS) test, which is typically done using rat liver cells or human fibroblasts. In this *in vitro* assay, the radioactively based thymidine is added to the culture medium to determine its uptake. The amount of thymidine incorporated into the cells that are treated with a test chemical is compared with untreated controls, and differences in thymidine incorporation are used as a measure for DNA repair.

Chromosomal effects involve the exposure of cell cultures and microscopic examination for chromosome damage. The most commonly used cells are human lymphocytes and Chinese hamster ovary (CHO) cells. The CHO cells have a low chromosome number (22), which makes for easier identification of chromosome damage.

## Tumor Promotion

The screening of chemicals as possible promoters of carcinogenesis has been done using RAS transfected BALB 3T3 (Bhas 42) cells to determine whether they lose contact inhibition in cell culture in response to a suspected promoter. In addition, tumor promoters have also been studied in cell culture by examining the transfer of the dye Lucifer yellow between SV-40 transformed hamster fibroblasts.

## Cytotoxicity

There have been a number of *in vitro* tests developed that measure cytotoxicity with either cellular death as an end-point or the disruption of a physiological process (e.g., disruption of enzyme function) or cellular structure (leakage of cellular macromolecules across the cell membrane). The neutral red assay is an example of an *in vitro* test designed to provide an indication of cell membrane integrity as an end-point. In this test cells are cultured in plastic Petri dishes and treated with various concentrations of a test chemical. The neutral red dye, which is added to the cell culture after rinsing out the test chemical, is accumulated and stored by cells. The amount of dye retained by the cells indicates the number of living cells in the dish. A general test like the neutral red assay thus provides some indication of cellular responses to chemicals that can then be interpreted as an indication of acute toxicity.

Other tests for cytotoxicity may measure leakage of cellular contents into the surrounding culture medium as an indication of a loss of normal cell membrane function. For example, human lymphocytes can be used to measure the leakage of large molecules such as the enzyme lactate dehydrogenase and DNA from the cell into the surrounding culture medium as an indicator of cytotoxicity. Under normal circumstances these macromolecules are too large to cross the cell membrane of intact cells. Disruption of the sodium potassium ATPase enzyme transport system, which is critical for normal distribution of ions across the cell membrane in CHO cells, can be used as another method to assess for cytotoxic effects from exposures to chemical agents.

## Eye Irritation

There are a number of *in vitro* surrogates for in vivo eye irritation tests. One procedure is the use of mouse fibroblast cells in cell culture and measuring zones of color change in cells that have been overlaid with agarose and then treated with test material. The zones are visualized by loss of neutral red from previously stained cells. The assay may have some use in assessing irritation of test substances, especially detergent or surfactant-based products as an alternative to the Draize rabbit eye test.

Another *in vitro* test to assess the effects of chemicals on the eye involved the culture of bovine whole lenses. Chemicals are assessed for their ability to alter the refractive index and transparency of the lens tissue using computer-assisted laser scanning.

## Cardiac Muscle Toxicity

Myocardial muscle preparations obtained from isolated 10-day-old chick embryos can be used in cell culture to test for the cardiotoxicity of chemicals. These cells contract spontaneously in cell culture and can be used to assess for any changes in mechanical and electrical activity as determined using appropriate microelectrode and video techniques. Inhibition of spontaneous beating activity, leakage of lactate dehydrogenase, alterations of membrane potential, and changes in cell morphology can be used as end-points to measure toxicity.

## Nephrotoxicity

The kidney is composed of a number of different types of cells with different functions. Nephrotoxicants may be selective in affecting one or more specific types of kidney cells, without affecting other adjacent cells. Some *in vitro* techniques that assess nephrotoxicity are based on exposure of specific renal cell types that can be isolated and exposed separately to various chemicals over a wide range of concentrations. Toxicity is assessed by measuring changes in aspects of cellular biochemistry in treated and control cells, including, for example, protein synthesis, glucose, and fatty acid metabolism. Decreases in these parameters are considered to be end-points of cytotoxicity and may indicate nephrotoxicity *in vivo* and selective cellular toxicity *in vitro,* further providing information about the potential sites of injury *in vivo.* The kidneys from one laboratory animal can provide enough cells to test a number of different chemicals for their nephrotoxic potential.

## Hepatotoxicity

The liver is the major internal organ for metabolism of xenobiotics and is also a major target organ for toxicity as well. A number of liver cell lines are available for study; however, their usefulness as a model to predict *in vivo* hepatotoxicity largely depends on the ability of the cells to maintain their normal metabolic functions. Cytotoxicity of xenobiotics in a number of different hepatoma (liver tumor) cell lines has been used as a method to test xenobiotics for liver toxicity using colony formation as an indicator of toxicity.

Six hepatoma cell lines have been used for such studies:

1. JM2: A rat hepatoma cell line that does not show monooxygenase activities.
2. MH1C1: A rat hepatoma cell line that shows basal and inducible levels of monooxygenases.
3. HepG2: A human hepatoblastoma cell line that shows basal and inducible levels of monooxygenases.
4. Hepa 1c1c7: A murine hepatoma cell line that shows basal and inducible levels of monooxygenases.
5. 7777: A rat hepatoma cell line that shows basal and inducible levels of monooxygenases.
6. HTC: A rat hepatoma cell line that does not show monooxygenase activities.

### Endocrine Toxicity

Biopsies obtained during surgery from a human thyroid gland can be used as a source of thyroid cells. These cells can be maintained in culture for several weeks and still retain their morphological characteristics and physiological functions. The cells can be used to assess for toxicity of xenobiotics and drugs on thyroid function.

### Respiratory Toxicity

Inhaled particulates may produce irritation and fibrosis in the respiratory system through the activation of alveolar macrophages and the release of mediators of inflammation. Alveolar macrophages can be isolated and exposed to particulates in cell culture to assess cytotoxicity measured by cell death. Cellular injury can be determined by measuring cellular membrane damage as determined by vital dye exclusion and leakage of the enzyme lactate dehydrogenase (LDH). Although alveolar macrophages are generally obtained from the lungs of rodents, human macrophages may be collected from patients who are undergoing bronchoscopy.

### Reproductive Toxicity

Bovine ejaculated spermatozoa can be used to study the cytotoxic effects of chemicals. Swimming activity, velocity, ATP content, and cellular structure can be used as end-points to measure the cytotoxic effect of test compounds. Another example of an *in vitro* test is the use of cultured human cumulus granulosa cells as a marker for reproductive toxicity. Human granulosa cells that remain after the *in vitro* fertilization of oocytes can be cultured for several days and exposed to human chorionic gonadotropin to obtain a baseline for progesterone under control conditions. Cells are then exposed to test compounds in the presence of human chorionic gonadotropin, and the production of progesterone is compared with their control values.

### Ecological Toxicity Tests

Numerous tests are available that can screen environmental media for potential toxicity. One such bioassay that is used to test for soil contamination is the Allium test. *Allium cepa* (onion) may be used to detect soils that alter root growth and chromosomes. The root tip, which comes into contact with the soil and therefore any pollutants contained within this medium, is contrasted with comparably treated control soil preparations. Observations on the root tip system shows that it is particularly sensitive to the harmful effects of environmental contaminants and can be quantified through the measurement of growth inhibition. In addition, the chromosomes contained within the root system in these actively dividing cells can be used to assess for damage that may possibly indicate a mutagenic or genotoxic effect. In addition to soil as the environmental medium to be tested, environmental water samples may also be used as well to prepare soils for testing in the laboratory.

The protozoan *Tetrahymena thermophila* can be used to study the effect of chemicals on its proliferation rate as a measure for toxicity. This organism is found in freshwater environments and has a relatively short generation time (approximately 4 hours), making it an ideal organism for study. Effects of chemicals on the swimming speed of this protozoan may be detected as well using video-imaging analysis. Proliferation rate, maximum cellular density, and swimming speed are indicators of physiological status of the organism and are used to assess for differences in organisms that have been treated with the test chemical and those that have not.

The development and refining of alternative methodologies to the use of animals for toxicity testing has been and will continue to be an important area of concern for toxicologists. In closing this chapter, however, it must be emphasized that any alternative methodology to the use of whole animals is by its nature a much more simplistic system for addressing concerns about toxicity outcomes and thus leaves open a greater gap in our knowledge about what it means in context to human health effects.

## Websites

Chemical Toxicity Database:
http://wwwdb.mhlw.go.jp/ginc/html/db1.html

National Toxicology Program:
http://ntp-server.niehs.nih.gov/

The Centers for Disease Control:
http://www.cdc.gov/

The Department of Health and Human Services:
http://www.hhs.gov/

The Environmental Protection Agency:
http://epa.gov/

The Food and Drug Administration:
http://www.fda.gov/

The National Toxicology Program:
http://ntp.niehs.nih.gov/

U.S. Department of Labor Occupational Safety & Health Administration:
http://osha.gov/

U.S. FDA Center for Food Safety and Applied Nutrition:
http://www.cfsan.fda.gov/

## Bibliography

Auletta, C. S. (2004). Current in vivo assays for cutaneous toxicity: local and systemic toxicity testing. *Basic and Cinical Pharmacology and Toxicology, 95,* 201–208.

Bernauer, U., Oberemm, A., Madle, S., & Gundert-Remy, U. (2005). The use of in vitro data in risk assessment. *Basic and Clinical Pharmacology and Toxicology, 96,* 176–181.

Brennan, F. R., & Dougan, G. (2005). Non-clinical safety evaluation of novel vaccines and adjuvants: new products, new strategies. *Vaccine, 23,* 3210–3222.

Guzelian, P. S., Victoroff, M. S., Halmes, N. C., James, R. C., & Guzelian, C. P. Evidence-based toxicology: a comprehensive framework for causation. *Human and Experimental Toxicology, 24,* 161–201.

Pellizzer, C., Bremer, S., & Hartung, T. (2005). Developmental toxicity testing from animal towards embryonic stem cells. *ALTEX : Alternativen zu Tierexperimenten, 22,* 47–57.

Reynolds, V. L. (2005). Applications of emerging technologies in toxicology and safety assessment. *International Journal of Toxicology, 24,* 135–137.

Travis, K. Z., Pate, I., & Welsh, Z. K. (2005). The role of the benchmark dose in a regulatory context. *Regulatory Toxicology and Pharmacology, 43,* 280–291.

U.S. National Library of Medicine, National Institutes of Health, Environmental Health, and Toxicology Specialized Information Services (SIS). (2005). *Toxicology tutorial III.* Retrieved October 2, 2005 from http://www.sis.nlm.nih.gov/enviro/toxtutor.html.

# APPENDIX
# 20

## Example of a Template for a Subchronic Toxicity Study in Rodents for FDA Review

Subchronic Toxicity Study in Rodents
Date of Submission:
Title of Petition or Notification:
Name and Address of Petitioner or Notifier:

I.  Identification of Study
    A.  Study File Location:
    B.  Study Title/Report Number:
    C.  Name and Address of Testing Facility:
    D.  Date of Study Report:
    E.  Dates Study Conducted:
    F.  Study Objective:
    G.  Comments:

II.  Good Laboratory Practice
    A.  Good Laboratory Practice (GLP) Compliance?
    B.  Quality Assurance (QA) Statement?
    C.  Availability and Location of Original Data/Specimens/Test Substance:

III. Executive Summary

IV. Materials and Methods
    A.  Test Substance
        1.  CAS name:
        2.  Other name(s):
        3.  CAS registry number:
        4.  Molecular structure: http://www.chemfinder.com
        5.  Purity:
        6.  Impurities:
        7.  Stability:
        8.  Comments:

B. Test Substance as Administered
   1. Batch/lot number:
   2. Route:
   3. Vehicle used:
   4. Tested adequately for concentration?
   5. Tested for homogeneity?
   6. Tested for stability?
   7. Problems with storage?
C. Animal Diet
   1. Feed
      a. Type:
      b. Name:
      c. Availability:
      d. Analysis for contaminants:
      e. Comments:
   2. Water
      a. Source:
      b. Availability:
      c. Analysis for contaminants:
      d. Comments:
D. Test Animals
   1. Species/strain/substrain:
   2. Sex:
   3. Age range at initiation of study:
   4. Weight range at initiation of study:
   5. Quarantine/acclimation?
   6. Physical examination times:
   7. Number per cage:
   8. Environmental conditions:
   9. Comments:
E. Experimental Design
   1. Targeted dose levels:

| Test Group | Conc. in Diet (ppm or mg/kg) | Dose to Animals (mg/kg body weight/day) | Number of Males | Number of Females |
|---|---|---|---|---|
| Control | | | | |
| Low | | | | |
| Mid | | | | |
| High | | | | |

2. Total number of animals:
3. Duration of study (including recovery period, if any):
4. Length of exposure to test substance:
5. Were animals randomized?
6. Recovery period:
7. Comments:

F. Body Weight and Feed Intake
   1. Parameter examined:

| Examined | Not Examined |
|---|---|
| | Feed Intake* |
| | Feed Spillage* |
| | Water Intake* |
| | Body Weight* |
| | Body Weight Changes* |

*These parameters are recommended in REDBOOK for subchronic toxicity studies.

2. Comments: (e.g., list frequency)

G. Cage-Side Observations
   1. Parameter examined:

| Examined | Not Examined |
|---|---|
| | Appearance* |
| | Abnormal Stool* |
| | Morbidity* |
| | Mortality* |
| | Neurotoxicity Screening (specify parameters)*, ** |

*These parameters are recommended in REDBOOK for subchronic toxicity studies. Add additional parameters tested.

**The parameters for neurotoxicity screening may include, but are not limited to, the following:
- Changes in skin, fur, eyes, mucous membranes, gait, posture, and response to handling
- Occurrence of secretions/excretions or other evidence of autonomic activity such as lacrimation, piloerection, pupil size change, unusual respiratory pattern
- Presence of clonic or tonic seizure
- Stereotype behaviors such as excessive grooming and repetitive circling
- Bizarre behavior such as self-mutilating and walking backward
- Gross tumor development

2. Comments: (e.g., list frequency)

H. Ophthalmological Examination

   1. Parameter examined:

   2. Comments: (e.g., list frequency)

I. Hematology

   1. Fasting duration prior to blood collection:

   2. When in the study were the blood samples collected?

   3. How were the blood samples drawn?

   4. Dose groups and number of animals tested:

   5. Parameter examined:

| Measurement Related to | Examined | Not Examined |
|---|---|---|
| Red Blood Cells | | Hematocrit (Hct)* |
| | | Hemoglobin Conc. (Hb)* |
| | | Mean Corp. Hb. (MCH)* |
| | | Mean Corp. Hb. Conc. (MCHC)* |
| | | Mean Corp. Volume (MCV)* |
| | | Total Erythrocyte Count (RBC)* |
| White Blood Cells | | Basophils, Eosinophils*, Lymphocytes* |
| | | Macrophage/Monocytes* |
| | | Neutrophils* |
| | | Total Leukocytes (WBC)* |
| Clotting Potential | | Activated Partial-Thromboplastin Time* |
| | | Clotting Time* |
| | | Platelet Count* |
| | | Prothrombin Time* |
| Others | | Bone marrow cytology* |
| | | Reticulocyte counts* |

*These parameters are recommended in REDBOOK for subchronic toxicity studies. Add additional parameters tested.

   6. Comments:

J. Clinical Chemistry

   1. Fasting duration prior to blood collection:

   2. When in the study were the blood samples collected?

   3. How were the blood samples drawn?

   4. Dose groups and number of animals tested:

   5. Parameter examined:

| Measurement Related to | Examined | Not Examined |
|---|---|---|
| Electrolyte Balance | | Calcium* |
| | | Chloride*,** |
| | | Phosphorus* |
| | | Potassium*,** |
| | | Sodium*,** |
| Carbohydrate Metabolism | | Glucose*,** |
| Liver Function: | | |
| A) Hepatocellular (Recommend at least 3 out of 5 RED BOOK PARAMETERS) | | Alanine Aminotransferase (ALT or SGPT)*,** |
| | | Aspartate Aminotransferase (AST or SGOT)* |
| | | Glutamate Dehydrogenase* |
| | | Sorbitol Dehydrogenase* |
| | | Total Bile Acids* |
| B) Hepatobiliary (Recommend at least 3 out of 5 RED BOOK PARAMETERS) | | Alkaline Phosphatase (ALP)*,** |
| | | Gamma-Glutamyl Transferase (GGT)*,** |
| | | Total Bile Acids* |
| | | Total Bilirubin* |
| | | 5' Nucleotidase* |
| Kidney Function | | Creatinine*,** |
| | | Urea Nitrogen*,** |
| Others (acid-base balance, cholinesterases, hormones, lipids, methemoglobin, and proteins) | | Albumin (A)* |
| | | Globulin (G, calculated) or A/G Ratio* |
| | | Total Cholesterol* |
| | | Cholinesterase* |
| | | Total protein*,** |
| | | Fasting Triglycerides* |

*These parameters are recommended in REDBOOK for subchronic toxicity studies. Add additional parameters tested.

** These parameters should generally be given priority when adequate volumes of blood samples cannot be obtained from test animals.

6. Comments:

K. Urinalysis

   1. When were urine samples collected?

   2. Parameter examined:

| Examined | Not Examined |
|---|---|
| | Glucose*, Microscopic evaluation for sediment and presence of blood/blood cells*, pH*, Protein*, Specific Gravity*, Volume* |

* These parameters are recommended in REDBOOK for subchronic toxicity studies.

      3. Comments:

L. Other Tests

      1. Observations:

      2. Comments:

M. Necropsy (Interim Sacrifice)

      1. Was there an interim sacrifice?

      2. Dose groups and number of animals:

      3. Organs/Tissues weighed:

| Examined | Not Examined |
|---|---|
| | Adrenals*, Brain*, Epididymides*, Heart*, Kidneys*, Liver*, Spleen*, Testes*, Thyroid/parathyroid*, Thymus*, Ovaries*, Uterus* |

\* These parameters are recommended in REDBOOK for subchronic toxicity studies.

      4. Comments:

N. Necropsy (Terminal)

      1. Organs/Tissues weighed:

      2. Comments:

| Examined | Not Examined |
|---|---|
| | Adrenals*, Brain*, Epididymides*, Heart*, Kidneys*, Liver*, Spleen*, Testes*, Thyroid/parathyroid*, Thymus*, Ovaries*, Uterus* |

\*These parameters are recommended in REDBOOK for subchronic toxicity studies. Add additional parameters tested.

O. Gross Pathology Observations

      1. Organs/Tissues Examined:

      2. Comments:

P. Histopathology Observations

      1. Organs/Tissues were collected from which dose groups?

      2. Organs/Tissues were examined from which dose groups?

      3. How were the organs/tissues prepared for histopathology observation?

      4. Organs/Tissues collected:

| System | Examined | Not Examined |
|--------|----------|--------------|
| Digestive | | Salivary Gland*, Esophagus*, Stomach*, Duodenum*, Jejunum*, Ileum*, Cecum*, Colon*, Rectum*, Gall Bladder* (in case of mice), Liver* (middle, left and triangular lobes), Pancreas* |
| Respiratory | | Nasal Turbinates*, Trachea*, Lung* (with main-stem bronchi) |
| Cardiovascular | | Aorta*, Heart* |
| Reticulo- Endothelial/ Hematopoietic | | Bone Marrow* (sternum), Lymph Nodes* (1 related to route of administration, and 1 from a distant location), Spleen*, Thymus* |
| Urogenital | | Kidneys*, Ovaries* and fallopian tubes*, Corpus Uteri*, Cervix Uteri*, Prostate*, Seminal Vesicle* (if present), Testes*, Urinary Bladder*, Vagina* |
| Neurological | | Brain* (at least 3 different levels), Spinal-Cervical*, Spinal-Lumbar*, Spinal-Midthoracic*, Sciatic Nerve*, Harderian Gland* (if present) |
| Glandular | | Adrenals*, Mammary Glands*, Pituitary Glands*, Thyroid/Parathyroid Glands*, Thymus*, Zymbal's Gland* (if present) |
| Other | | Bone (Femur)*, Eyes*, Skeletal Muscle*, Skin*, Epididymis* |

*These parameters are recommended in REDBOOK for subchronic toxicity studies. Add additional parameters tested.

    5.  Comments:

Q.  Statistical Methods

    1.  Methods of statistical analysis:

| Methods of Statistical Analysis | Parameters Tested |
|---------------------------------|-------------------|
| | |
| | |
| | |
| | |

2. Comments:

V. Results
   A. Dose Verification
      1. Were doses verified?

| Dose Group | Targeted Concentration (ppm or mg/kg) | Concentrations Found in Feed (ppm or mg/kg) | Standard Deviation | N* |
|---|---|---|---|---|
| Low | | | | |
| Mid | | | | |
| High | | | | |

* Number of measurements.

      2. Verified by:
      3. Comments:
   B. Feed Consumption Changes
      1. Observations:
      2. Comments:
   C. Intake Of Test Substance
      1. Observations:

| Dose Group | Daily Dose (mg/kg body–weight/day) |
|---|---|
| Control | 0 |
| Low | |
| Mid | |
| High | |

      2. Comments:
   D. Feed Efficiency
      1. Was feed efficiency calculated?
      2. Comments:
   E. Body Weight Changes
      1. Observations:
      2.Comments:
   F. Cage-Side Observations
      1. Observations:
      2. Comments:

G. Mortality
    1. Observations:
    2. Comments:

H. Ophthalmological Examination
    1. Observations:
    2. Comments:

I. Hematology
    1. Observations:

| SEX | Males | | | | Females | | | |
|---|---|---|---|---|---|---|---|---|
| **DAILY DOSE** (mg/kg bodyweight/day) | **0** Control | | | | **0** Control | | | |
| **NUMBER OF ANIMALS** | | | | | | | | |
| **Red Blood Cells** | | | | | | | | |
| Hematocrit (Hct)　　　% | | | | | | | | |
| Hemoglobin Conc. (Hb)　g/l | | | | | | | | |
| Mean Corp. Hb. (MCH) | | | | | | | | |
| Mean Corp. Hb. Conc. (MCHC) | | | | | | | | |
| Mean Corp. Volume　　l/l (MCV) | | | | | | | | |
| Total Erythrocyte Count (RBC)　　　$10^{12}$/l | | | | | | | | |
| **White Blood Cells** | | | | | | | | |
| Basophils | | | | | | | | |
| Eosinophils | | | | | | | | |
| Lymphocytes　　　$10^9$/l | | | | | | | | |
| Macrophage/ Monocytes | | | | | | | | |
| Neutrophils　　　$10^9$/l | | | | | | | | |
| Total Leukocytes (WBC)　$10^9$/l | | | | | | | | |
| **Clotting Potential** | | | | | | | | |
| Activated Partial- Thromboplastin Time | | | | | | | | |
| Clotting Time | | | | | | | | |
| Platelet Count　　　$10^9$/l | | | | | | | | |
| Prothrombin Time | | | | | | | | |
| **Others** | | | | | | | | |
| Bone marrow cytology | | | | | | | | |
| Reticulocyte counts　　$10^{12}$/l | | | | | | | | |

(Specify a method of statistical analysis): * $p < 0.05$, ** $p < 0.01$

2. Comments:

J.  Clinical Chemistry

   1. Observations:

| SEX | Males | | | | Females | | | |
|---|---|---|---|---|---|---|---|---|
| **DAILY DOSE** (mg/kg bodyweight/day) | 0 Control | | | | 0 Control | | | |
| **NUMBER OF ANIMALS** | | | | | | | | |
| **Electrolyte Balance** | | | | | | | | |
| Calcium        mmol/l | | | | | | | | |
| Chloride       mmol/l | | | | | | | | |
| Phosphorus    mmol/l | | | | | | | | |
| Potassium     mmol/l | | | | | | | | |
| Sodium        mmol/l | | | | | | | | |
| **Carbohydrate Metabolism** | | | | | | | | |
| Glucose        mmol/l | | | | | | | | |
| **Liver Function:** | | | | | | | | |
| **A) hepatocellular** | | | | | | | | |
| Alanine Aminotransferase (ALT or SGPT)      U/l | | | | | | | | |
| Aspartate Aminotransferase (AST or SGOT)      U/l | | | | | | | | |
| Glutamate Dehydrogenase      U/l | | | | | | | | |
| Sorbitol Dehydrogenase   U/l | | | | | | | | |
| **Liver Function:** | | | | | | | | |
| **B) hepatobiliary** | | | | | | | | |
| Alkaline Phosphatase (ALP)      U/l | | | | | | | | |
| Gamma-Glutamyl Transferase (GGT)      U/l | | | | | | | | |
| Total Bile Acids    mmol/l | | | | | | | | |
| Total Bilirubin     mmol/l | | | | | | | | |
| 5' Nucleotidase      U/l | | | | | | | | |
| **Kidney Function** | | | | | | | | |
| Creatinine      mmol/l | | | | | | | | |
| Urea Nitrogen     mg/dL | | | | | | | | |

| SEX | Males | | | | Females | | | |
|---|---|---|---|---|---|---|---|---|
| **DAILY DOSE** (mg/kg bodyweight/day) | 0 Control | | | | 0 Control | | | |
| **NUMBER OF ANIMALS** | | | | | | | | |
| **Others** | | | | | | | | |
| Albumin (A)              g/l | | | | | | | | |
| Globulin (G, calculated)  g/l | | | | | | | | |
| A/G Ratio | | | | | | | | |
| Total protein            g/l | | | | | | | | |
| Total Cholesterol      mmol/l | | | | | | | | |
| Fasting Triglycerides  mmol/l | | | | | | | | |
| Cholinesterase           U/l | | | | | | | | |

(Specify statistical method of analysis): * p < 0.05, ** p < 0.01

    2.  Comments:

K.  Urinalysis

    1.  Observations:

| SEX | Males | | | | Females | | | |
|---|---|---|---|---|---|---|---|---|
| **DAILY DOSE** (mg/kg bodyweight/day) | 0 Control | | | | 0 Control | | | |
| **NUMBER OF ANIMALS** | | | | | | | | |
| Glucose               mmol/l | | | | | | | | |
| Microscopic evaluation for sediment and presence of blood/ blood cells | | | | | | | | |
| pH | | | | | | | | |
| Protein                g/l | | | | | | | | |
| Specific Gravity | | | | | | | | |
| Volume               l/time | | | | | | | | |

2. Comments:
L. Other Tests
   1. Observations:
   2. Comments:
M. Organ Weights
   1. Observations:

| SEX | Males | | | | Females | | | |
|---|---|---|---|---|---|---|---|---|
| **DAILY DOSE** (mg/kg bodyweight/day) | **0** Control | | | | **0** Control | | | |
| **NUMBER OF ANIMALS** | | | | | | | | |
| **BODY WEIGHT (gram)**[a] | | | | | | | | |
| **BRAIN** | | | | | | | | |
| Absolute Weight[a]   gram | | | | | | | | |
| Per Body Weight[a]   % | | | | | | | | |
| **ADRENALS** | | | | | | | | |
| Absolute Weight[a]   gram | | | | | | | | |
| Per Body Weight[a]   % | | | | | | | | |
| Per Brain Weight[a]   % | | | | | | | | |
| **EPIDIDYMIDES** | | | | | | | | |
| Absolute Weight[a]   gram | | | | | | | | |
| Per Body Weight[a]   % | | | | | | | | |
| Per Brain Weight[a]   % | | | | | | | | |
| **HEART** | | | | | | | | |
| Absolute Weight[a]   gram | | | | | | | | |
| Per Body Weight[a]   % | | | | | | | | |
| Per Brain Weight[a]   % | | | | | | | | |
| **KIDNEYS** | | | | | | | | |
| Absolute Weight[a]   gram | | | | | | | | |
| Per Body Weight[a]   % | | | | | | | | |
| Per Brain Weight[a]   % | | | | | | | | |
| **LIVER** | | | | | | | | |
| Absolute Weight[a]   gram | | | | | | | | |
| Per Body Weight[a]   % | | | | | | | | |
| Per Brain Weight[a]   % | | | | | | | | |

| SEX | Males | | | | Females | | | |
|---|---|---|---|---|---|---|---|---|
| **DAILY DOSE** (mg/kg bodyweight/day) | 0 Control | | | | 0 Control | | | |
| **NUMBER OF ANIMALS** | | | | | | | | |
| **SPLEEN** | | | | | | | | |
| Absolute Weight[a]  gram | | | | | | | | |
| Per Body Weight[a]  % | | | | | | | | |
| Per Brain Weight[a]  % | | | | | | | | |
| **TESTES** | | | | | | | | |
| Absolute Weight[a]  gram | | | | | | | | |
| Per Body Weight[a]  % | | | | | | | | |
| Per Brain Weight[a]  % | | | | | | | | |
| **THYROID and PARATHYROID** | | | | | | | | |
| Absolute Weight[a]  gram | | | | | | | | |
| Per Body Weight[a]  % | | | | | | | | |
| Per Brain Weight[a]  % | | | | | | | | |
| **THYMUS** | | | | | | | | |
| Absolute Weight[a]  gram | | | | | | | | |
| Per Body Weight[a]  % | | | | | | | | |
| Per Brain Weight[a]  % | | | | | | | | |
| **OVARIES** | | | | | | | | |
| Absolute Weight[a]  gram | | | | | | | | |
| Per Body Weight[a]  % | | | | | | | | |
| Per Brain Weight[a]  % | | | | | | | | |
| **UTERUS** | | | | | | | | |
| Absolute Weight[a]  gram | | | | | | | | |
| Per Body Weight[a]  % | | | | | | | | |
| Per Brain Weight[a]  % | | | | | | | | |

[a]Group means at the end of terminal necropsy are shown.
(Specify methods of statistical analysis): * $p < 0.05$, ** $p < 0.01$

    2. Comments:

  N. Gross Pathology Changes Observed

    1. Observations:

    2. Comments:

O. Histopathology Changes Observed

1. Observations:

| | NUMBER OF ANIMALS WITH, GROSS, NON-NEOPLASTIC, OR NEOPLASTIC LESIONS | | | | | | | |
|---|---|---|---|---|---|---|---|---|
| **SEX** | **Males** | | | | **Females** | | | |
| **DAILY DOSE** (mg/kg bodyweight/day) | **0** Control | | | | **0** Control | | | |
| **NUMBER OF ANIMALS EXAMINED** | | | | | | | | |
| *DIGESTIVE SYSTEM* ORGAN/TISSUE # | | | | | | | | |
| Gross lesion | | | | | | | | |
| Non-neoplastic lesion | | | | | | | | |
| Non-neoplastic lesion | | | | | | | | |
| non-neoplastic lesion | | | | | | | | |
| neoplastic lesions | | | | | | | | |
| neoplastic lesions | | | | | | | | |
| neoplastic lesions | | | | | | | | |
| *RESPIRATORY SYSTEM* ORGAN/TISSUE # | | | | | | | | |
| gross lesion | | | | | | | | |
| non-neoplastic lesion | | | | | | | | |
| non-neoplastic lesion | | | | | | | | |
| non-neoplastic lesion | | | | | | | | |
| neoplastic lesions | | | | | | | | |
| neoplastic lesions | | | | | | | | |
| neoplastic lesions | | | | | | | | |
| *CARDIOVASCULAR SYSTEM* ORGAN/TISSUE # | | | | | | | | |
| gross lesion | | | | | | | | |
| non-neoplastic lesion | | | | | | | | |
| non-neoplastic lesion | | | | | | | | |
| non-neoplastic lesion | | | | | | | | |
| neoplastic lesions | | | | | | | | |
| neoplastic lesions | | | | | | | | |
| neoplastic lesions | | | | | | | | |

| | NUMBER OF ANIMALS WITH, GROSS, NON-NEOPLASTIC, OR NEOPLASTIC LESIONS | | | | | | | |
|---|---|---|---|---|---|---|---|---|
| **SEX** | **Males** | | | | **Females** | | | |
| **DAILY DOSE** (mg/kg bodyweight/day) | 0 Control | | | | 0 Control | | | |
| **NUMBER OF ANIMALS EXAMINED** | | | | | | | | |
| ***RETICULO-ENDOTHELIAL/ HEMATOPOIETIC SYSTEM*** **ORGAN/TISSUE** [#] | | | | | | | | |
| gross lesion | | | | | | | | |
| non-neoplastic lesion | | | | | | | | |
| non-neoplastic lesion | | | | | | | | |
| non-neoplastic lesion | | | | | | | | |
| neoplastic lesions | | | | | | | | |
| neoplastic lesions | | | | | | | | |
| neoplastic lesions | | | | | | | | |
| ***UROGENITAL SYSTEM*** **ORGAN/TISSUE** [#] | | | | | | | | |
| gross lesion | | | | | | | | |
| non-neoplastic lesion | | | | | | | | |
| non-neoplastic lesion | | | | | | | | |
| non-neoplastic lesion | | | | | | | | |
| neoplastic lesions | | | | | | | | |
| neoplastic lesions | | | | | | | | |
| neoplastic lesions | | | | | | | | |
| ***GLANDULAR SYSTEM*** **ORGAN/TISSUE** [#] | | | | | | | | |
| gross lesion | | | | | | | | |
| non-neoplastic lesion | | | | | | | | |
| non-neoplastic lesion | | | | | | | | |
| non-neoplastic lesion | | | | | | | | |
| neoplastic lesions | | | | | | | | |
| neoplastic lesions | | | | | | | | |
| neoplastic lesions | | | | | | | | |

(Specify methods of statistical analysis): *$p < 0.05$, **$p < 0.01$

# Organs/tissues listed under section IV.P.

In general, data at end of dosing period can be shown; however, if there were additional noteworthy findings at earlier time points, these should be included. Note severity of lesions as needed.

2. Comments:

P. Neurotoxicity

  1. Observations:

| | NUMBER OF ANIMALS | | | | | | | |
|---|---|---|---|---|---|---|---|---|
| **SEX** | **Males** | | | | **Females** | | | |
| **DAILY DOSE**<br>(mg/kg bodyweight/day) | **0**<br>Control | | | | **0**<br>Control | | | |
| **NUMBER OF ANIMALS EXAMINED** | | | | | | | | |
| *OBSERVATIONS OF NERVOUS SYSTEM TOXICITY* + <br>observation<br>observation<br>observation | | | | | | | | |
| *GROSS- AND HISTO-PATHOLOGY CHANGES IN THE NEUROLOGIC SYSTEM* # **ORGAN/TISSUE**<br>gross lesion<br>non-neoplastic lesion<br>non-neoplastic lesion<br>non-neoplastic lesion<br>neoplastic lesions<br>neoplastic lesions<br>neoplastic lesions | | | | | | | | |

+ See under section IV.G for the types of observation for nervous system toxicity: List noteworthy findings. If additional parameters (other than those in the Template) showed noteworthy changes, these should be added to the tables. In general, include data at the end of the dosing period. However, if one observes additional noteworthy findings at earlier time points, these should be included. Footnotes should be used as needed to provide additional information about the tests or the results. Note the severity of the abnormal observations using the following scales; + Mild, ++ Moderate, and +++ Marked or other scales, as appropriate.

# Organs/tissues listed under section IV.P

2. Comments:

VI. Evaluation and Comment on Study

VII. Summary and Conclusions
   A. Brief Summary of Major Findings from the Study:
   B. Relationship Between Dose and Incidence/Severity of Lesions or Abnormalities:
   C. Was There a Target Organ?
   D. NOEL
      1. Was there a no observed effect level?
      2. Comments:

# CHAPTER 21

# Uses and Limitations of Product Labeling for Public Safety

## Purpose of Product Labeling

Labeling is the main method of communication between a manufacturer and the user of the product. The information attached to the product package is what most consumers look at; however, labeling includes all other information received from the manufacturer about the product when it is purchased, including pamphlets or brochures and package inserts.

Labeling for the manufacturer is a way to advertise and sell the product. To the user, it provides directions on how to use the product safely and effectively. To medical personnel, it is a source to identify toxicants for treatment in the case of poisoning. To the federal government, it is a means for control and assurance that standards are met and adequate information is provided to safeguard the public. If a product is found to pose an unacceptable risk to people or the environment, it can be restricted in its use or removed from the market. For example, the use of dichlorodiphenyltrichloroethane (DDT), chlordane, and other pesticides has been banned in the United States.

## Use of Product Labels by Consumers

Consumers generally assume that chemical products are safe if used according to the label directions. They generally read product labels for the following reasons:

- If the product is new to them
- To understand the directions for safe and effective use
- If there are children or pets in the household
- If there is a concern for a potential hazard if used incorrectly
- An accidental exposure has occurred

## Limitations of Product Labels

If you observe the product label from household products, many of them are difficult to read because of the small size of the type and inadequate color contrast. For some products, such as formulations, a good deal of information is provided on the label attached to the container. Many products contain a fold-out label, and some consumers may feel obligated to buy the product if they open it up. These small attached booklets contain a large amount of information, and many consumers may be discouraged from reading it. Additionally, many products fail to provide comprehensive ingredient information, including full chemical names and Chemical Abstracting Service (CAS) numbers.

Some products are proprietary formulations, and one or more ingredients may not be listed. This information, although perhaps of limited value to most consumers, becomes important in the event of a poisoning incident. It is always preferable for medical personnel to know exactly what is contained in the product as quickly as possible. Consumers may recognize what an "active ingredient" is but may not fully understand what is meant by "inert ingredients." In the case of pesticides, statements such as "it is a violation of federal law to use this product in a manner inconsistent with its labeling" should be clarified. Over the past decade there have been some good changes in product labeling; for example, the "statement of practical treatment" has been replaced by "first aid information." Consumers may also misinterpret some statements such as "hazards to humans and animals" to mean hazardous to humans and animals. Although the difference between the terms *danger* and *caution* or *warning* is relatively clear, there is no clear distinction between the last two terms.

## Federal Requirements

Federal law requires that the manufacturers of household products warn consumers about their products' hazards to humans, animals, and the environment. Hazardous household products are identified by the Federal Hazardous Substance Act (FHSA). A product or substance is hazardous when it contains one or more of the following properties:

- Flammable
- Explosive/reactive

- Corrosive/caustic
- Toxic/poisonous/sensitizer
- Radioactive

The FHSA is administered by the Consumer Product Safety Commission and covers most consumer products other than foods, drugs, cosmetics, pesticides, and tobacco products. A hazardous substance under the FHSA includes "any substance or mixture of substances which is toxic if such substance or mixture of substances may cause substantial personal injury or substantial illness during or as a proximate result of any customary or reasonably foreseeable handling or use, including reasonably foreseeable ingestion by children." The Act defines the term *toxic* in a very broad statutory definition as "any substance which has the capacity to produce personal injury or illness to man through ingestion, inhalation, or absorption through any body surface." The Act does not require that manufacturers of consumer products adhere to any specific federally approved label but does require the clear use of identification of specific label components, including

- *Brand or trade name.*
- *Common and/or chemical name:* common names of the chemical ingredients; chemical name if there is no common name; both chemical and common names may appear on the label (e.g., bleach and sodium hypochlorite).
- *Amount of contents* (e.g., weight or volume).
- *Description of hazard and precautionary statements:* description of the principal hazard involved in using the product, such as
  - Do not eat, drink, or smoke while using this product, and wash hands thoroughly when finished; may be harmful if swallowed.
  - Harmful vapor—work in a well-ventilated area. (A shortcoming of labels is that they do not specify how much ventilation is adequate or (in many cases) what personal protective equipment should be used.)
  - Flammable—avoid excessive heat and open flames.
  - Avoid skin contact—can be absorbed through the skin—wear long sleeves and gloves
  - Avoid eye contact—product is an "irritant" to the eyes; avoid splashing and wear protective goggles.
  - Avoid use if pregnant (indicates a concern that the product could injure the developing fetus).
  - Keep out of the reach of children.

- *Signal word:* informs the consumer about the level of the hazard. The signal word *danger* appears on products that are extremely flammable, corrosive, or highly toxic (additionally the word *poison* will appear on these products). The signal words *warning* (moderately hazardous) or *caution* (slightly hazardous) appear on all other hazardous substances. The word *nontoxic* lacks a regulatory definition, but it is often used by the manufacturer as a marketing tool. The absence of a signal word implies a nonhazardous product.
- *Name and address of manufacturer, distributor.*

- *Instructions for safe handling and use* (e.g., warnings about where to avoid the use of the product; the amount to be mixed with water; what not to mix with the product).
- *First aid instructions* (e.g., do not induce vomiting; if redness persists see a physician; seek medical help immediately).

The labeling of pesticides, even for household use, falls under the Federal Insecticide, Fungicide, and Rodenticide Act (FIFRA). Here, signal words associated with the level of toxicity (based on laboratory studies and oral consumption) include *slightly toxic* (caution), *moderately toxic* (warning), and *highly toxic* (danger)

- Caution: slightly toxic, more than 1 ounce can be fatal. Any product marketed as a pesticide must at least bear the word *caution* on the label.
- Warning: moderately toxic, 1 teaspoon to 1 ounce can be fatal.
- Danger or poison: Highly toxic, a few drops to 1 teaspoon can be fatal.

## FIFRA and Pesticides

As a general statement, pesticides are an important public health intervention to control vectors of disease and increase the yields of agricultural products on a global scale. In addition, pesticide use protects the public and our property from species that can produce physical injury to both. Because of the extent of pesticide use, however, great concerns exist regarding the potential health risks to the public and the environment. Special concern exists about exposures in more susceptible individuals, including pregnant women, the very young or elderly, and those with certain disease states. This is reflected in part by the level of product label detail for these chemicals.

The U.S. Environmental Protection Agency (EPA) under FIFRA regulates pesticide sale and use in the United States. Pesticides must be registered with the EPA for use, whether that use is residential or commercial and no matter who is applying the pesticide. To obtain a registration number, a pesticide must undergo extensive testing and characterization of its chemical, physical, and toxicological properties. Manufacturing production aspects, toxicology test results, and information on environmental fate are examples of the necessary data requirements to apply for registration. These must be provided by the manufacturer. The EPA also conducts risk assessments for pesticides. FIFRA was amended in 1996 by the Food Quality Protection Act (FQPA) to take into account prenatal, infant, and child exposures to pesticides, recognizing that they require additional margins of safety (10-fold) for exposures because of their unique potential health risks and vulnerabilities associated with toxicant insults.

## Pesticide Product Labeling

To comply with EPA guidelines, mandatory statements must appear on pesticide product labels. These mandatory statements include the actions that are necessary to ensure the proper use of the product and to help prevent adverse effects on the applicator, bystanders, and the environment. Examples of mandatory statements include directions for the use of the pesticide and precautions needed for the user to take or to avoid specific actions. Examples of *mandatory statements* may include the following:

- Wear chemical-resistant gloves when applying this product.
- Do not apply in windy conditions.
- Keep away from open flames, sparks, and heat.
- Do not induce vomiting.
- Do not use indoors.

In addition to mandatory statements, *advisory statements* must be provided on the labeling as well. The statements must not conflict with the mandatory statements and must not be misleading or false or violate any regulatory provisions. Advisory statements include the following:

- This product is best applied within 2 hours of mixing.
- Spray around the baseboards for optimum coverage.
- For best results, apply the granules at the base of the ant mound.
- Common household latex gloves provide adequate protection.
- This product may discolor carpet.

The required information on pesticide product labeling is as follows:

- *The name and address of the manufacturer or registrant* must appear on the label so that the purchaser of the product knows who manufactured or sold it and can contact them if necessary for any additional information, including material safety data sheets (MSDSs) that are not normally a part of labeling for consumer purchases of pesticide products but can be obtained by request.
- A *"restricted use" statement* (not applicable to the consumer) must appear where a product should only be applied commercially or has a high level of restrictions on its use. A restricted use pesticide "ensures" that only trained and certified companies and applicators can purchase and use the product. Restriction may be due to the high toxicity of the product or the level of concern to the public and environment if the product is misapplied. EPA considers restricted use as a risk reduction measure. It also provides a better degree of assurance that the individual applying the product has a level of training and understanding of pesticides greater than would be typically present in the general population. Restricted use is clearly marked on the front label of the package or container (Figure 21.1).
- The *product name, brand, or trademark* must be plainly visible on the front label of the product container. A brand name is the name that we typically recognize and the one that is used by the manufacturer in the advertising campaign for the product. The consumer product label typically describes what the product does. So although we may not recognize the chemicals and what they do in a pesticide formulation, a brand name of "Weeds B' Gone" tells the consumer that this product is to be used for the treatment of weeds and not fire ants. Other similar products (brands) may contain many of the same chemicals in their formulations, which are recognized on the product labels. Although many of us have used the brand name "Roundup" in our yards to remove unwanted vegetation, recognizing that the active

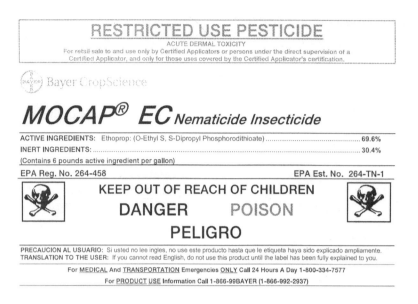

**FIGURE 21.1** Example of typical labeling of a restricted use pesticide. *Source:* With permission of Bayer Crop Science.

ingredient is glyphosate allows the consumer a greater selection of brands, especially when the patent for a new product runs out. The brand name can also give us information concerning the formulation of the product and where it is intended to be used. For example, a brand name followed by WSP, G, T&O, or R&F indicates a water-soluble powder, a granule formulation, to be used on turf and ornamental plants, and range and field, respectively.

- A *statement of ingredients* must be on the product label and include the percentage of active and "inert" ingredients. The chemical name for the active ingredients must appear on the label. Where common names are used, the technical name must appear as well. Although the inert ingredients can be listed, there is no requirement for this currently. The choice of a manufacturer not to disclose these may in part be related to a proprietary formulation for the active ingredients. The terms *inactive* and *inert* should not be taken to mean that they are synonymous. Chemicals in a formulation that are deemed inert by the manufacturer may merely indicate that they do not change the chemical properties of the active ingredients. For example, surfactants or organic solvents may be considered by the manufacturer to be inert; however, they still may be important from the standpoint of exposures and human toxicity, especially in view of the fact that very often it is the inert ingredients that represent the larger percentage of the volume or weight of the product. Inert should not be taken to mean not toxic. In addition, the product label must also show the weight or volume in the container.
- The *EPA registration number* and *EPA establishment number* appear on the front of the label. The first three numbers of the registration number identify the company that produced the pesticide. The establishment number identifies where the pesticide was manufactured or labeled. The establishment number is important because it identifies the responsible parties in the event of a problem with the product, recalls, and so on.

*Precautionary statements* include

- Hazards to humans and domestic animals
- First aid (statement of practical treatment)
- Environmental hazards and physical/chemical hazards

*An appropriate signal word* must appear on the front label of the pesticide container. The label must provide the user with the nature of the hazard that the product poses, whether it is flammable, corrosive, toxic, and so forth. There may be more than one hazard present. The label must provide information on emergency first aid measures and also state if exposures may require medical attention and at what level (e.g., seek medical attention immediately); the label must inform physicians about antidotes for poisoning.

Signal words for toxicity must convey the degree of potential toxicity pose by the product:

- Caution: slightly toxic
- Warning: moderately toxic
- Danger: highly toxic or hazardous in some manner

The word *danger* generally indicates that the product can cause illness from all routes of exposure or may produce severe local tissue injury such as eye and skin irritation. Based on acute toxicity tests ($LD_{50}$ or $LC_{50}$ values) and skin and eye irritant tests from laboratory animals, the designation of dangerous must appear on the label when:

- Acute oral: 50 mg/kg or less
- Acute dermal: 200 mg/kg or less
- Acute inhalation: 0.05 mg/l or less for a 4-hour exposure
- Primary eye irritation: a corrosive effect (irreversible destruction of ocular tissue) or corneal injury or irritation persisting for more than 3 weeks
- Primary skin irritation: a corrosive effect (tissue destruction extending into the dermis)

The term *poison* and the skull and crossbones symbol must be present as well on the front label of the container of products that have the designation *danger*.

The level of fatality certainty can include such statements:

- Fatal if swallowed, inhaled, or absorbed through skin. Do not breathe vapors or mists. Do not get in eyes or on skin or clothing. The front of the label requires a statement of medical treatment.
- May be fatal if swallowed, inhaled, or absorbed through the skin. Do not breathe vapors or mists. Do not get in eyes or on skin or clothing.

Statements using the terms *warning* or *caution* also indicate the conditions under which the product may produce injury to humans, domestic animals, and the environment and may contain precautions to take when applying (e.g., may be toxic to fish).

The statement "Keep Out Of Reach Of Children" must appear on every pesticide product on the front label of the package.

The manufacturer's "Directions for Use" is information that must be followed to minimize exposure risk. These are not suggestions, but rather they are required and legal instructions to follow. Individuals that have used a particular product in the past are less apt to read the directions again. Label directions provide the appropriate information concerning, for example

- The type of pests that the product is registered to control for
- Where the product should be applied
- When the product should be applied
- How much of the product should be used
- Directions for mixing if necessary
- The frequency of application

All pesticide labels must have a *misuse statement* on the label that generally reads "use of this product in any manner inconsistent with its labeling is a violation of federal law." The directions for the proper use of a pesticide product are not advice; they are a legal requirement.

Federal law permits the use of pesticides at concentrations and application frequency less than that listed on the label. Knowingly applying a pesticide formulation at higher concentrations and frequencies is in effect a violation of federal law. The application of two or more pesticides that have been mixed together is permitted as long as the amount in the mixture for each is at or below the manufacturer's lower or upper values.

A statement for the *storage and disposal* of pesticides is a labeling requirement as well. Generally, a statement to the effect of "store in a cool dry area away from heat or open flame" is present. In addition, the statement to not reuse empty containers is found on the label as well as information for the proper disposal of any unused product. The toll-free number, 1-800-CLEANUP, provides a regional link to Earth 911, a national effort to provide information concerning disposal sites in your area where the product can be collected.

A "Statement of Warranty" is provided that describes the conditions of sale and limitation of warranty and liability. This might be found as well under the precautionary statement section as "Notice: Buyer assumes all responsibility for safety and use not in accordance with directions."

In summary, a pesticide product label is in effect a legal agreement between the registrant of the product, the user of the product, and the EPA.

## Product Labels Are Not Material Safety Data Sheets

The product label is not a material safety data sheet (MSDS). The manufacturers of pesticides and other consumer products can provide an MSDS upon request. MSDSs are not generic and may vary with respect to the accuracy and amount of information contained within them. They should essentially be viewed as documents that contain additional product information that could not be contained within the confines of a typical container label. An MSDS contains information on

- Product identification
- Composition information and/or ingredients
- Hazardous identifications

- First aid
- Fire-fighting measures
- Accidental release measures
- Handling and storage
- Exposure controls and personal protection
- Physical and chemical properties
- Stability/reactivity
- Toxicological information
- Ecological information
- Disposal
- Transport
- Regulatory information
- Other

The legal requirement for the chemical products that we use at home, with respect to the types of information disclosed by the manufacturer, is contained in the product label. Occupationally, there is an additional legal requirement through Ocupational Safety and Health Administration (OSHA) HazCom (short for hazard communication) that the employer must conform to as well. Employees that work either directly or indirectly with chemicals must have access to the appropriate MSDS if requested. The employer is legally obligated to maintain or have access to these documents for all products that are used in that particular occupational setting. At least in principle, the same bleach that one would use at home must have an accompanying MSDS if used at work. The product label and the MSDS should be in reasonable harmony with each other. If an MSDS for a pesticide recommends certain personal protective equipment and the product label requires the use of specific items of personal protection, then a pesticide applicator *must* follow the label. Similarly, if a product label indicates "caution," then this should be consistent with the values obtained through toxicity testing in experimental animals. Although the actual $LD_{50}$ values can be found in MSDSs, they are not present on product labels.

# Federal Drug Administration Requirements for Labeling

We have seen a great increase in use of both prescription and over-the-counter (OTC) drugs in the United States and worldwide. This is due, in part, to a growing number of older people who probably account for half of all medicines used. People frequently rely on OTC preparations to "self-medicate" themselves or their children. Many OTC preparations were once available by prescription only and thus today are relied on to treat many conditions (e.g., pain, allergy, acid reflux, colds, and bronchial asthma). Thousands of generic preparations are available and, when placed on the shelves side-by-side with major brand names, they are more attractive due to their reduced costs. The enormous market of OTC drugs has been associated with medicine misuse, in part because of failure to recognize the potential risks associated with their use. Part of the blame for this has been largely attributed to the difficulty of reading and understanding product labels. Failing eyesight accompanying old age and reading and language difficulties are examples of conditions that can place individuals at increased risk for medicine misuse. An individual with arthritis, for example, who develops a cold and decides to obtain relief from an OTC cough-and-cold product may not recognize that the product contains aspirin, which would increase nonsteroidal anti-inflammatory drug (NSAID) intake if he or she is already on a prescription or OTC formulation for arthritis. In its review of the readability of OTC drug labels, the Food and Drug Administration (FDA) found studies in which a significant number of people 60 and older could not read the print on some labels and some labels even required eyesight much better than normal.

Similarly, label information is frequently difficult to read and often confusing to interpret for health professionals. Each year, hundreds of thousands of preventable adverse events occur, many from confusing label information. Research shows that prioritizing the warning information has a greater impact on reducing such events. Today, the new prescription label provides the most important information about a prescription product in a format that is more readily accessible and clearer to physicians.

It has been said that providing health care professionals and patients with clear and concise information about prescriptions will help ensure safe and optimal use of drugs, which translates into better health outcomes for patients and more efficient health care delivery. Improving the package insert to make it more useful for health care providers makes it easier for them to explain the benefits and risks of medications to their patients.

In January 2006 the FDA conducted a major overhaul to the format of prescription drug information, commonly referred to as the package insert. The purpose of this information is to enable the physician to better manage the risks associated with medication use and to better communicate this information to the patient. Unfortunately, many of us just leave the physician's office with a prescription and perhaps a sample of the product. At the pharmacy we are almost always given an amber bottle with dispensed pills or other container for liquid formulations from the manufacturer, both with a pharmacy label that says, for example, "take 1 pill daily" or "take as directed." A small warning such as "drowsiness may occur. . . . alcohol may intensify this effect" may be present on the label as well. I have rarely seen a manufacturer's insert for the patient enclosed. Label enclosures are generally provided by the pharmacy, and we hope that they accurately reflect the "full prescribing information" that the physician has access to. These inserts typically contain

- Ingredient name
- Common uses
- Things to do before using this medicine
- Instructions on how to use this medicine
- Cautions
- Possible side effects
- Overdose
- Additional information

"Americans are overwhelmed with the complexity of health information. We have hit a point of information overload and the public health message is being diluted," said Surgeon General Richard H. Carmona, MD. "This is of great concern when it comes to making sure a patient knows how to use prescription drugs safely and effectively. This problem is compounded by prescription medication information that reads more like legal disclaimers than useful or actionable health information."

The FDA's recent revision of prescription drug labeling requires that *new and recently approved* products

- Are organized so that physicians can readily locate important safety and prescribing information
- Meet specific graphical requirements
- Show the date of initial product approval, making it easier to determine how long a product has been on the market
- Provide a toll-free number and Internet reporting information for suspected adverse events to encourage more widespread reporting of suspected side effects
- Include addition of a new "Patient Counseling Information" that places greater emphasis on the importance of communication between health care professionals and patients as a guide for discussions about the potential risks involved in taking a specific treatment and steps for managing those risks
- Contain a "highlights" section to provide immediate access to the most important prescribing information about benefits and risks and to serve as a concise summary of information about specific areas including: Boxed Warning, Indications and Usage, and Dosage and Administration (refers the health care professional to the appropriate part of the *Full Prescribing Information*)
- Provide a table of contents for easy reference to detailed safety and efficacy information
- Have the Full Prescribing Information reorganized to give greater prominence to the most important and most commonly referenced information
- Have the Indications and Usage and the Dosage and Administration sections moved to the beginning of the Full Prescribing Information
- Include a summary outlining the most important information about a product prominently displayed at the top of the page

The new requirement also requires drug manufacturers to include a list of all substantive changes made on an annual basis to ensure that the most up-to-date information is available before prescribing. The agency has encouraged drug manufacturers to consider complying with the new labeling requirements as early as possible. All drugs approved within the past 5 years are included, as well as older drugs for which there is a major change in the prescribing information; for example, approval of a new use will gradually be converted to the new prescribing information format.

"The new label design makes it easier for doctors to get access to important information about drug safety and benefits, and this in turn will help them have more meaningful discussions with their patients" (Acting Commissioner of Food and Drugs Andrew von Eschenbach, MD). "This redesigned label is a big step in our commitment to giving health professionals the tools and information they need to optimize their clinical practice and choose among a growing number of effective treatments to make more personalized prescribing decisions for their patients."

The FDA began requiring drug manufacturers in 2005 to submit to them prescription drug information that follows a new electronic format. The intent is to allow both the public and health care professionals easy access to package inserts for all FDA-approved medicines in the United States using a standard format ("structured product labeling"). Electronically managed drug information allows the user to readily search for specific information such as dosage and administration, warnings, active and inactive ingredients, and how the drug is supplied.

The American public has already seen changes in the product labels for many OTC drugs. Most OTC medicines are subject to rules known as monographs, which require certain labeling information for certain types of drugs (e.g., antacids, antihistamines, pain relievers). The consideration for label changes by the FDA began in the 1990s in response to concerns from consumers, health professionals, industry, and other interested groups:

- There are about 100,000 OTC drug products on the market.
- Consumers self-treat four times more health problems than doctors treat.
- Sixty percent to 95% of all illnesses are initially treated with self-care, including self-treatment with OTC drugs

Proper use of OTC drugs has become more important as prescription drugs increasingly switch to OTC use as their safety profiles become better established. How many times have we heard in pharmaceutical advertising campaigns "now available without prescription"? It therefore becomes increasingly important to effect changes in product labels to make them simpler and more easily understood while still retaining the important information concerning use and safety.

It is important to recognize that just because the drug is OTC does not imply that it is necessarily safer (a common misperception) than a prescribed drug for the same use. When proprietary drugs enter into the OTC market, as we have seen for so many in the past, it becomes especially important that the public has available accurate, clear, and concise information about the product. Debra Bowen, MD, director of the FDA's division of OTC drug products, has said about the pharmacologically active agents that have side effects as well as beneficial effects: and ".... to use them correctly and not get into trouble from using them, people are going to have to read the label and make sure they're appropriately selecting and using them with other drugs they may be taking." Clearly, this is a recognition that we must somehow try to better regulate the "self-medication" of the American public.

The FDA rules already require OTC drug labels to include information consumers need for safe and effective use; however, use of this information requires consumers to first read the entire label and understand what they have read. William Gilbertson, PharmD, and the associate director for the FDA's OTC drug monographs, said, "We want the label to be easier to read so people will indeed read it . . . and we want it to be easier to understand so people will react correctly." Today, most product labels contain a questions section with a toll-free number to obtain additional information in both English and Spanish.

A person allergic to or intolerant of an ingredient in a drug product (e.g., lactose) needs to know whether the product contains it. Although active ingredients are usually listed on OTC drug products, current rules do not require labels for all drugs to list inactive ingredients. Although there is a clearly marked warnings section on OTC product labels, these generally address the "do not use with any other product containing . . .". Any "inactive" ingredients for which there is information concerning allergic responses should be clearly stated in this section as well.

The FDA proposed a new look for product labels of OTC drugs (Figure 21.2). For those of us old enough to remember what old OTC product labels looked like, the differences are readily apparent. The standardization of OTC product labels makes comparisons between products easier, thus facilitating the selection of the most appropriate choice of product by the consumer, in the absence of cost considerations. Although it is still too early to assess for effectiveness, this simple approach, which more readily educates the public concerning the hazards of the medications they take, may reduce the number of adverse event incidents from their use/misuse.

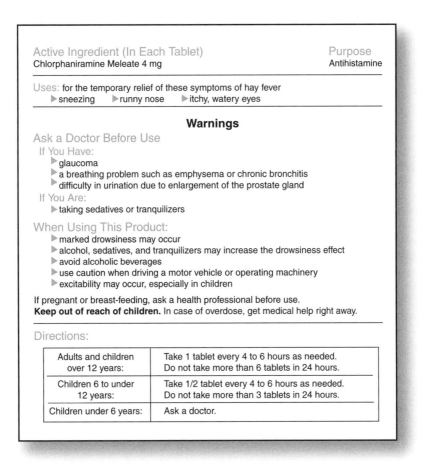

**FIGURE 21.2**    Example of OTC product label. *Source:* Courtesy of U.S. Food and Drug Administration.

## Websites

American National Standards Institute:
http://www.ansi.org/

California Department of Health Services Food and Drug Branch:
http://www.dhs.ca.gov/ps/fdb/PDF/FDNews_Fd-LABEL2_CRL_030201.PDF

Clinical Data Interchange Standards Consortium:
http://www.cdisc.org/

Gateway to Government Food Safety Information:
http://www.foodsafety.gov/

HL7:
http://www.hl7.org/

U.S. EPA Regulating Pesticides:
http://www.epa.gov/oppfead1/labeling/lrm/

U.S. FDA:
http://www.fda.gov/default.htm

U.S. FDA Center for Drug Evaluation and Research:
www.fda.gov/cder/regulatory/physLabel/

U.S. FDA Center for Food Safety and Applied Nutrition:
http://www.cfsan.fda.gov/list.html

U.S. FDA Data Standards Council:
http://www.fda.gov/oc/datacouncil/

U.S. FDA Structured Product Labeling Resources:
http://www.fda.gov/oc/datacouncil/spl.html

U.S. HHS Office of the National Coordinator for Health Information Technology (ONC):
http://www.hhs.gov/healthit/chiinitiative.html

U.S. National Library of Medicine, National Institutes of Health, Environmental Health, and Toxicology Specialized Information Services (SIS). (2005). *Toxicology tutorial I.* Retrieved October 2, 2005 from http://www.sis.nlm.nih.gov/enviro/toxtutor.html

# Toxicology Principles in the Management of Acute Poisonings

The basic principles of toxicology come into play in the rational management of individuals that have become ill from chemicals through either intentional or unintentional exposures. Among the important toxicological principles that are applied in evaluating the poisoned individual are

- Exposure and aspects related to reducing absorption
- Dose–response considerations
- Target tissue and systemic effects
- Chemical interactions
- Chemical antagonism as a management approach
- Acute versus chronic effects

Clinical toxicology is the area of specialization that deals with these issues as they relate to drug overdoses (prescription and over-the-counter preparations), chemical exposures to nonclinically useful chemicals from accidental or intentional exposures, and overdoses of illicit substances. Illicit technically includes not only illegal drugs but legally purchased prescription drugs used by another individual for whom it was not intended.

Regional poison control centers receive thousands of calls daily from individuals seeking advice as to whether or not they should seek medical attention from an accidental or unintentional exposure. The directors of poison control centers are commonly certified in pediatrics (or another specialty) and emergency medicine, including specific training in toxicology. Approximately 80% of all exposures are treated on the site where they occurred, generally the patient's home with phone advice and assistance from local poison control experts. Most poisonings involve everyday household items such as cleaning supplies, medicines, cosmetics, and personal care items.

In 2004 poison control centers in the United States reported approximately 2.2 million poisonings, 1,183 of which resulted in death. For individuals who seek medical attention (approximately 600,000 sought treatments in health care facilities) most did not require specific treatment, only clinical observation. About 10% of hospital admissions required some measure to reduce absorption or enhance the elimination of the chemical and 5% needed intensive supportive care.

## Management of Acute Poisoning

In the management of an individual who may have been acutely poisoned, the medical staff must

- Make a rapid assessment of the patient with respect to the level of consciousness, ventilation, blood pressure, and other physiological assessments as deemed necessary
- Consider the need for a clinical chemistry assessment for determining blood levels of certain drugs or illicit substances
- Consider whether it is possible or necessary to limit further absorption of the chemical or attempt to increase its elimination
- Consider whether an antidote is available, appropriate, or necessary
- Consider contacting their regional poison information center for additional advice

Clinical assessment is made to determine the need for specific treatments when the chemical has been identified. Examples include:

- Salicylates: to assess the severity of poisoning and the need for alkaline diuresis or hemodialysis
- Acetaminophen: to assess the severity of poisoning and the need for administration of N-acetylcysteine
- Iron: to assess the severity of poisoning and the need for administration of deferoxamine
- Theophylline: to assess the severity of poisoning and the need for charcoal hemoperfusion
- Lithium: to assess the severity and the need for hemodialysis
- Barbiturates: to assess the need for charcoal hemoperfusion
- Methanol: to assess the severity of poisoning and the need for administration of ethanol or hemodialysis

- Ethylene glycol: to assess the severity of poisoning and the need for administration of ethanol or hemodialysis
- Ethanol: to facilitate the monitoring of treatment of ethylene glycol and methanol poisonings

## Reducing Toxicant Absorption

Absorption is a requirement for systemic toxicity. For respiratory exposures, the only ways to reduce absorption is by eliminating the chemical from the breathing zone or shortening the exposure time. The absorption of chemicals that have been spilled onto the skin can be reduced in many instances, the extent of which depends on the nature of the chemical (e.g., lipid vs. water solubility), its concentration, and the duration of contact time. The washing of skin with soap and water, for example, as quickly as possible after a spill of a residential use organophosphate pesticide formulation, further reduces skin absorption. This is especially important for undiluted liquids from the product container and for solid preparations as well. Shortened exposure time coupled with dilution reduces the amount absorbed. This is commonly referred to as "decontamination."

For oral consumption, reduction of absorption may be accomplished (depending on the chemical) through gastric lavage and activated charcoal. For chemicals already absorbed into the blood and in severe cases of intoxication, charcoal hemoperfusion may be a clinical option. Gastric lavage is used when a patient has ingested life-threatening amounts of a toxic agent up to 1–2 hours previously. It is not used for corrosive substances because of increased risk of esophageal and gastric perforations or petroleum compounds because of risk of chemical pneumonitis. Activated charcoal is often used to limit further absorption because it adsorbs a wide variety of drugs and toxic agents, if given within and hour or two of ingestion. It has been shown to be effective for many pharmaceuticals (e.g., aspirin, paracetamol, digoxin, phenobarbitone, and theophylline) as well as many nonpharmaceutical chemicals.

## Reducing Toxicity by the Use of an Antidote

An antidote can simply be defined as a clinical treatment using a chemical(s) to counteract the effects of another. An antidote for any chemical can only be developed upon a thorough understanding of the toxicokinetics and toxicodynamics of the offending agent. Because a potential antidote may have additional risks associated with its use, the toxicological properties must be determined as well. The ultimate therapeutic goal is to reduce toxicity by interacting with the toxicant in ways that

- Directly inhibit its effect through modification of its chemical properties
- Inhibit its effect by altering its physical properties
- Reduce effects at its sites of action
- Facilitate its elimination
- Provide for replacement of endogenous protective (e.g., glutathione) or required (e.g., oxygen) chemicals

Examples of common poisonings and their antidotes are provided in Table 22.1.

**Table 22.1**    Examples of Common Poisonings and Their Antidotes

| Poison | Antidote |
| --- | --- |
| Acetaminophen | N-acetylcysteine |
| Anticholinergics | Physostigmine |
| Benzodiazepines | Flumazenil |
| Beta-blockers | Glucagons |
| Calcium channel blockers | Calcium, glucagons |
| Carbamates | Atropine |
| Carbon monoxide | Oxygen |
| Cyanide | Sodium nitrite/sodium thiosulfate |
| Digoxin | Digoxin immune Fab |
| Ethylene glycol | Ethanol, fomepizole |
| Heavy metals | DMSA, BAL, CaEDTA, penicillamine |
| Iron | Deferoxamine |
| Lead | DMSA, BAL, CaEDTA, penicillamine |
| Methanol | Ethanol, fomepizole |
| Nitrates/nitrites | Methylene blue |
| Opiates | Naloxone |
| Organophosphates | Atropine, pralidoxime |
| Snakes (pit viper) | Crotalidae antivenin, CroFab |

BAL = British anti-Lewisite ; CaEDTA = calcium chelate of ethylenediamine tetraacetic acid; CroFab = Crotalidae Polyvalent Immune Fab (Ovine); DMSA = Dimercaptosuccinic acid.

# Route of Exposure Influences Toxicity: An Example Using Cocaine

Cocaine hydrochloride (the water-soluble form of cocaine) is snorted or injected intravenously, whereas crack cocaine is smoked. The route of exposure can profoundly influence the level of toxicity for the same dose. When cocaine is injected, the entire dose is delivered systemically in seconds and a peak plasma level is obtained so rapidly that the individual experiences a "rush" or "flash" that produces increased feelings of alertness, euphoria, well-being, energy, confidence, and sexuality. The user becomes more restless and irritable and visual, tactile, and auditory hallucinations may occur.

Topical application onto the nasal mucosa results in a much slower absorption due to local vasoconstriction and a lower peak plasma level. Smoking crack cocaine delivers the substance directly to the pulmonary circulation, where it is delivered to the heart and into the brain. Not all the cocaine that is smoked is available for delivery, so the delivered dose is less than that for intravenous use.

Cocaine, like amphetamines, is sympathomimetic and produces not only behavioral effects but also increases in heart rate, blood pressure, muscle tension, and core body temperature. These effects are associated with its toxicity. The resulting tachycardia and hypertension may result in myocardial infarction and cerebrovascular hemorrhage, coronary vasospasms, and cardiac arrhythmias. Many individuals have the signs and symptoms of a myocardial infarction. The most potentially serious toxicity results from intravenous use; this is followed by respiratory and then nasal exposures.

Overdose of cocaine is usually rapidly fatal, with victims dying within minutes from arrhythmias, seizures, and respiratory depression. In 2004 approximately 40,000 cases of illicit stimulant and other street drug use resulted in 214 fatalities. For the same year, 102,000 cases of pesticide exposures (all pesticides) resulted in eight fatalities. The management of individuals with severe cocaine intoxication includes measures to antagonize the sympathetic effects of this substance.

## Intentional and Unintentional Exposures in the American Population

In 2004 approximately 84% of reported poisonings (2 million cases) resulted from unintentional exposures to chemicals, with approximately 200 deaths as outcomes. This category of exposures includes

- Therapeutic error
- Misuse
- Animal bites and stings
- Food poisonings
- Occupational and environmental exposures
- Adverse reactions
- Unspecified

Intentional exposures resulted in less than 20% of reported poisonings, however; over 900 deaths occurred. Intentional exposure to nonclinically important chemicals for the purpose of obtaining a "high" continues to be a problem of enormous public health concern. Marijuana is the most commonly used illicit drug and is used by approximately 15 million Americans. Approximately 2 million persons currently use cocaine, and there are 200,000 current heroin users. Among youngsters aged 12–17 years, inhalant use is higher than the use of cocaine. Current illicit drug use is highest among young adults 18 to 25 years old, with over 20% using drugs. The costs of illicit substance use, from the suppliers to the users, through law enforcement and the court system and the associated medical costs for treatment of acute poisonings and rehabilitation programs are staggering. This may very well represent the number one preventable public health problem in the country.

## Inhalant Use

The use of commonly obtained chemicals that can be inhaled to produce central nervous system (CNS) effects has become a serious problem, especially in low income communities and those who have become isolated, such as Native American reservations. The problem is most prevalent among teenagers and especially boys, where "huffing" gasoline, glues, paints, and other products containing volatile organic has become commonplace. The problem is also evident in more affluent communities to the extent that some items on the shelves in stores now require proof that the purchaser is over 18 years of age. It is doubtful that this will have significant impact on the problem; however, it does recognize that one exists.

Inhalants can be

- Volatile organics contained in such products as lacquer thinners, gasoline, typing correction fluid, lighter fluids, and glues that may be collected in a common paper bag so that the vapors can be concentrated and inhaled.
- Aerosols with fluorocarbons and other propellants that can be released along with other chemicals such as alcohols, ketones, and n-hexane (found in such common products as cans of spray paint) when inhaled directly have the potential to produce significant neurological, cardiovascular, and liver toxicity.
- Anesthetic agents such as chloroform, methyl trichloroethylene, and ether that may be present in common products (e.g., special cleaners, grease dissolvers).
- Nitrites such as isobutyl, butyl, and amyl nitrite that are found in many commonly available household products and have similar effects to nitrites that are used clinically as vasodilators.

These chemicals when inhaled in a concentrated fashion can cause dizziness, hypotension, euphoria, ataxia, a feeling of drunkenness, impaired judgment, perceptual disturbances, CNS depression of respiration, and even death. The mechanism of action is unclear but is related to the highly lipophilic nature of many of these chemicals and the likelihood that they alter the fluidity of cellular membranes, especially within the CNS, thereby affecting normal impulse and synaptic activity.

## Toxicities Associated with "Street Drugs"

The most common toxicities associated with street drugs result from stimulants, depressants, hallucinogens, and narcotics. Common stimulants include

- Methamphetamine ("speed," "crystal," "ICE")
- Methylenedioxymetamphetamine (ecstasy, MDMA, XTC)
- Methylenedioxyamphetamine (MDA)
- Methylphenidate (Ritalin®, used to treat attention deficit and hyperactivity disorders, especially in children)
- Phenmetrazine (used to treat obesity)
- Cocaine (in all its forms)

Overdoses of amphetamines are managed by reducing sympathetic effects through the use of depressants such as diazepam.

Depressants (sedative hypnotics) include barbiturates such as pentobarbital (yellow jackets), phenobarbital (purple hearts), amobarbital (blue angels), and secobarbital (red devils). The benzodiazepines include flurazepam (sleeping pills), flunitrazepam ("date rape drug"), diazepam (Valium®), alprazolam (Xanax®), chlordiazepoxide (Librium®), clonazepam (anticonvulsant), and methaqualone (Quaalude or "downers").

Flunitrazepam (Rohypnol®) is an example of a clinical drug (a benzodiazepine) that has become a popular street drug, especially among teenagers and young adults. Clinically, it is used in the short-term management of insomnia and as a sedative hypnotic and preanesthetic medication. It is 10 times more potent than Valium®. Its effects begin within 30 minutes, peak within 1–2 hours, and, depending on the dose, may persist for 8 hours or longer. It produces a marked decrease of blood pressure, urinary retention, visual disturbances, gastrointestinal disturbances, memory impairment, dizziness, confusion, and behavior opposite to depression such as excitability or aggressive behavior in some users. Intoxications can result in death from respiratory failure and cardiovascular collapse, especially in combination with alcohol. On the street the drug is referred to as rophy, circles, Mexican Valium, roofies, roopies, ropies, and ruffies. Being under its influence is referred to as being "roached out."

The drug gamma-hydroxybutyrate (GHB) is an increasingly abused and potentially lethal drug. GHB is a CNS depressant most often abused for the purpose of feeling euphoric and uninhibited. In the United States GHB can be prescribed in a very low dose as an experimental treatment for narcolepsy. However, those who abuse GHB (also known as "G" or "liquid ecstasy") may require emergency medical attention when they overdose or experience withdrawal symptoms. GHB and other "club drugs" are often abused by young people at all-night parties and "raves." In some European countries GHB is prescribed as a treatment for alcoholism, although the medical evidence to support its use is wanting. GHB, usually in combination with alcohol, has been linked to more than 60 deaths, mostly among young adults. The number of reported GHB-related deaths may be an underestimate because GHB does not remain in the body very long and is usually not tested for at autopsy.

The general progression of effects from depressants are relief from anxiety → sedation → hypnosis → confusion, ataxia and delirium → surgical anesthesia → depression of vasomotor and respiratory centers in the brainstem → coma → death. Treatment of overdose of benzodiazepines includes flumazenil, a benzodiazepine receptor blocker.

A number of hallucinogens are illegally used, and although these drugs differ in mechanisms of action, chemical similarities, CNS target receptors, and seriousness of toxic effects, they are often considered together because of the common form of intoxication that includes hallucinations, delusions, and illusions that occasionally result in death due to dangerous behaviors.

Common hallucinogens include

- Cannabis: marijuana, delta-9-THC
- Anticholinergics: atropine, scopolamine, mandrake root, jimson weed
- Indolamines: lysergic acid diethylamide (LSD), morning glory seed (LSM), psilocybin, psilocin, ibogaine, dimethyltryptamine (DMT)
- Phenylethylamines: mescaline, bufotenin, dimethoxymethyl-amphetamine (DOM)
- Dissociative anesthetics: ketamine, phencyclidine (PCP)

Common narcotic intoxications involve the use of morphine, heroin, hydromorphone, oxymorphone, codeine (methylmorphine), dihydrocodeine, hydrocodone (Dicodid®, Hycodan®), and oxycodone (Percodan®). The designer opioid (MPTP)1-methyl-4-phenyl-1,2,3,6-tetrahydropyridine is a meperidine/heroin-like drug that was synthesized in the 1980s. It produces Parkinson-like symptoms in the young adults who used it. It is used experimentally as a model in rodents to produce the disease by destroying certain regions of the brain (e.g., substantia nigra) that produce dopamine and other neurotransmitters that coordinate neuromuscular activity.

## Websites

Agency for Toxic Substances and Disease Registry (ATSDR):
http://www.atsdr.cdc.gov/

American Association of Poison Control Centers:
http://www.aapcc.org

American College of Medical Toxicology:
http://www.acmt.net/main/

Centers for Disease Control and Prevention (CDC):
http://www.cdc.gov/

Food and Drug Administration (FDA):
http://www.fda.gov/

MEDLINEplus:
http://medlineplus.gov/

Medwatch Homepage:
http://www.fda.gov/medwatch/report/hcp.htm

National Institute on Drug Abuse:
http://www.nida.nih.gov/DrugPages/DrugsofAbuse.html

National Institute of Environmental Health Sciences (NIEHS):
http://www.niehs.nih.gov/

National Institutes of Health (NIH):
http://www.nih.gov/

Poisonous Plants Informational Database:
http://www.ansci.cornell.edu/plants/

U.S. Department of Health and Human Services:
http://www.dhhs.gov/news/press/2003pres/20030905.html

World Health Organization:
http://www.who.int

# Bibliography

U.S. National Library of Medicine, National Institutes of Health, Environmental Health, and Toxicology Specialized Information Services (SIS). (2005). *Toxicology tutorial II*. Retrieved October 2, 2005 from http://www.sis.nlm.nih.gov/enviro/toxtutor.html.

Watson, W. A., Litovitz, T. L., Rodgers, G. C., Jr., Klein-Schwartz, W., Reid, N., Youniss, J., Flanagan, A., & Wruk, K. M. (2004). Annual report of the American Association of Poison Control Centers Toxic Exposure Surveillance System. *American Journal of Emergency Medicine, 23,* 589–666.

# CHAPTER 23

# Risk Assessment and the Perception of Risk

## Overview of Risk

Risk is the probability that harm will be produced under a specific set of conditions. It is a combination of two considerations: the probability or likelihood that an adverse event will occur and the consequences or level of harm that will result. Risk assessment is a methodology to assist us in evaluating human health effects and environmental consequences from the exposure to chemicals. Just as the dose–response assessment for several chemicals would allow one to rank them as to their relative toxicities, risk assessments should be used as a tool for the allocation of public health resources aimed toward recognizing, prioritizing, and reducing human health risk and environmental problems. In theory, it should be recognized for its value and limitations in public health programs and in the making of rational management decisions, which are always based in part on financial considerations. As public health professionals it is our responsibility when communicating risk that the results are clearly and accurately presented, so that everyone can hopefully understand the difference between a hazard as perceived through risk assessment versus a risk "perceived as real."

Regulatory bodies that recommend or set limits for exposures to chemicals are faced with challenges. Underestimating risk could potentially result in setting a standard that could lead to overexposure of the population, whereas overcalculating the risk may result in unnecessary costs to the public to manage them. There have been serious concerns about the benefits to the public from the extremely costly cleanups of some areas deemed as hazardous. A further challenge to our regulatory agencies is in recognizing that apart from often limited human data, inferences concerning risk must be made from animal toxicity studies that use high exposure levels. The question then becomes *not* what the risks are from ozone exposure at 10 ppm, but rather what are they at exposures more likely to be encountered in the environment on the best day? Additionally, in real life we are exposed to a multitude of chemicals at any one time that can interact in complex and sometimes unpredictable ways in the body and in the environment.

## Risk Assessment

Risk assessment has been used by regulators for well over 50 years, although early on it probably was not recognized as a methodology. It essentially assumed that all chemicals had the potential to be hazardous to health at a level that exceeded the "threshold." The "process" of risk assessment became one in which

- A chemical hazard is recognized.
- Its potential to produce injury is assessed by evaluating it at different levels of exposure using laboratory animals as human surrogates and through collection of any human data from epidemiological or clinical sources, including information from poisonings.
- A quantitative dose response for a toxic end-point is determined.
- Analytical data as to the environmental concentrations of chemical or amounts of chemical(s) are collected.
- Recognizing that toxicity testing in laboratory animals was often the sole basis for evaluating chemical hazards, "safety factors" are used to compensate for the uncertainties of extrapolation from laboratory animals to human populations.
- Safety factors are set at exposure levels several orders of magnitude lower than the thresholds observed in the laboratory.
- Intake assumptions considering all routes of exposure are made for humans.
- All information is assessed to characterize the existence and magnitude of the risk to the health of the public.

In 1983 the National Academy of Sciences (NAS) published standard terminology and concepts for risk assessments. At this point it would be helpful to define a number of terms that are commonly associated with risk:

- *Hazard:* the ability of the chemical to produce an adverse response
- *Risk:* the probability that the hazard will occur under defined conditions of exposure

- *Risk assessment:* a quantitative process by which hazard, exposure, and risk are determined
- *Risk management:* the process of selection of the most appropriate actions based on the results of social, economic, and other concerns

Overall, the components of the process of risk assessment are the identification of the hazard, an exposure assessment, toxicity or dose–response assessment, risk characterization, risk communication, and risk management (Figure 23.1). Risk communication and management are not considered as components of the risk assessment process proper but can be viewed as the application of the process.

## Hazard Identification

Hazard identification involves the evaluation of the chemical for its toxic potential. Information is collected from animal studies and human data where available. The latter may come from, for example, epidemiological studies, case studies, or other published information on accidental or intentional poisonings. Additional resources may be available from regional poison control centers. Information may indicate that a particular chemical is associated with a particular health effect (e.g., cancer, kidney toxicity, birth defects). This information is analyzed by taking a "weight of evidence" approach to determine the nature of the toxicity that is consistently produced at the lower doses. This is taken to be the primary hazard of the chemical. So although we all recognize that lead can also result in toxicities to other tissues, its primary hazard is its neurotoxicity.

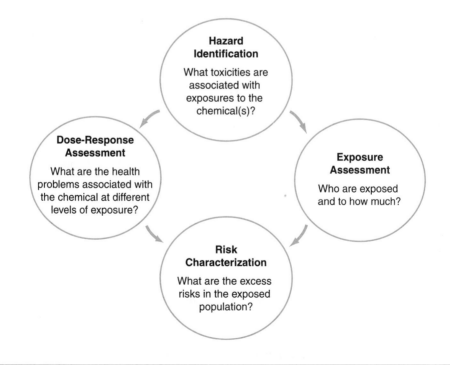

**FIGURE 23.1**   Components of risk assessment.

Although human data would be the most desirable with respect to making rational decisions concerning risk from exposure to a particular chemical(s), it may not be readily available or reliable. Often the most reliable epidemiological data come from retrospective occupational studies of workers who have been using identified chemicals, often for long periods of time. Their use has been causally linked to the development of specific types of injuries. We recognize, for example, the human neurotoxic effects of the solvent carbon disulfide from studies of workers in the rayon industry. Unfortunately, whereas the hazards have been identified, information concerning the nature of the exposures is often difficult to determine and thus to move the risk assessment process forward would require quantitative dose–response information that would then be essentially limited to laboratory studies. In addition to toxicity tests using whole animals, supporting data from *in vitro* studies, using human cells in culture for example, can also assist in the risk assessment process.

## Dose–Response Assessment

The dose–response assessment is a quantification of the hazard assessment. At this point in the risk assessment process, qualitative and quantitative toxicity information is collected. Quantitative dose–response relationships in humans are extremely difficult to obtain; however, when human exposures are available, they may at least provide the strongest evidence for causality between exposure to a particular chemical and the development of a specific type of injury. Generally, information for quantitative risk assessment is provided by empirical data arrived at through animal studies. Under controlled laboratory conditions, animals may be exposed to specific chemicals, either individually or in combinations, and quantitative exposure–response data may be generated.

The least desirable toxicological end-point for quantitative dose–response information, which may sometimes be the only end-point, is lethality. For noncarcinogens a threshold response will be obtained. The application of this information is, of course, subject to the limitations of extrapolating animal data to the human situation. The extrapolations of generally high experimental doses to doses more representative of human exposures are arrived at by "adjusting" the experimental data because a surrogate for humans was used and to address additional uncertainties concerning human safety. For carcinogens, risk estimations are arrived at differently than for noncancer end-points. This is because the idea that carcinogens, at least for legislative purposes, are considered not to have a threshold dose but rather are considered to have risk at any dose or concentration. A plot of dose versus response yields a straight line through the origin, indicating some degree of risk at any dose.

## Exposure Assessment

This is a critical aspect of the risk assessment process, because there is no risk if there is no exposure. A hazardous underground storage tank poses no risk for chemical exposure unless it is leaking, or there has been a spill, or until you can identify the chemicals contained in the storage tank in the soil, water, or air at concentrations above "background levels." If not, then an industrial or hazardous waste worker or the nearby community would not be at current risk for exposure to these chemicals. The exposure assessment establishes who, what, when, where, and how:

- What are the contaminants? The chemical nature of the substances must be determined and if we are dealing with a single chemical or a mixture of substances.
- Where are the contaminants located? The location and transport away from the source must be addressed. This is a very complex aspect of the exposure assessment that must consider physicochemical properties and biological factors:
  - Partitioning between media (air-to-soil, water-to-soil, air-to-water)
  - Vapor pressures
  - Bioconcentration
  - Degradation
  - Biotransformation
- What are the concentrations? Adequate sampling and quantitative analyses are required. Risk characterization is only as good as the risk assessor's confidence in the sampling and analytical methodologies.
- Who is at risk for exposure? The consideration may be limited to a select group of individuals such as hazardous substance workers or it may involve the residents of a community. Here there are considerations of differences in vulnerabilities of groups such as the elderly, children, individuals with certain medical conditions, women in their reproductive years, and pregnant women.
- How would an exposure result? Considerations as to exposures from air, soil, and water where sampling data indicate a point source (e.g., children in direct soil contact) and contamination of the groundwater and freshwater drinking supplies from current or future transports are examples.
- When would an exposure occur? Exposures may be limited to direct contact with the soil during the times when a child might be outdoors and playing, or it may occur each time an individual consumes water obtained from a well or municipal drinking water supply.
- What are the pathways of exposure? Consideration is given for all possible exposure pathways, including oral, respiratory, and dermal. Additionally, environmental media as the source for exposure include the consideration of air, soil, groundwater, surface water, and transfer to the infant via breast milk.

## Noncancer Risk Assessment

For chronic intake of noncarcinogens, the acceptable daily intake (ADI) has been traditionally used to calculate the amount of the chemical to which an individual may be exposed on a daily basis over the course of his or her lifetime (or other defined long-term period of time) without developing any apparent toxicity. Although the ADI has been frequently used by such agencies as the U.S. Food and Drug Administration (FDA), federal agencies use other indices for assessing noncancer end-points as well, such as the minimal risk levels (MRLs) of the Agency for Toxic Substances and Disease Registry (ATSDR) and the reference dose (RfD) used by the Environmental Protection Agency (EPA). They are all basically similar in that they essentially express the highest experimental dose that does not produce an adverse effect (referred to as the NOAEL) or the lowest dose at which an adverse affect was produced (referred to as the LOAEL) divided by a value (generally 100 or greater) to account for uncertainty (safety factors).

A typical dose–response curve for noncarcinogens is illustrated in Figure 23.2. In practice, the most sensitive toxicity end-point should be selected for human risk assessments; however, there may be occasions when lethality is used as an end-point because of little additional information being available or lack of confidence in it.

The product of uncertainty factors is multiplied together and divided into the NOAEL or LOAEL to derive the ADI, MRL, or RfD. Uncertainty (safety) factors include

- Factor (FH): Human variability factor (10×)
- Factor (FA): Animal data extrapolation to humans (10×)
- Factor (FL): LOAEL use in place of the NOAEL (10×).
- Factor (FS): Subchronic data (10×)
- Factor (FD): Doubt as a modifying factor (0.1 – 10×)

The use of modifying factors provides an additional safety element to compensate for the quality of the published studies that are relied on by the risk assessor. If studies are limited or the risk assessor is doubtful about the quality of a particular study, then a modifying factor can be used. The level of modification is subject to the opinions of the assessor. Thus the ADI can be expressed as

$$ADI = NOAEL \div cumulative\ safety\ factors$$

The RfD allows the risk assessor to use the LOAEL if the NOAEL has not been established. The general formula for deriving the RfD is

$$RfD = NOAEL\ or\ LOAEL \div UFl \times UF2 \times UF3$$

where UF represents uncertainty factors. As an example, the following data were obtained from laboratory rats for chemical "X":

NOAEL = 15.5 mg/kg/day (chronic study)
LOAEL = 62.7 mg/kg/day (subchronic study)

Using the NOAEL:

RfD = NOAEL ÷ FA × FH × FD = 15.5 mg/kg/day ÷ 10 × 10 × 10 =
0.015 mg/kg/day (15 μg/kg/day)

Using the LOAEL:

RfD = LOAEL ÷ FA × FL × FH × FS = 62.7 mg/kg/day ÷ 10 × 10 × 10 × 10 =
0.0063 mg/kg /day (6.3 μg/kg/day)

The smaller value would be selected as the RfD for humans.

A *hazard quotient* is the ratio of an exposure over a period of time to the RfD for the substance. A value greater than or equal to 1 indicates a risk of noncancer adverse health effects.

Hazard quotient = dose (mg/kg/day) ÷ RfD (mg/kg/day)

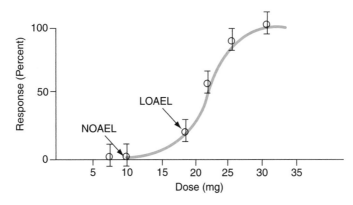

**FIGURE 23.2** Threshold curve showing NOAEL and LOAEL.

If the hazard quotient is greater than 1, then individuals are exposed to more of the substance than is acceptable under current public policy. This should not be taken to imply that illness will develop; it merely suggests an increased likelihood that an adverse effect may result. The *hazard index (HI)* is the summation of more than one hazard quotient for multiple substances and exposure routes and is calculated when a potential for more than one chemical to produce the same or similar adverse response exists.

The MRL, like the ADI, is an estimate of what is deemed to be a likely safe human exposure to chemical(s) over a defined period of time. The ATSDR uses the MRL to assess for safety acutely (2 or less weeks of exposure) and chronically (365 or more days of exposure). It is essentially similar to the EPA's RfD, with UFs that can be lower than 10 times, generally either 1 or 3, based on the judgment of the assessor.

Occupational standards and guidelines such as permissible exposure limits (PELs), threshold limit values (TLVs), and the National Institute for Occupational Safety and Health (NIOSH) recommended exposure levels are arrived at by the application of the same principles of risk assessment to the workplace. Here the difference is that "the worker" is viewed somewhat differently than "the general public" with respect to human variability. These standards and guidelines represent levels of exposure that are considered as safe daily exposures for workers, and one standard applies to all.

## Cancer Risk Assessment

By the end of World War II, scientists were reevaluating their views about cancer and its causes. The link between cancer and radiation was firmly established. By the 1950s, the idea that carcinogens produced toxicity through cellular mechanisms that differed somehow from most toxicants became an area of special concern to federal regulatory agencies. The idea held by some scientists that carcinogen-induced injury occurred through "nonthreshold" mechanisms resulted in a profound influence on public health policymaking. It was the idea that any exposure to a carcinogen increased the risk of developing cancer and that safe limits for exposure could therefore not be established for these types of chemicals. This drove regulators into knee-jerk reactions. The enactment in 1958 of the Delaney clause to the Food and Color Additive Amendments of the Federal

Food, Drug and Cosmetic Act (FFDCA) is an example. This specifically forbid the addition of any chemical classified as a carcinogen, whether it be human or animal, to the American food supply. Other additives, where a toxicity threshold could be established, were permitted as long as there was a sufficiently large margin of safety.

Similar regulatory positions were taken by the EPA and enacted through the Safe Drinking Water Act (SDWA). As analytical detection methodologies improved, more and more chemicals that have been shown to be carcinogenic in laboratory animals were found in environmental media. For regulators, the setting of environmental standards for chemicals could not take a below the detection limit position due to the continuing improvement of analytical methodologies. Thus faced with the dilemma of low-dose exposures to carcinogens, regulators still needed some way to assess for cancer risk. The way out of this dilemma was simply to make assumptions even in the absence of direct information concerning human carcinogenicity. The assumptions, of course, cannot be at odds with the known scientific literature. Humans and laboratory animals were assumed to be equally at risk from exposures to carcinogens; from a regulatory standpoint it is better to use scientific information from a human surrogate or to overestimate low-dose risks rather than to conclude that nothing can be concluded.

The public does not want to hear that their officials can arrive at no conclusions. It is always preferable to say that a risk is insignificant or acceptable, even at the possibility of engaging with the public to better define what those words actually imply. Cancer risk assessment evaluates information from human or animal studies that suggest that a chemical is a carcinogen. An assessment is made as to the likelihood of it being a human carcinogen. Many chemicals have already been classified as to their cancer risk to humans based on the "weight of evidence" as a definite, probable, or possible human carcinogen. Review of Chapter 11 provides more detailed information concerning carcinogen classification by regulatory and nonregulatory agencies.

Mathematical models are used in quantitative risk assessments to draw inferences about cancer risk based on the extrapolation of data in laboratory animals from generally high experimental doses to levels that would be more likely encountered in the environment. Many of these models assume a linear dose–response and a zero threshold dose. Many state and municipal risk assessments use the EPA "cancer slope factor," which estimates probability that an individual will develop cancer that is causally related to exposure to a carcinogen over the course of a lifetime. The cancer slope factor is expressed as mg/kg/day.

A number of cancer risk assessment models can yield different lifetime cancer risks. As an example, for the pesticide chlordane (not in use today) the results of a lifetime risk of $1 \times 10^{-6}$ (one cancer death per 1 million individuals) from its consumption in drinking water have been calculated using several models:

- *One-hit model* (0.03 µg/l) assumes that even one molecule of a carcinogen is sufficient to produce cancer (this is not widely accepted by the scientific community and is inconsistent with the more probable multistage hypothesis for chemical carcinogenesis).
- *Multihit model* (2 µg/l) is consistent with the multistage process of carcinogenesis and assumes several mutagenic events are required before cancer is produced.
- *Probit model* (50 µg/l) is infrequently used in cancer risk assessments and assumes a log normal distribution of susceptibility in the population.

- *Linearized multistage model* (0.07 µg/l) assumes linear extrapolation with a zero dose threshold from the upper confidence level of the lowest dose that produced cancer as determined from laboratory or epidemiological studies. It produces a cancer slope factor that can be used to predict cancer risk at a specific dose and is used by the EPA and other state agencies (Figure 23.3).

In 1980 the EPA issued the following: "It should be emphasized that the linearized multistage procedure leads to a plausible upper limit to the risk that is consistent with some mechanisms of carcinogenesis. Such an estimate, however, does not necessarily give a realistic prediction of the risk. The true value of the risk is unknown and may be as low as zero."

Another form of modeling is the *physiologically based toxicokinetic model,* which is becoming more popular. However, its use requires extensive physiological and toxicokinetic data input and the use of very sophisticated computer programs for the extrapolation of cancer risk.

## Risk Characterization

Fundamental to the process of risk assessment is the characterization of the relationship between a specific chemical, a causally related adverse health outcome, and its severity in exposed populations. Risk characterization is the final step in a risk assessment process whereby cancer and noncancer risks are estimated, uncertainties and modifying factors are addressed, and all information is combined and summarized in a way that is meaningful to those engaged in decision-making for managing the risk. Because most risk assessments have uncertainties, these need to be clearly identified. Quantitative exposure assessments are often difficult to produce, and estimates are frequently made based on exposure scenarios and assumptions with respect to the intake of a chemical through multiple routes of exposure. Risk characterization therefore often becomes an estimation under different scenarios of exposure. To reduce the inherent difficulties about variation in human populations, some assumptions have to be made; for example:

- 20 m³/day is the *average inhalation rate of an adult*
- 2 l/day is the *average water consumption rate of an adult*
- 70 kg is *the average weight of an adult male*

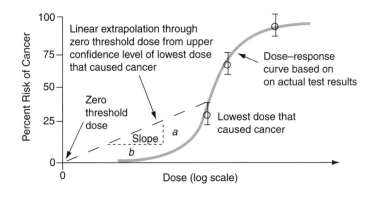

**FIGURE 23.3**    Linear multistage extrapolation of dose–response for carcinogens. *Source:* Courtesy of the Toxicology and Environmental Health Information Program of the National Library of Medicine, U.S. Department of Health and Human Services.

While there are differences in intake assumptions for young children (e.g., oral consumption of a chemical from soil is greater than for an adult), assumptions are clearly not applicable to all individuals.

In many situations risk characterization must consider simultaneous exposure to more than one chemical. An airborne exposure to several volatile organic chemicals that are each neurotoxic must take into consideration that while the concentration of each alone may place individuals at minimal risk, the additive concentration may place them at significant risk.

In risk characterization the best estimates for exposure to noncarcinogenic chemicals, based on different scenario exposures, is compared with levels of exposure deemed to be safe for that chemical, such as the ADI or the RfD, obtained from acute, subchronic, and chronic laboratory toxicity studies. For exposed human populations, acute effects are considered those that occur over the course of a few days to a few weeks, whereas chronic effects occur over the course of a year or more.

For cancer, the increased likelihood that an individual will develop it sometime during the course of an average life span of 70 years is estimated by multiplying the cancer slope factor (mg/kg/day) for the substance by the daily intake (mg/kg/day) over a lifetime. A "general level of concern" of one in a million ($1 \times 10^{-6}$) has been established for carcinogens by the EPA.

## Risk Management

Rational management decisions frequently must be made in the absence of a complete picture. Overestimation of risk could result in risk management decisions that may be very costly and time-consuming. Significant underestimation of risk may leave communities or sensitive individuals vulnerable to exposures that are excessive.

The management of risk is not typically considered a part of the risk assessment process proper; it is the application of the characterization of risk that is used as the basis for interaction between the risk manager and risk assessors, the community, industry, academia, and government in ways that hopefully produce the most rational decisions for dealing with public health concerns (Figure 23.4).

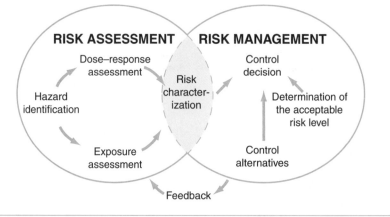

FIGURE 23.4    Risk characterization as a basis for decision making. *Source:* Courtesy of the Toxicology and Environmental Health Information Program of the National Library of Medicine, U.S. Department of Health and Human Services.

## *Ecological Risk Assessment*

One of the difficulties in attempting to characterize the risk to ecosystems or the resident populations and communities is the great diversity of animal and plant species that are present. Perhaps of all the chemicals that impact ecosystems, pesticides as a group of chemicals deserve special consideration, because they have been developed and are used with the specific intent of controlling by killing species deemed to be undesirable. Unfortunately, other species are adversely affected as well. The EPA requires a risk assessment for any new pesticide, or new formulations of existing ones, as part of the registration process and may require it as well for the reregistration of existing ones, should new information on adverse effects become available. Additionally, they may require changes to be made on the product label when there are any significant changes in the way the product is used, to ensure a "reasonable certainty of no harm."

The EPA produces a registration eligibility decision document that contains information on and a decision whether or not to register or reregister a pesticide. The EPA bases its decision on risk assessments that are conducted by contributions made from the Human Health Effects Division (HED) and the Ecological Fate and Effects Division (EFED). A typical representation of the organization of information for a pesticide in the registration eligibility decision (RED) document is as follows:

- Use characterization
- Exposure characterization
- Environmental fate assessment
- Data gaps and uncertainties in the exposure assessment
- Environmental fate and transport data
- Water resources assessment
- Major conclusions
- Drinking water exposure assessment
- Monitoring study summaries
- Modeling
- Exposure to nontarget terrestrial animals
- Exposure to nontarget freshwater aquatic animals
- Ecological effects characterization
- Environmental risk assessment
- Ecological incidents summary
- Summary
- References
- Appendices

Like human health risk assessments, hazard identification is the starting point for ecological risk assessments. The EPA considers two types of hazards: acute toxicity and reproductive/developmental toxicity for vertebrates and invertebrates. For plants, they rely on tests such as root growth, growth reduction, and seed germination. They require a minimum of one species of fish and one species of an aquatic invertebrate to be tested by the manufacturer in support of a petition to register their product. For the reregistration of a pesticide, the EPA relies on additional published information if necessary.

Acute lethality tests from vertebrate and invertebrate organisms are used to calculate $LC_{50}$ values, and the most sensitive species tested is considered to be the most susceptible for risk characterization. For plants, a growth reduction by 25% is considered, as an example, to be a sufficient indicator of plant toxicity. Chronic toxicity is the concentration that causes no adverse effects on reproduction or development of animals. The no observed adverse effect concentration (NOAEC) for the most sensitive species is used as a chronic toxicity end point in the characterization of risk. Because of the complexity of ecosystems, sampling data can be limited and the EPA often uses modeling for exposure assessments, especially in aquatic ecosystems.

Risk is characterized by dividing the level of exposure as a point estimate with a toxicological end-point such as the $LC_{50}$ or NOAEL for the most sensitive species. This ratio is judged to be either above or below their "level of concern." This is "deterministic" risk characterization. In the risk characterization additional considerations may be important, such as whether or not a particular species may be one that is endangered. Another way that the EPA can characterize risk is through the use of "probabilistic" techniques, whereby a species sensitivity distribution for a given toxicity end-point (e.g., $LD_{50}$) is obtained through the use of logistic regression modeling and actual (or modeled) environmental exposure levels.

## Toxicant Interaction and Chemical Mixtures

Toxicants in the body may act independently of each other. Toxicants may also affect the body's response to other toxicants and to the "normal" chemicals present by producing an effect that may be one that is more or less intense than predicted. Prediction of a response is largely based on the known toxicological effects of each chemical independently. For example, warfarin (an anticoagulant) is bound to plasma albumin (an important blood protein produced by the liver), so that only 2% of the administered warfarin is in the free (unbound) and active state. Other drugs that compete for albumin binding sites can elevate the level of free warfarin, thus causing potentially fatal hemorrhage.

Most toxicological studies have been concerned with the effects from exposures to an individual chemical agent. This "single chemical exposure" scenario is unrealistically simplistic and actually represents an exposure situation that can only be reasonably achieved under controlled laboratory conditions. We are never really exposed to a single chemical alone because multiple chemicals are introduced into our bodies through air, water, food, and medications. Within each medium, numerous chemicals may be simultaneously introduced into the body. We are thus actually exposed to "mixtures" of chemicals that at any time may be from multiple exposure pathways. The EPA defines a chemical mixture as either

- *Complex,* in that it contains "so many components that any estimation of its toxicity based on its components toxicities contains too much uncertainty and error to be useful," or

- *Simple,* which contains "two or more identifiable components but few enough that the mixture toxicity can be adequately characterized by a combination of the components' toxicities and the components' interactions."

## Types of Interactions

Human health risk assessments generally consider multiple chemicals as simple mixtures and any combined toxicity as the result of the summation of individual toxicities derived primarily from single chemical studies in laboratory animals. This "components approach" may not truly represent a realistic picture for potential toxicity; however, it is the primary foundation upon which regulatory decisions have been largely based. Different chemicals may act or interact in a number of different ways to produce their effects in the body:

- Independent effects
- Physiologically similar or additive effects
- Antagonistic effects
- Synergistic effects
- Potentiation effects

Independent chemical action occurs when chemicals produce their dose-dependent effects through different physiological mechanisms of action. As an example, consider the presence of the metal cadmium and the organophosphate pesticide malathion. The combined presence of these two chemicals in the body is such that one does not affect the toxicity of the other, thus resulting in independent toxicities and not a combined toxicity. The cadmium may produce renal injury and the malathion may produce some changes in nervous system physiology. These are independent toxicities.

When two or more chemicals interact in the body to produce physiologically similar actions, a combined toxicity results that is dependent on factors related to the type of exposure and combined dose of the chemicals. So if one is exposed to two different organophosphate pesticides, a similar physiological response results from the "additive" effect of the two pesticides. If either one or both of the pesticides are taken in combination with the drug atropine, then an "antagonistic" effect results such that the atropine would tend to reduce the toxicity of the organophosphates. Antagonistic relationships are especially important in clinical toxicology because they often form the basis for the rational management of poisoned individuals by the use of an appropriate "antidote."

A chemical(s) that may have no toxic effect can increase the magnitude of toxicity from another chemical when they are present together. This is referred to as *potentiation.* As an example, in the presence of isopropyl alcohol, which alone does not produce significant liver injury, there is a greatly increased hepatotoxicity from carbon tetrachloride.

When chemicals interact in a way that the resulting toxicity of any one chemical is greatly increased beyond what could be reasonably predicted based on the toxicities of each chemical independently, then we can recognize what is commonly referred to as a "synergistic" effect. Here, the toxicity could not be predicted from the contributions of the individual chemicals.

The EPA defines synergism as ". . . the effect of the combination is greater than suggested by the component toxic effects." As an example, both ethyl alcohol and carbon tetrachloride are toxic to the liver individually; however, their combined effect results in more injury than the summation of their individual effects.

## Government Concerns About Chemical Interactions

There is a relatively new focus on chemical mixtures in toxicology and regulatory policy in the United States. The need for better predictive methodologies and toxicity studies for chemical mixtures to which the public is likely exposed is reflected in the toxicology literature and government initiatives of the past decade. The relevance of chemical interactions has received and will continue to receive governmental attention from a regulatory perspective, especially when dealing with population exposures to environmentally relevant concentrations of chemicals. Several examples are provided:

- There have been amendments to the Federal Insecticide, Fungicide, and Rodenticide Act (FIFRA) and the Federal Food Drug and Cosmetic Act (FFDCA) through the Food Quality Protection Act (FQPA) in 1996 and 2003 by the setting of standards for exposures to similarly acting pesticides in foods. The FQPA is an early attempt by the government to recognize and regulate the potential for combined toxicity by developing pesticide tolerances.
- In 1996 amendments were made to the Safe Drinking Water Act (SDWA) to require "new approaches for studying the adverse effects of contaminant mixtures in drinking water" such as the disinfection byproducts that may be present in municipally treated drinking water.
- The EPA via the Clean Air Act (CAA) is concerned about the effects of multiple air pollutant affects and has been directed to include information on chemicals that may interact to "produce an adverse effect on public health or welfare."
- The EPA and the ATSDR have developed guidance documents and chemical interaction profiles for assessing human health impact from chemical mixtures. For Superfund, the EPA acknowledges that a simultaneous exposure to a mixture of chemicals, each contributing to a subthreshold response, could nonetheless result in a cumulative adverse health effect.

## Approaches for Assessing Toxicant Interactions

The EPA has indicated that for chemicals with similar toxicokinetics and effects (same target organ or mechanism of action) and for which a lack of interaction has been demonstrated by laboratory studies, the dose addition methodology for assessing toxicant interaction is suggested. This methodology ranks the potency of each chemical in a mixture relative to a common chemical using, for example, the relative potency factor (RPF) or the hazard index (HI). The HI is recommended where there are insufficient data concerning the mechanism of action of the chemical.

The EPA describes the RPF methodology as the scaling of the potency of a chemical relative to an index chemical. The index chemical has been well studied toxicologically and is considered to be representative of the chemicals constituting the mixture. As an example, the organophosphate pesticide chlorophos is an index chemical for chemicals that act through the inhibition of the enzyme cholinesterase. In this method, the inhibition of cholinesterase relative to chlorophos is determined for each chemical, and the predicted toxicity of the mixture is determined by summation. With the HI methodology, there is similarly the assumption that total toxicity of the chemicals is additive; however, the chemicals are scaled to RfDs or reference concentrations (inhalation).

The EPA defines an RfD as an estimate of a daily oral exposure to the human population (including sensitive subgroups) that is likely to be without significant risk of adverse effects during the lifetime of the individual. The RfD is based on the empirically determined NOAEL for the most sensitive end-point of toxicity for the chemical. The most sensitive end-point of toxicity is also referred to as the *critical effect*. This is arrived at by acute, subacute, and chronic studies in laboratory animals. By dividing the concentration of the chemical by the RfD (C/RfD), the HI is calculated for each chemical. This ratio is a measure of relative potency, and by adding together the contributions from each chemical of the mixture, the HI for the whole mixture can be determined. The EPA suggests that when using this approach "exposure data should be at relatively low levels (near NOAEL), at which interaction effects are not expected."

The concern about the combined toxicities from exposure to multiple chemicals should not be viewed as a research interest exclusive to toxicologists, but rather it should be studied as a multidisciplinary approach to better assess the role of lifestyle factors, preexisting diseases, health care availability, occupational history, physical and biological agents, cultural practices, and others factors on the public health impact from chemical interactions. Low-level exposures to chemicals may not result in any clinically apparent toxicity. Subclinical physiological changes as end-points of toxicity require the application of sophisticated genetic, biomonitoring, computer modeling, and biochemical methodologies that could assist regulatory decision making.

## Responding to Public Concerns

As a toxicologist for the state, you have been asked to conduct a risk assessment in response to public outcry from the use of specially treated lumber in play equipment at state and municipal parks. Local officials have already restricted access to the equipment because of public concerns about its safety, concerns raised in response to a journalist's news column and its airing on local TV. The concern is about the use of copper chromated arsenate (CCA) in the treatment of the wood. This is an especially charged area for parents who already have arrived at the conclusion that these playgrounds are dangerous to their children and perhaps to them as well. Their risk assessment is based on two words: "arsenic" and "children." You are initially troubled because this preservative has been used for many decades, so why the concern at this point? There has been no accepted link between children playing on these wooden structures and illness, other than the accidental physical injuries that kids sustain while playing. In fact, your own children have play equipment made from CCA-treated lumber.

You have been asked to attend a municipal meeting with local government officials, news media, lumber distributors, and parents to discuss your findings and to make any recommendations to correct what is perceived to be a serious community health problem. You conduct your risk assessments following standard methodologies, knowing that the information will be shared with all stakeholders, including the manufacturers of these treated lumber products. Important information includes the following facts:

- Arsenic is ubiquitously present in the earth's crust.
- In North America the average soil concentration of arsenic is about 5 ppm.
- Arsenic is a known human carcinogen.
- The known noncarcinogenic toxicity of arsenic is well known.
- The sources of arsenic identified through sampling were from soil and treated lumber.
- The amount of arsenic present in the soil falls within the range typically seen in the area where playgrounds are not present.
- You cannot assess whether or not any significant arsenic present in the soil came from the lumber.

Cancer and noncancer risk assessments, using several scenarios, were developed based on sampling results and showed a mean value of arsenic in the soil at 3.46 mg/kg and 22 μg/100 cm$^2$ of wood surface. Additional soil sampling in close-by residential areas yielded values comparable with those obtained at the playground in question. In your assessments you used a scenario that would produce the maximum level of risk. You assumed

- All of the arsenic from soil was bioavailable.
- All arsenic from the treated lumber was bioavailable.
- Children used the playground on a daily basis.
- You considered children between 2 and 6 years old in your assessment, because they are the most likely to consume the largest amount of soil and have the greatest hand-to-mouth contact.
- The weight of the average child was 20 kg.
- An ingestion of 100 mg soil/day.

Four routes of exposure were considered for both cancer and noncancer risk:

- Skin absorption from the soil
- Skin absorption from direct contact with the wood
- Ingestion of soil
- Ingestion from direct oral contact with wood

For your calculations, you relied on information from the ATSDR to obtain an arsenic cancer slope factor of 1.5 mg/kg/day and an RfD of 0.0003 mg/kg/day (0.3 μg/kg/day). Your conclusions were that for the average child of about 20 kg body weight who ingests 100 mg of soil every day of the year from the playground and lives to be 70 years old, the risk for developing cancer from exposure to arsenic at the playground is 6 in 10,000,000. Additionally, because you obtained a hazard quotient of 0.06, you conclude that there was no increased risk of noncancer toxicity. In communicating this, you may wish to point out that there may be a wide variation in the amount of arsenic as sampled from playground lumber depending on its age, condition, and whether or not it has been additionally sealed against water permeation. Your sampling was limited and may not accurately reflect the conditions in other areas with similar playground equipment.

You may further discuss the levels of risk that you arrived at in comparison with other risks more readily identified with by the public, such as a lifetime risk of being struck by lightening as 100 to 1,000 times more likely to occur than developing cancer from treated lumber under these conditions of exposure. A recommendation that you might make is to have CCA–treated play equipment sealed against water intrusion into the surface of the wood, as an additional measure of protection. This measure would be cost-effective when compared with other alternatives such as removing it or replacing it with one of a different composition. Replacement costs for equipment for all municipal playgrounds may be beyond the resources of the local government. To further emphasize the level of risk to children at play, you might add that your own kids play on similarly treated equipment.

## Websites

Integrated Risk Information System (IRIS):
http://toxnet.nlm.nih.gov/cgi-bin/sis/htmlgen?IRIS

International Toxicity Estimates for Risk (ITER):
http://toxnet.nlm.nih.gov/cgi-bin/sis/htmlgen?iter

National Toxicology Program:
http://ntp-server.niehs.nih.gov/

NIOSH:
http://www.cdc.gov/Niosh/homepage.html

Occupational Safety and Health Administration (OSHA):
http://www.osha.gov/

Registry of Toxic Effects of Chemical Substances:
http://www.cdc.gov/niosh/97-119.html

Right to Know Hazardous Substance Fact Sheets:
http://www.state.nj.us/health/eoh/rtkweb/rtkhsfs.htm

The Society for Risk Assessment:
www.sra.org/

Toxicology Excellence for Risk Assessment:
www.tera.org/

Toxikon Multimedia Project:
http://www.uic.edu/com/er/toxikon/

TOXLINE:
http://toxnet.nlm.nih.gov/cgi-bin/sis/htmlgen?TOXLINE

U.S. Environmental Protection Agency Superfund Risk Assessment:
www.epa.gov/superfund/health/risk/index.htm

## Bibliography

Benjamin S. L., & Belluck, D. A. (2001). *A practical guide to understanding, managing, and reviewing environmental risk assessment reports.* Boca Raton, FL: CRC Press.

Calabrese, E. J., & Kenyon, E. M. (1991). *Air toxics and risk assessment.* Chelsea, MI: Lewis Publishers.

Isselbacher, K. J. (1996). *Science and judgment in risk assessment* (student edition). New York: Taylor & Francis.

Klaassen, C. D. (2001). *Casarett & Doull's toxicology. The basic science of poisons.* New York: McGraw-Hill.

Klaassen, C. D., & Watkins, J. B. (2003). *Casarett & Doull's essentials of toxicology.* New York: McGraw-Hill.

Newman, M. C., & Strojan, C. (1998). *Risk assessment: logic and measurement.* Chelsea, MI: Ann Arbor Press.

Pastorok, R. A., Bartell, S. M., Ferson, S., & Ginzburg, L. R. (Eds.) (2001). *Ecological modeling in risk assessment: chemical effects on populations, ecosystems, and landscapes.* Boca Raton, FL: CRC Press.

Simon-Hettich, B., Rothfuss, A., & Steger-Hartmann, T. (2006). Use of computer-assisted prediction of toxic effects of chemical substances. *Toxicology, 224,* 156–162.

U.S. National Library of Medicine, National Institutes of Health, Environmental Health, and Toxicology Specialized Information Services (SIS). (2005). *Toxicology tutorial III.* Retrieved October 2, 2005 from http://www.sis.nlm.nih.gov/enviro/toxtutor.html.

Woolley, A. A. (2003). *Guide to practical toxicology: evaluation, prediction and risk.* New York: Taylor & Francis.

# CHAPTER 24

# Making Informed Decisions

## Difficulties in Decision Making

". . . because as we know, there are known knowns; there are things we know we know. We also know there are known unknowns; that is to say we know there are some things we do not know. But there are also unknown unknowns—the ones we don't know we don't know." This quote by former Secretary of Defense Donald Rumsfeld, though essentially true, was widely ridiculed. Decision makers in toxicology face many of the same uncertainties mentioned in the quote and sometimes may face comparably unsympathetic audiences as did Mr. Rumsfeld. As public health professionals, we make decisions that generally take the form of recommendations that can have enormous potential impact, because we are dealing with populations and not single individuals. Making informed decisions involves quantifying the various knowns, recognizing that there are unknowns, and determining courses of action that might be taken along with the consequences of each. This is true for both human health decisions and the decisions that may affect ecosystems.

The way in which chemicals are used has become a growing area of concern, especially as more of them are identified with some form of chronic toxicity. Epidemiological and laboratory studies have revealed associations between chemical exposures and health effects such as cancer and birth defects. To assist decision making, federal agencies developed procedures for identifying health hazards and estimating human health risks resulting from chemical exposures. These agencies have concerns about the demands for health protection by the public for a growing list of toxic chemicals that have been detected in the environment.

Chemical use is intended to provide benefit, whether it is for a pharmaceutical or a pesticide. And chemical exposures, whether intentional or unintentional, should ideally not produce injury. Where there is use, there are inevitably exposures, and therefore standards and guidelines must be in place to protect health and environment. In addition, standards need to be set at levels that can be met. We would like to see human exposure levels for all non-beneficial chemicals set as low as feasibly possible. Here, as elsewhere, decisions need to be made concerning safety, in the absence of all information that we ideally would want to have. Regulatory decisions have to balance the costs and benefits that may be imposed by any regulatory policies that are enacted. Considerations for the small business, which may not have the resources for costly engineering modifications to reduce airborne concentrations of chemicals to levels well below regulatory exposure standards, have to enter into the equation or these small businesses may be forced to close their doors. The arrival of any regulatory policy should be a dynamic process to include input from decision makers as well as all stakeholders, as early on in the process as is feasible, rather than a scratching of heads wondering "when did this come about" or "how did they arrive at that decision"?

## Risk Assessment in the Federal Government: Managing the Process

The opinions of toxicologists, whether they are employed in academia, industry, or government, have an important influence on federal agencies having primary authority to regulate substances and activities that pose health risks, including U.S. Food and Drug Administration, U.S. Environmental Protection Agency, Occupational Safety and Health Administration, the Consumer Product Safety Commission, and the Departments of Agriculture, Defense, Energy, and Transportation.

The response of the executive branch and the Congress to concerns about the federal regulatory policymaking procedures was a study conducted by the National Research Council (NRC), which resulted in a 1983 report entitled *Risk Assessment in the Federal Government: Managing the Process*. An important concern underlying the reason to conduct this 1983 study was to discuss the common perception that policymakers unduly influence the risk assessment process. A relationship between assessment and management needed to be discussed to better draw clearer lines of separation between the two. The goal was to improve risk assessment, and thus regulatory decision making, by providing a framework around which federal agencies could establish risk assessment methodologies to meet their institutional goals and objectives and to consider the merits of separating policymaking decisions from the analytic functions of developing risk assessments.

Additionally, the study considered the feasibility of all agencies having uniform guidelines for risk assessment within a centralized agency rather than conducting separate assessments within each agency. This would prove to be difficult because of differences in various laws and areas of regulatory control between the different agencies; an earlier attempt to standardize federal carcinogen guidelines was short-lived.

Review of the "process" in 1983 essentially led to the formalization of the procedural steps that were necessary for all agencies to follow in conducting formal risk assessments:

- Hazard identification for identifying if a substance is or is not causally linked to a particular health effect
- Dose–response assessment for determining the relationship between exposure level and the probability of occurrence of the health effects in question
- Exposure assessment for determining the extent of human exposure both before and after regulatory action that might be taken
- Risk characterization for describing the nature and possibly magnitude of the risks posed and any uncertainties considered in arriving at the characterization

Recommendations to the federal regulatory agencies from the NRC 1983 study included the following:

- Before deciding whether a substance should be regulated as a health hazard, a written, comprehensive, and publicly accessible risk assessment needs to be prepared to clearly distinguish between the scientific and the policy basis for any conclusions.
- Clear conceptual distinctions must be made between the risk assessment characterization and risk management considerations.
- Inference guidelines must be uniformly developed and should be sufficiently comprehensive, detailed, and flexible, with a clear distinction between science and policy.
- Before adopting any final guidelines, a panel of experts should be in place to provide recommendations for procedural guidelines rather than regulations.
- A central board on risk assessment should be established to periodically review guidelines, inference uncertainties, research needs, and agency experience.
- An independent science advisory panel should review an agency's risk assessment, which should be made publicly available, before any major regulatory actions or decisions not to regulate are made.
- Have a joint risk assessment prepared by an appropriate third party such as the National Toxicology Program (NTP) when more than one agency shares an interest and jurisdiction over a potentially regulated health hazard.
- The risk assessments should describe all components of hazard identification, dose–response assessment, and risk characterization, with detailed guidance on how to consider each of these components.
- The guidelines should include how to present the assessment results and the associated uncertainties.
- Cancer risks should be considered a priority of initial assessment guidelines, with assessment of other health risks to follow. This recommendation reflects the relative abundance of experimental and human carcinogen data available at the time, though the report also provides recommendations concerning evaluating and regulating other health effects.

The risk assessment recommendations were subsequently adopted by many agencies. The EPA was the only federal agency to develop carcinogenic, developmental toxicity, mutagenicity, and chemical mixture effects risk assessment guidelines. In response to The Clean Air Act Amendments of 1990, the NRC conducted a review of the EPA risk assessment procedures in helping the agency evaluate approximately 200 additionally named hazardous air pollutants in the 1990 legislation. The objective was to determine whether current procedures were sufficiently adequate or should be improved to address the new concerns of the 1990 amendment. The 1994 report of the NRC recommended the following to the EPA:

- Provide qualitative and quantitative risk characterizations to decision makers and the public to include sources and magnitude of uncertainties associated with the estimates.
- Modify the current approach to risk assessment to include recommendations addressing validity, flexibility, quantitative and qualitative techniques, and risk communication.
- Use an iterative approach to risk assessment. This includes using stratified levels of increasing complexity to evaluate substances, with a goal of not spending resources that yield little additional value to the health of the American public.

## Making the Best Decisions

Arriving at a decision is a long and painstaking process, especially when those decisions will likely result in the implementation of policies and regulations that will greatly impact on the health of the public and environment. As public health professionals, this must always be our primary consideration above and beyond all other concerns with respect to costs and implementation. Our next priority is to frame our decisions into a range of regulatory and nonregulatory options so they can be implemented. It is here that we need to recognize considerations of cost and other factors that affect implementation. There is no escaping the fact that we become an integral part of the management of risk, based on our assessments and conclusions regarding public health issues.

Our decisions should

- Be based on the weight of evidence about potential health and environmental risks, which should be clearly articulated in the context of a public health or environmental concern
- Recognize that we can never truly "prevent" risk but rather must reduce or minimize it in ways that are consistent with the best available scientific, technical, and socioeconomic information
- Recognize there are political, social, legal, and cultural considerations
- Consider the views and opinions of those affected by any decisions that we make "on their behalf"
- Be made with an understanding of the range of regulatory and nonregulatory options available for implementation

# The CRAM Report

The Presidential/Congressional Commission on Risk Assessment and Risk Management report on the accomplishments of the Commission on Risk Assessment and Risk Management (1997 CRAM Report) provides a framework for risk management (Figure 24.1) that is conceptually divided into a number of stages:

- Define the problem and put it into context.
- Analyze the risks associated with the problem in context.
- Examine options for addressing the risk.
- Make decisions about which options to implement.
- Take actions to implement the decisions.
- Conduct an evaluation of the action.

Peer review is an important component for decision making, but other components important in making informed decisions include economic, legal, social, political, and budgetary factors as well as the opinion of the public and their values (Figure 24.2). This has been conceptualized by the EPA into a decision-making framework that is clear, consistent, and reasonable and where input from multiple sources is evaluated before decisions are made.

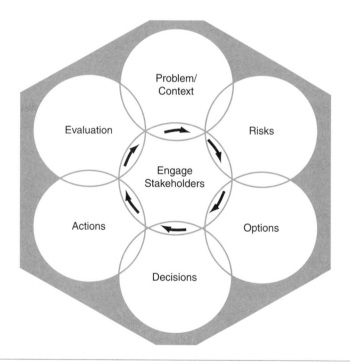

**FIGURE 24.1** Risk management framework. *Source:* Courtesy of U.S. Food and Drug Administration.

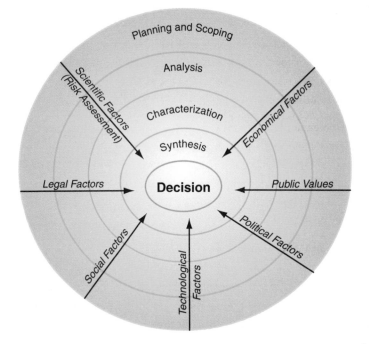

FIGURE 24.2    Risk management decision framework. *Source:* Courtesy of EPA.

## Websites

National Toxicology Program:
http://ntp.niehs.nih.gov/

U.S. Consumer Product Safety Commission:
www.cpsc.gov

U.S. Department of Agriculture:
http://www.usda.gov/wps/portal/usdahome

U.S. Department of Defense:
http://www.defenselink.mil/

U.S. Department of Energy:
http://www.doe.gov/

U.S. Department of Labor Occupational Safety & Health Administration:
www.osha.gov

U.S. Department of Transportation:
http://www.dot.gov/

# Bibliography

Klaassen, C. C. (Ed.) (2001). *Casarett and Doull's toxicology: the basic science of poisons.* New York: McGraw-Hill.

Kurtzman, D. (2003). *Donald Rumsfeld wins "Foot in Mouth Award."* Retrieved from http://political humor.about.com/b/b/o47299.htm.

National Research Council. (1983). *Risk assessment in the federal government: managing the process.* Washington, DC: National Academy Press.

National Research Council. (1994). *Science and judgment in risk assessment.* Washington, DC: National Academy Press.

National Research Council. (1996). *Understanding risk: informing decisions in a democratic society.* Washington, DC: National Academy Press.

Ohanian, E. V., Moore, J. A., Fowle, J. R., Omenn, G. S., Lewis, S. C., Gray, G. M., & North, D. W. (1997). Workshop overview. Risk characterization: a bridge to informed decision making. *Fundamental and Applied Toxicology, 39,* 81–88.

The Presidential/Congressional Commission on Risk Assessment and Risk Management (1997). *Framework for environmental health risk management* (Vol. 1). Retrieved from http://www.riskworld.com/Nreports/1997/risk-rpt/pdf/EPAJAN.PDF (Volumes 1 and 2 available at http://www.riskworld.com/Nreports/nr7me001.htm).

U.S. Environmental Protection Agency. (2002). *Risk characterization handbook.* Retrieved from http://www.epa.gov/osa/spc/pdfs/rchandbk.pdf (another link to the PDF file is http://www.epa.gov/osa/spc/2riskchr.htm).

U.S. National Library of Medicine, National Institutes of Health, Environmental Health, and Toxicology Specialized Information Services (SIS). (2005). *Toxicology tutorial III.* Retrieved October 2, 2005 from http://www.sis.nlm.nih.gov/enviro/toxtutor.html.

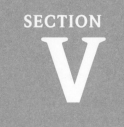

SECTION

V

# Glossary of Terms

## A

**Absorbed Dose**
The amount of a substance that actually enters into the body. The absorbed dose is usually expressed as milligrams of substance per kilogram (mg/kg) of body weight.

**Absorption**
The movement and uptake of substances into cells or across tissues by way of processes of active transport, diffusion, or osmosis.

**Acceptable Daily Intake (ADI)**
The dose of a chemical to which a person can be exposed daily over a period of time (usually lifetime) without suffering apparent harmful effects.

**Acetylcholine**
A neuromuscular transmitter that regulates synaptic and neuromuscular function.

**Acetylcholinesterase**
An enzyme that catalyzes the hydrolysis of acetylcholine to choline and acetic acid that is present in nervous tissue, muscle, and red blood cells.

**ACGIH**
American Conference of Governmental Industrial Hygienists. It is a nongovernmental professional society for industrial hygienists that publish threshold limit values (TLV) and biological exposure indices (BEI) for physical and chemical agents.

**Active Transport**
The movement of a substance across a cell membrane that requires the expenditure of energy.

**Acute Dose**
The amount of a substance administered or received over a relatively short period of time (minutes or hours), usually within a 24-hour period.

**Acute Effect**
An effect that occurs after a single or brief exposure to a toxic agent. Generally, acute effects are evident within several days but often occur within minutes or hours.

**Acute Toxicity**
Any poisonous effect produced within a short period of time after an exposure, usually within 24 to 96 hours.

**Adenine (A)**
One of the nitrogenous bases, and a member of the base pair AT (adenine-thymine) of DNA.

**Adsorption**
The process of attracting and holding a substance to a surface. For example, a substance such as an herbicide may adsorb onto a soil particle.

**Adverse Effect**
A biochemical change, functional impairment, or pathological lesion that affects the performance of the whole organism or reduces an organism's ability to respond to an additional environmental challenge.

**Adverse Reactions to Drug Reports**
A report that is voluntarily submitted by physicians to the FDA after a drug has been approved and in use. Adverse reactions to drugs in clinical trials are subject to mandatory report. http://www.fda.gov/medwatch/report/hcp.htm.

**Aerosols**
Aerosols are airborne particulates. They may be solid or liquid droplets.

**Allele**
The variant form of a genetic locus; a single allele for each locus is inherited from each parent (e.g., the locus for blood type or eye color).

**Allergy**
An immune hypersensitivity reaction of body tissues to allergens, typically harmless substances, that can affect the skin (e.g., urticaria), respiratory tract (e.g., asthma), gastrointestinal tract (vomiting and nausea), or produce a systemic circulatory response (anaphylactic response).

**Allogeneic**
The variation of alleles within the same species.

**Alternative Splicing**
Combinations of exons to make variations of a complete protein, accomplished by recombination during mRNA splicing in eukaryotic cells.

**Alveoli**
The thin-walled air sacs at the ends of the tracheobronchial tree in which oxygen and carbon dioxide are exchanged between inhaled air and the pulmonary capillary blood.

**Ambient**
Surrounding conditions (e.g., ambient air, ambient water, ambient soil).

**Ames Test**
A test for mutagenesis using the bacterium, *Salmonella typhimurium*. Developed in the 1970s by Bruce Ames to investigate new and old environmental chemicals.

**Amino Acid**
The building blocks of proteins. A class of 20 or so molecules that are combined to form proteins. Amino acids share a common amino portion of the molecule ($NH_2$) and a carboxyl (COOH) portion. The sequence of amino acids in a protein and hence the type of protein function are determined by the genetic code.

**Anemia**

A condition in which there is reduced or impaired red blood cells or hemoglobin resulting in an inadequate capacity of the blood to transport oxygen to body tissues. Often characterized by fatigue, weakness, and dyspnea.

**Aneuploidy**

Any deviation from an exact multiple of the haploid number of chromosomes. This may involve missing or extra chromosomes or parts of chromosomes. Hypoploidy (fewer than normal) can result in Turner's syndrome, whereas hyperploidy (more than normal) like trisomy 21 results in Down's syndrome.

**Anoxia**

A complete lack of oxygen in the body tissues. Used interchangeably with hypoxia (a diminished oxygen supply).

**Antagonism**

An interaction between two chemicals in which the observed effect is less than the predicted effect when those chemicals are considered independently.

**Antibody**

An antibody is a protein molecule (immunoglobulin with a unique amino acid sequence) that only interacts with a specific or closely related foreign substance (antigen). Some act directly to destroy the antigen, whereas others simply make it easier for that antigen to be destroyed by leukocytes. The antibody is induced (a response of the immune system) as a result of prior exposure to the antigen.

**Anticholinergic Effects**

Neurological effects (e.g., dry mouth, confusion, constipation, visual disturbances, etc.) resulting from the blockage of acetylcholine, which transmits impulses across nerve junctions.

**Antidote**

A treatment to counteract a poison.

**Aplastic**

Diminished or absent cell production, as in aplastic anemia.

**Apoptosis**

Programmed cell death, also called "cellular suicide," is an orderly process by which the organism disposes of unnecessary or damaged cells.

**Asphyxiant**

A relatively nontoxic gas that in high concentrations in the air results in insufficient oxygen, which can cause hypoxia. Simple asphyxiants like nitrogen displace or consume atmospheric oxygen, whereas chemical asphyxiants like carbon monoxide disrupt absorption or transportation of oxygen within the body.

**Atypia**

State of being not typical.

**Autoimmunity**

An immune response that recognizes the constituents of the body's own cells as foreign and thus induces hypersensitivity to its own tissues. Implicated in diseases like rheumatoid arthritis and lupus.

**Autoradiography**

A technique that uses x-ray film to visualize and quantitate radioactively labeled molecules or molecular fragments; following separation by gel electrophoresis, the technique is used to analyze length and number of DNA fragments.

**Autosomal Dominant**

Refers to a gene located on nonsex chromosomes that is expressed whenever present. The chance of passing the gene to offspring is 50% for each pregnancy.

**Autosome**

A eukaryotic chromosome not involved in sex determination. The diploid human genome consists of a total of 46 chromosomes: 22 pairs of autosomes and 1 pair of sex chromosomes (the X and Y chromosomes).

**Average Daily Intake**

The amount of a chemical which a person consumes over a period of a day. It is determined by multiplying typical concentration of the chemical in drinking water, air, and food by an average daily intake factor such as 2 liters of water per day.

**Axon**

The elongated extension of a neuron that usually conducts impulses away from the cell body.

# B

**Base**

Generic term describing the nitrogenous molecule that forms the informational portion of DNA and RNA (adenine, thymine, guanine, cytosine, uracil).

**Base Pair**

Two nitrogenous bases (a purine and a pyrimidine) held together by weak bonds. In DNA the pairs consist of adenine and thymine or guanine and cytosine; in RNA uracil replaces thymine. Two strands of DNA are held together in the shape of a double helix by the bonds between base pairs.

**Base Sequence**

Refers to the order of base pairs in DNA and RNA; the sequence determines the shape of the protein produced.

**Basement Membrane**

The layer upon which the epithelium rests. The term actually refers to the combination of basal lamina and lamina reticularis or two basal laminae. The basement membrane consists of an electron dense layer (lamina densa, composed of collagen) sandwiched between two electron lucid layers (lamina lucida) and is approximately 0.1–2 μm in thickness.

**Basophil**

Also called a granular leukocyte; basophils make up less than 1% of circulating white blood cells. They are active in inflammation and participate in allergic response. Basophils contain histamine and heparin.

**B Cells**

Also known as B lymphocytes, B cells play an important role in humoral immunity because they synthesize and secrete antibodies that protect us from infection, viruses, and so on.

**Benchmark Dose (BMD) or Concentration (BMC)**

A dose or concentration that produces a predetermined change in response rate of an adverse effect (called the benchmark response or BMR) compared with background.

**Benchmark Response (BMR)**

An adverse effect, used to define a benchmark dose from which an RfD (or RfC) can be developed. The change in response rate over background of the BMR is usually in the range of 5–10%, which is the limit of responses typically observed in well-conducted animal experiments.

**Benign Tumor**

A tumor that grows only at the site of origin and does not invade adjacent tissues or metastasize. Characterized by slow growth and expansion. It is generally treatable.

**Benzene**

The simplest ringed compound consisting of 6 carbon and 6 hydrogen atoms. It is a colorless and flammable liquid widely used in organic synthesis, as a solvent, and as a motor fuel. Exposure to benzene can increase the risk of cancer and lead to anemia and a decrease in blood platelets.

### Bias

In experimental design, systematic error that may be introduced in sampling by selecting or encouraging one outcome over another. May lead to incorrect conclusions.

### Bioaccumulation (also referred to as Bioconcentration)

The buildup of a substance in a biological organism such that the level in the organism is greater than in environmental media. Occurs when the rate of uptake exceeds the rate of elimination.

### Bioactivation

Describes the metabolic process whereby a parent chemical is metabolized to a chemical with enhanced biological activity. The bioactivation of a precarcinogen to a carcinogen is an example of a bioactivation.

### Bioassay

An assay for determining the potency (or concentration) of a substance that causes a biological change in experimental animals.

### Bioavailability

The physical and/or biological state of a substance that renders it capable of being absorbed into the body.

### Biodegradation

Breakdown of a chemical into smaller less complex molecules by microorganisms in environmental media (e.g., soil, water, sediment).

### Bioinformatics

The science of management and analysis of biological data using advanced computing techniques. Particularly important in analyzing genomic research data.

### Biological Half-Life

The time required to reduce the quantity of a substance in a biological medium (e.g., plasma) by 50%.

### Biomarker

Cellular or molecular indicators of events occurring in biologic systems due to a xenobiotic. The types of indicators are exposure, effects, or susceptibility.

### Biopsy

A procedure used to remove cells or tissues for diagnostic evaluation. Some of the biopsy material may also be used for research purposes.

### Bioremediation

The use of biological organisms, particularly microorganisms, to aid in removing hazardous substances from an area.

### Biotechnology

Biological techniques developed through basic research and now applied to research and product development. In particular, biotechnology refers to the use by industry of recombinant DNA, cell fusion, and new bioprocessing techniques. Biotechnology features prominently in pharmaceuticals and medical research.

### Biotransformation

Conversion of a chemical from one form to another by a biological organism. Examples include enzyme-mediated metabolism of xenobiotics. Biotransformation and metabolism are often used to mean the same thing.

### Birth Defect

An abnormality present at birth resulting from a genetic mutation or some other non-genetic factor.

**BMDL or BMCL**

A statistical lower confidence limit on the dose or concentration at the BMD or BMC, respectively.

**Body Burden**

The accumulation of a chemical in the body. The chemical does not necessarily produce adverse effects.

**Bone Marrow**

The tissue within the internal open space of bones (e.g., shaft of long bones) in which the blood-forming elements like erythrocytes, leukocytes, and thrombocytes are produced.

**BRCA1**

Identified in 1994, BRCA1, or "Breast Cancer 1," is a mutation in chromosome 17. This mutation is present in about two-thirds of heritable breast cancers and a smaller number of heritable ovarian cancers. Only about 5% of the female breast cancers in the world are attributable to having the BRCA1 mutation.

**BRCA2**

Identified in 1995, BRCA2, or "Breast Cancer 2," is a mutation in chromosome 13. This mutation is present in male and female heritable breast, ovarian, and prostate cancers. Less than 5% of cancers of the male and female breast, ovary, and prostate are attributable to the BRCA2 mutation.

**Bronchioles**

The very small branches of the tracheo-bronchial tree of the respiratory tract that ultimately terminate in the alveoli. Each human lung has approximately 30,000 bronchioles.

# C

**Cancer**

A group of approximately 100 diseases characterized by uncontrolled cellular growth and divisions. Most cancers are named for the type of cell or the organ of origin. When cancer spreads (metastasizes), the new tumor has the same name as the original (primary) tumor.

**Cancer Slope Factor**

An EPA key risk assessment parameter, extrapolated from available data to estimate the probability that an individual will develop cancer if exposed to a specified amount of chemical (mg/kg) every day over the course of a lifetime.

**Candidate Gene**

A gene located in a chromosome region and suspected of being involved in a disease. The gene product, a protein, has properties suggestive of involvement in the disease process.

**Carbohydrate**

Any of a variety of compounds of carbon, hydrogen, and oxygen (as sugars, starches, and celluloses) most of which are formed by green plants and which constitute a major class of animal foods. Starch, sugar, and cellulose are the most common.

**Carcinogen**

Something that produces cancer, generally by either directly or indirectly, effecting changes in DNA.

**Carcinogenesis**

A multistep process resulting in the formation of cancer from normal cells or tissues.

**Carcinogenic**

The ability of a chemical or other agent to cause cancer.

**Carcinoma**
Term used to denote a cancer derived from epithelial cells. Found in body tissues that cover or line surfaces of organs, glands, or body structures. Approximately 80% of cancers are carcinomas.

**Case-Control Study**
A type of epidemiological study that compares the exposure histories of individuals who have particular signs, symptoms, or disease with that of normal individuals.

**Catecholamine**
Any of various biologically active amines (e.g., epinephrine, norepinephrine, and dopamine) that can function as hormones and neurotransmitters.

**cDNA Library**
A collection of DNA sequences, generated in the laboratory using mRNA sequences, that code for genes.

**Ceiling Level**
The maximum allowable level of exposure of a chemical in the workplace for a specific period of time (usually 15 minutes).

**Cell**
The smallest structural and functional unit of any living organism that carries on the biochemical processes of life.

**Cell Transformation**
The change of a cell from one form to another; usually denotes the change from normal to malignant.

**Central Nervous System (CNS)**
The brain and spinal cord.

**Centriole**
A cylinder-shaped organelle composed of microtubules found in the nucleus of a cell.

It forms the spindle during nuclear division and ensures that the duplicated chromosomes are equally divided between the daughter cells.

**Centromere**
A specialized chromosome region to which spindle fibers attach during mitotic and meiotic division.

**Chemotherapy**
The treatment of cancer with drugs formulated to destroy cancer cells. These drugs often are called "anticancer" drugs. They destroy cancer cells by inhibiting growth and multiplication. Healthy cells can also be harmed, especially those that divide quickly. Harm to healthy cells is what causes side effects.

**Cholestasis**
A liver condition in which excretion of bile salts via the bile duct is inhibited, resulting in bile salts backing up into liver cells. Blockage can occur in the bile ducts or in the liver.

**Cholinergic Effect**
Neurological effects (a parasympathetic response) resulting from the transmission by acetylcholine of impulses across synaptic or neuromuscular junctions.

**Chromatin**
A complex of nucleic acid and basic proteins (such as histone) in eukaryotic cells that is usually dispersed in the interphase nucleus and condensed into chromosomes in mitosis and meiosis.

**Chromatography**
An analytic method that separates and identifies the components of a complex mixture exploiting differential movement through a two-phase system. It is based on the physicochemical principles of adsorption, partition,

ion exchange, exclusion, or a combination of these principles.

**Chromosomal Deletion**
The loss of a portion of a chromosome's DNA.

**Chromosomal Inversion**
Chromosome segments that are reversed with respect to the rest of the chromosome.

**Chromosome**
The self-replicating genetic structure of cells containing the cellular DNA that bears in its nucleotide sequence the linear array of genes. In prokaryotes, chromosomal DNA is circular, and the entire genome is carried on one chromosome. Eukaryotic genomes consist of a number of chromosomes whose DNA is associated with different kinds of proteins.

**Chromosome Aberration**
Changes in chromosome structure or number.

**Chromosome Region p**
Term for the short arm of a chromosome.

**Chromosome Region q**
Term for the long arm of a chromosome.

**Chronic Dose**
Exposure to a substance gradually over a long period of time (months to years).

**Chronic Effect**
An effect that appears a long time after an exposure (the latency period) or an effect that results from a long-term (chronic) exposure.

**Chronic Exposure**
Repeated exposure by the oral, dermal, or inhalation route for more than approximately 10% of the life span in humans. This time period corresponds to 90 days to 2 years in commonly used mammalian laboratory species.

**Chronic Myelogenous Leukemia (CML)**
A malignant bone marrow cancer causing rapid growth and accumulation of myeloid precursors (blood forming cells) in the bone marrow, peripheral blood, and body tissues.

**Chronic Toxicity**
The capacity of a substance to cause adverse human health effects as a result of chronic exposure.

**Cirrhosis**
A chronic degenerative disease of the liver in which hepatic cells are replaced by fibrous cells.

**Clone**
An exact replica made of biological material such as a DNA segment (e.g., a gene or other region), a whole cell, or a complete organism.

**Cloning**
Using specialized DNA technology to produce many identical copies of a single gene or segment of DNA to generate enough material for further study. This process, used by researchers in the Human Genome Project, is referred to as cloning DNA. The resulting cloned (copied) collections of DNA molecules are called clone libraries. A second type of cloning capitalizes on the natural process of cell division to make multiple copies of an entire cell. The genetic makeup of these cloned cells, called a cell line, is identical to the original cell. A third type of cloning produces complete, genetically identical animals such as the first mammal successfully cloned, Dolly the Sheep.

**Codon**
The sequence of three nucleotides responsible for encoding an amino acid.

**Cohort Study**

An epidemiology study in which a group (the cohort) of individuals with exposure to a chemical and an unexposed cohort are followed over time to compare disease occurrence.

**Complementary DNA (cDNA)**

DNA that is synthesized in the laboratory from a messenger RNA template that is often used as a mapping probe.

**Complementary Sequence**

Nucleic acid base sequence capable of forming a double-stranded structure with another DNA fragment following base-pairing rules (A pairs with T and C with G). The complementary sequence to GTAC, for example, is CATG.

**Computational Biology**

The use of algorithmic tools to analyze biological systems.

**Congenital**

A trait present at birth; may stem from genetic or nongenetic factors.

**Conjugation**

The metabolic process in which chemical groups are attached to foreign substances in the body, usually rendering them more water soluble and easier to eliminate.

**Connective Tissue**

The general term referring to one of the primary tissues of the body that makes up the supporting or framework tissue. Derived from the mesenchyme (this in turn from the mesoderm); the varieties of connective tissue are cartilage and bone; areolar or loose; adipose; dense, regular or irregular, white fibrous; elastic; mucous; and lymphoid tissue. The blood and lymph may be regarded as connective tissues with a liquid as the ground substance.

**Conserved Sequence**

An invariant base sequence in a DNA molecule (or the amino acid sequence in a protein) that has remained essentially unchanged throughout evolution.

**Consumer Product Safety Commission (CPSC)**

Created in 1972, it is a federal agency responsible for protecting the public from toxicants and other hazards present in consumer products through voluntary and mandatory standards, research, product bans, and recalls.

**Control Group**

A study group of animals or humans that are treated the same as the exposed groups but without receiving the exposure in question.

**Cornea**

The transparent anterior surface of the eye covering both the pupil and the iris.

**Corpus Callosum**

The great band of commissural fibers uniting the cerebral hemispheres of higher mammals including humans. Also called the commissura magna cerebri.

**Corpus Luteum**

The zona granulosa and theca cells remaining in the ovary after ovulation and some surrounding capillaries and connective tissue evolve into the corpus luteum. Secretes progesterone.

**Corrosion**

Direct chemical action resulting in irreversible damage such as ulceration, necrosis, and scar formation at the site of contact.

**Cortex**

The outer or superficial part of an organ or bodily structure (e.g., kidney, adrenal gland) as distinguished from the deeper layers.

**Covalent Bond**
The joining together of atoms or radicals that results from sharing electrons.

**Critical Effect**
The first adverse effect, or its known precursor, that occurs in the most sensitive relevant species as the dose rate of an agent increases.

**Cross-Sectional Study**
A type of epidemiology study that assesses the prevalence of a disease or clinical parameter among one or more exposed groups (e.g., the prevalence of liver conditions among solvent-exposed workers).

**Crossing Over**
Reciprocal breaking and rejoining of one maternal and one paternal chromosome during meiosis; the exchange of corresponding sections of DNA, and the rejoining of the chromosomes. This process can result in an exchange of alleles between chromosomes.

**Cutaneous**
Referring to the skin (dermal).

**Cytogenetics**
The study of chromosomes, the visible carriers of DNA, the hereditary material. Cytogenetics is a fusion science that combines cytology (the study of cells) and genetics (the study of inherited variation).

**Cytology**
Cytology is the study of the structure and function of cells.

**Cytoplasm**
The cellular contents within the plasma membrane, excluding the nucleus. It consists of a continuous aqueous solution and the organelles and inclusions suspended in it.

**Cytosine ($C_4H_5N_3O$)**
The pyrimidine member of the base pair GC (guanine and cytosine) in DNA.

**Cytotoxic**
Any substance or process that has the capacity to harm or destroy cells.

# D

**Decigram**
Metric unit of mass equal to 1/100th of a gram.

**Deletion**
A loss of a portion of the DNA from a chromosome that may lead to a disease or abnormality.

**Demyelination**
The destruction or loss of the myelin sheath (insulation) around a nerve.

**Dendrite**
Any of the usually branching protoplasmic processes that conduct electrochemical impulses toward the body of a nerve cell.

**Deoxyribonucleotide**
Nucleic acid found in the nucleus of a cell associated with genetic transmission.

**Deoxyribose ($C_5H_{10}O_4$)**
The aldopentose (a type of sugar) that is one component of DNA (deoxyribonucleic acid).

**Dermal Sensitization Test**
An assay for immune hypersensitivity of the skin.

**Dermal Toxicity**
Adverse effects, ranging from mild irritation to corrosivity, hypersensitivity, and skin cancer, resulting from direct contact or internal distribution of a xenobiotic to the skin.

**Detoxification**
The metabolic process in which the parent substance is transformed to a metabolite that has lessened toxicity.

**Developmental Toxicity**
Adverse effects on the developing organism that may result from exposure before conception (either parent), during prenatal development, or postnatally until the time of sexual maturation. The major manifestations of developmental toxicity include death of the developing organism, structural abnormality, altered growth, and functional deficiency.

**Differentiation**
The process by which immature cells transform into specialized adult cells. In cancer, differentiation refers to how mature (developed) the cancer cells are in a tumor. Differentiated tumor cells resemble normal cells and grow at a slower rate than undifferentiated tumor cells, which lack the structure and function of normal cells and grow uncontrollably.

**Diploid**
The complete complement of genetic material consisting of paired chromosomes, one from each parental set. Most animal cells (except the gametes) have a diploid set of chromosomes. The diploid human genome has 46 chromosomes.

**Directed Evolution**
A laboratory process used to force mutations in isolated molecules or microbes to identify subsequent adaptations to novel environments.

**Directed Mutagenesis**
Specific alteration of cloned DNA and its reinsertion into an organism to study any effects of the change.

**Disposition**
The term used to describe the kinetics of a substance in the body. It encompasses absorption, distribution, metabolism, and elimination of a chemical.

**Distal**
Remote, farther from any point of reference, away from the point of origin or attachment as opposed to proximal.

**Distribution**
Movement of a substance from the point of entry to other parts of the body.

**DNA (deoxyribonucleic acid)**
The molecule that encodes genetic information. DNA is a double-stranded molecule held together by weak bonds between base pairs of nucleotides. The four nucleotides in DNA contain the bases adenine (A), guanine (G), cytosine (C), and thymine (T). In nature, base pairs form only between A and T and between G and C; thus the base sequence of each single strand can be deduced from that of its partner.

**DNA Probe**
A segment of labeled (radioactive or fluorescent tag) DNA used to locate a specific piece of DNA through the complementary binding.

**DNA Repair Genes**
Genes that code proteins whose function is DNA sequence correction.

**DNA Replication**
The use of existing DNA as a template for the synthesis of new DNA strands. In

humans and other eukaryotes, replication occurs in the cell nucleus.

### DNA Sequence
The relative order of nucleotide base pairs in a DNA fragment, gene, chromosome, or an entire genome.

### Domain
Refers to the discrete portion of a protein with its own function. Within the single protein, the combination of domains determines its overall function.

### Dominant
An allele that is almost always expressed, even if only one copy is present.

### Dominant Lethal Assay Test
A mutagenicity test that can detect heritable dominant lethal mutations present in the sperm as the result of exposure to a substance.

### Dosage
The cumulative expression of the quantity of a substance received that incorporates the size, frequency, and duration of doses (e.g., 5 mg every 8 hours for 10 days).

### Dose
The amount of a substance available for interactions with metabolic processes or biologically significant receptors after crossing the outer boundary of an organism. The POTENTIAL DOSE (or administered dose) is the amount ingested, inhaled, or applied to the skin. The APPLIED DOSE is the amount presented to an absorption barrier and available for absorption (although not necessarily having yet crossed the outer boundary of the organism). The ABSORBED DOSE is the amount crossing a specific absorption barrier (e.g., the exchange boundaries of the skin, lung, and digestive tract) through uptake processes. INTERNAL DOSE is a more general term denoting the amount absorbed without respect to specific absorption barriers or exchange boundaries. The amount of the chemical available for interaction with any particular organ or cell is termed the DELIVERED or BIOLOGICALLY EFFECTIVE DOSE for that organ or cell.

### Dose–Response Assessment
A determination of the relationship between the magnitude of an administered, applied, or internal dose and a specific biological response. Response can be expressed as measured or observed incidence or change in level of response, percent response in groups of subjects (or populations), or the probability of occurrence or change in level of response within a population.

### Dose–Response Curve
A graphical representation of the quantitative relationship between doses of a substance and specific biological effects.

### Dose–Response Relationship
The relationship between a quantified exposure (dose) and the proportion of subjects demonstrating specific biologically significant changes in incidence and/or in degree of change (response).

### Double Helix
Term used to describe the twisted-spiral staircase-like configuration that two linear strands of DNA assume when complementary nucleotides on opposing strands bond together.

### Draize Test
Product safety test for ocular irritation in which the test substance is placed on the eyes of white rabbits and observed over the course of several days for irritant effects.

**Drug Idiosyncrasy**
Unusual individual susceptibility or sensitivity to a drug.

**Dysplasia**
Premalignant change characterized by alteration in the size, shape, and organization of the cellular components of a tissue.

# E

**Ecology**
A term referring to the general environment.

**Ecotoxicity**
Studies of the toxic effects of chemicals on environmental organisms.

**ED$_{50}$**
Effective dose 50%. The estimated dose that causes some specific effect (usually desirable) for 50% of the population.

**ED$_{99}$**
Effective dose 99%. The estimated dose that causes some specific effect (usually desirable) for 99% of the population.

**Effective Dose (ED$_{10}$) or Effective Concentrations (EC$_{10}$)**
The dose or concentration corresponding to a 10% increase in an adverse effect, relative to the control response.

**Effluent**
The discharge of waste from a plant or other source into the environment.

**Electrolyte**
A substance that when dissolved in a suitable solvent or when fused becomes an ionic conductor.

**Electrophoresis**
The method of separating large molecules (such as DNA fragments or proteins) from a mixture of similar molecules using an electric current passed through a medium containing the mixture. The rate of movement of each type of molecule is dependent on its electrical charge and size. Agarose and acrylamide gels are the media commonly used for electrophoresis of proteins and nucleic acids.

**Embolus**
A mass, predominately blood clots but may also be fat that travels through the bloodstream, eventually obstructing blood flow through a smaller caliber vessel (e.g., stroke, pulmonary embolism, central retinal artery occlusion).

**Embryo**
An early stage of the development of the unborn offspring during which cell differentiation proceeds rapidly along with the formation of the major organs. In humans this stage occurs after fertilization from about 3 weeks until 8–9 weeks after conception.

**Embryonic Stem (ES) Cells**
A cell obtained from an embryo in the blastula phase that can replicate indefinitely, transform into other types of cells, and serve as a continuous source of new cells.

**Embryotoxic**
The harmful effects of a substance on the developing embryo.

**Endocrine**
The system in the body responsible for the manufacture and secretion of hormones. If the endocrine system is affected by certain drugs, resultant changes in hormones can affect growth, sexual development, and other physiological function.

**Endocytosis**
Cellular ingestion by phagocytosis (for solids) or pinocytosis (for liquids).

**Endonuclease**
An enzyme that catalyzes bond hydrolysis between nucleic acids in DNA and RNA.

**Endoplasmic Reticulum (ER)**
An organelle composed of interconnected vesicular and lamellar cytoplasmic membranes that functions primarily in intracellular transport of materials and as a site of lipid and lipoprotein production (smooth ER) or protein synthesis (rough ER). The smooth ER also contains a number of enzymes and other xenobiotic metabolizing components.

**Endothelium**
Mesodermally derived epithelium composed of a single layer of simple squamous cells that lines the heart and blood vessels. Capillaries are composed of endothelial cells.

**End-Point**
An observable or measurable biological event or chemical concentration (e.g., metabolite concentration in a target tissue) used as an index of an effect of a chemical exposure.

**Environmental Fate**
The fate of a biological or chemical pollutant after its release into the environment. It includes the movement and persistence of the substance in the physical and biological components of ecosystems.

**Environmental Protection Agency (EPA)**
Created in 1970, it is a federal agency responsible for regulation of most chemicals that can enter the environment. The EPA administers the following acts: the Federal Insecticide, Fungicide, and Rodenticide Act (FIFRA), the Toxic Substances Control Act (TSCA), the Resource Conservation and Recovery Act (RCRA), the Safe Drinking Water Act (SDWA), the Clean Air Act (CAA), and the Comprehensive Environmental Response, Compensation and Liabilities Act (CERCLA), also known as the Superfund Act.

**Enzyme**
A macromolecule, usually a protein, that speeds the rate of chemical reactions in the body without altering the direction or nature of the reaction. For example, salivary amylase in the mouth starts the process of breaking down carbohydrates in food.

**Enzyme Activation**
Conversion of an enzyme from an inactive to an active form.

**Enzyme Inhibitor**
A substance that inhibits the catalytic action of an enzyme.

**Eosinophilia**
Commonly associated with allergic reactions and is an increase in peripheral blood eosinophilic leukocytes to more than 450 cells/μl of blood.

**Epidemiology**
The study of the distribution and determinants of health-related states or events in specified populations.

**Epidermis**
The outer layer of the skin.

**Epithelium**
The thin layer of cells that covers the internal and external surfaces of the body, including the lining of vessels and other small cavities. It is the first cell encountered from toxicant exposure.

**Erythrocyte**
Red blood cell.

**Erythropoietin**
A glycoprotein hormone produced primarily by cells of the peritubular capillary endothe-

lium of the kidney, it is responsible for the regulation of red blood cell production.

**Escherichia coli**

A common gram-negative, facultative, anaerobe bacterium that has been studied intensively by geneticists because of its small genome size, normal lack of pathogenicity, and ease of growth in the laboratory. Some strains are used in *in vitro* mutagenicity tests.

**Estrogen**

Any of various natural steroids (as estradiol) that are formed from androgen precursors; that are secreted chiefly by the ovaries, placenta, adipose tissue, and testes; and that stimulate the development of female secondary sex characteristics and promote the growth and maintenance of the female reproductive system.

**Eukaryote**

Cell or organism with membrane-bound structurally discrete nucleus and other well-developed subcellular compartments. Eukaryotes include all organisms except viruses, bacteria, and blue-green algae.

**Evolutionarily Conserved**

A sequence in a DNA molecule or protein molecule that has remained mostly unchanged throughout evolution.

**Excretion**

Processes that eliminate substances (or metabolites) from the body.

**Exocytosis**

The release of cellular substances (as secretory products) contained in cell vesicles by fusion of the vesicular membrane with the plasma membrane and subsequent release of the contents to the exterior of the cell. Opposed to endocytosis.

**Exon**

The sequence of the gene that codes for the protein.

**Exonuclease**

An enzyme that clips nucleotides sequentially from free ends of a linear nucleic acid substrate.

**Exposure**

Contact made between a chemical, physical, or biological agent and the outer boundary of an organism. Exposure is quantified as the amount of an agent (i.e., potential or administered dose) available at the exchange boundaries of the organism (e.g., skin, lungs, gut).

**Exposure Assessment**

An estimate or analysis of the intensity, frequency, and duration of human exposures to an agent.

**Expressed Gene**

One whose coded information is converted into the structures present and operating in the cell, including transfer and ribosomal RNAs.

# F

**$F_0$ Generation**

The initial parent generation in a multigeneration reproductive study.

**$F_1$ Generation**

The first filial generation (offspring) in a multigeneration reproductive study. It arises from breeding individuals of the $F_0$ generation.

**$F_2$ Generation**

The second filial generation (offspring) in a multigeneration reproductive study. It arises from breeding individuals of the $F_1$ generation.

**Fascia**

Fascia, a connective tissue, is the packing material of the body. It envelopes the muscles, bones, and joints and holds us together supporting the body structure and giving us our shape. Fascia organizes and separates: it provides protection and autonomy for the individual muscles and viscera. It joins and bonds these separate entities and establishes spatial relationships. Chemically it is the collagen in the fascia that enables it to change.

**Federal Insecticide, Fungicide, and Rodenticide Act (FIFRA)**

An EPA-administered federal law that evaluates and registers pesticides.

**Femtogram (fg)**

An extremely minute mass, $1 \times 10^{-15}$ gram.

**Fertilization**

The process that unites two gametes to restore the somatic chromosome number and initiates the development of a new individual.

**Fetus**

An unborn or unhatched vertebrate, especially after attaining the basic structural plan of its kind and developing the main recognizable features of the adult animal; specifically, a developing human from approximately 3 months after conception to birth.

**Fibroblast**

A mesenchymally derived connective tissue cell that secretes proteins, especially molecular collagen, from which the extracellular fibrillar matrix of connective tissue forms.

**Fibrosis**

Refers to the presence of scar tissue or collagen fibers in any tissue resulting from processes including injury, inflammation, and infection. In the liver, fibrosis or scarring damages the architecture and thus the functionality of the organ. Fibrosis, combined with the liver's ability to regenerate, causes cirrhosis (regeneration within the scar tissue).

**Filial Generation (F$_1$, F$_2$)**

Each successive generation of offspring in a breeding program, designated F$_1$, F$_2$, etc.

**Flagellum**

A long tapering process that projects singly or in groups from a cell and is the primary organ of motility of many microorganisms. Similar in structure to cilia.

**Flow Cytometry**

Analysis of biological material by detection of the light-absorbing or fluorescing properties of cells or subcellular fractions such as chromosomes passing in a narrow stream through a laser beam. Samples are fractionated and analyzed using automated sorting devices to sort successive droplets of the stream into different fractions depending on the fluorescence emitted by each droplet.

**Food and Drug Administration (FDA)**

The federal agency that evaluates the safety of drugs, cosmetics, food additives, and medical devices.

**Forensics**

Identification using DNA. Examples include establishing paternity in child support cases, establishing the presence of a suspect at a crime scene, and identification of accident victims.

**Free Radicals**

An atom or a group of atoms with an unpaired electron. Byproducts of normal cellular chemical reactions, radicals are unusually reactive, strongly oxidizing species capable of causing a wide range of biological damage.

**Functional Genomics**

The study of genes, the proteins they code, and the actions of the proteins on the body's biochemical processes.

# G

**Gamete**

Mature male or female reproductive cell (sperm or ovum) with a haploid set of chromosomes (23 for humans). Also referred to as a germ cell.

**Gamma Ray**

A highly energized deeply penetrating photon that radiates spontaneously from the nucleus during fission and frequently accompanies radioactive decay. A form of electromagnetic radiation similar to light.

**Ganglion (pl. ganglia)**

A mass of nerve tissue, composed primarily of nerve-cell bodies, external to the brain or spinal cord.

**Gel Electrophoresis**

Type of electrophoresis that exploits the movement of charged molecules through an agarose or polyacrylamide gel.

**Gene**

The functional and physical unit of heredity composed of a sequence of DNA and occupies a specific position or locus.

**Gene Amplification**

Selective synthesis of DNA segment resulting in multiple copies; a characteristic of tumor cells.

**Gene Chip Technology**

Development of cDNA microarrays from a large number of genes. Designed to simultaneously assess the activity of all the genes on the chip.

**Gene Expression**

The process that takes a gene's coded information and converts it into the structures present and operating in the cell. Expressed genes include those that are transcribed into mRNA and then translated into protein and those that are transcribed into RNA but not translated into protein (e.g., transfer and ribosomal RNAs).

**Gene Family**

Group of closely related genes that make analogous products.

**Gene Library**

A collection of cloned DNA fragments from a variety of species.

**Gene Mapping**

Determination of the relative locations of genes on a DNA molecule (chromosome or plasmid) and of the distance, in linkage units or physical units, between them.

**Gene Mutation**

A change in the DNA sequence within a gene or chromosome; any alteration in the inherited nucleic acid sequence of the genotype of an organism.

**Gene Pool**

The total number of genes in a species.

**Gene Product**

The RNA or protein resulting from expression of a gene. The amount of gene product is used to measure how active a gene is; abnormal amounts can be correlated with disease-causing alleles.

**Gene Testing**

The examination of a sample of blood or other body fluid or tissue for biochemical, chromosomal, or genetic markers that indicate the presence or absence of genetic disease.

**Gene Therapy**

An experimental procedure that attempts to replace, manipulate, or supplement nonfunctional or malfunctioning genes with healthy genes.

**Genetic Code**

The sequence of nucleotides that determines the sequence of amino acids in protein synthesis. Coded in triplets (codons) along the mRNA, the sequence can be used to predict the mRNA sequence, and the genetic code can in turn be used to predict the amino acid sequence.

**Genetic Counseling**

An attempt to provide patients and their families with education and information about genetic-related conditions and help them make informed decisions.

**Genetic Engineering**

Altering the genetic material of cells or organisms in an effort to make new substances or perform new functions.

**Genetic Illness**

Sickness, physical disability, or other disorder that results from the inheritance of one or more deleterious alleles.

**Genetic Informatics**

Managing and analyzing biological data such as genomic research data through the use of advanced computer modeling.

**Genetic Map**

Map of relative positions of genetic loci on a chromosome.

**Genetic Marker**

A gene or other identifiable portion of DNA whose inheritance can be followed; a genetic landmark.

**Genetic Material**

Sum of the genetic information of an organism including DNA and RNA.

**Genetic Mosaic**

An organism containing different genetic sequence in different cells. Can result from mutation during development or fusion of embryos at an early developmental stage.

**Genetic Polymorphism**

Variations in DNA sequence among individuals, groups, or populations (e.g., genes for blue eyes vs. brown eyes).

**Genetic Predisposition**

A susceptibility to a genetic disease that might result in actual development of the disease.

**Genetic Screening**

Testing a group of people to identify those individuals with an elevated risk of having or passing on a specific genetic disorder.

**Genetic Testing**

Making a determination about an individual's predisposition to a particular health condition or to confirming a diagnosis based on an analysis of their genetic material.

**Genetic Toxicity**

Toxic effects stemming from damaged DNA and altered genetic expression.

**Genetics**

The study of inheritance patterns of specific traits in organisms.

**Gene Transfer**

Incorporation of novel DNA into the cells of an organism, generally accomplished using a vector such as a modified virus. Used in gene therapy.

**Genome**
Full complement of genetic material in the chromosomes of a particular organism; its size is generally reported as the total number of base pairs.

**Genome Project**
A research and technology-development driven attempt to map and sequence the genome of human beings and certain model organisms.

**Genomic Library**
A collection of clones constructed from a set of randomly generated overlapping DNA fragments representing the entire genome of an organism.

**Genomics**
The study of the structure and function of genes.

**Genotype**
The genetic constitution of an organism, not always manifested in its physical appearance (its phenotype).

**Germ Cell**
Gametes and progenitor cells that are haploid and have only one set of chromosomes (23 in all), whereas all other cells have two copies (46 in all).

**Germ Line**
Continuity of genetic information from one generation to the next.

**Globally Harmonized System of Classification and Labeling of Chemicals (GHS)**
GHS is a system that addresses classification of chemicals by types of hazard and proposes harmonized hazard communication elements, including labels and safety data sheets. It aims at ensuring that information on physical hazards and toxicity from chemicals is available to enhance the protection of human health and the environment during the handling, transport, and use of these chemicals. The GHS also provides a basis for harmonization of rules and regulations on chemicals at national, regional, and worldwide levels, an important factor also for trade facilitation.

**Glomerulus**
The highly vascularized structure in the kidney where much of the fluid portion of the blood (serum) is filtered and passes into the kidney tubules, thus eliminating toxins and many other materials present in the serum.

**Glucagon**
A protein hormone produced especially by the islets of Langerhans in the pancreas that promotes an increase in the sugar content of the blood by increasing the rate of glycogen breakdown in the liver.

**Glucose ($C_6H_{12}O_6$)**
An optically active sugar with an aldehydic carbonyl group; the sweet colorless soluble dextrorotatory form that occurs widely in nature and is the usual form in which carbohydrate is assimilated by animals. It is the only sugar normally found circulating in the blood.

**Glycoprotein**
A protein covalently linked to a carbohydrate. Glycoproteins play essential roles in the body. For instance, almost all the key molecules in the immune system involved in the immune response are glycoproteins.

**Goblet Cell**
An epithelial cell such as of intestinal columnar epithelium that secretes mucus and is distended at the free end.

**Goiter**

An enlargement of the thyroid gland and the most visible sign of iodine deficiency. The resulting bulge on the neck may become extremely large, but most simple goiters are brought under control before this happens. Occasionally, a simple goiter may cause some difficulty in breathing and swallowing.

**Golgi Apparatus**

A cytoplasmic organelle that consists of a stack of smooth membranous saccules and associated vesicles and that is active in the modification, storage, and transport of proteins.

**Gonadotropin**

A gonadotropic hormone. Examples include follicle-stimulating hormone (FSH) and human chorionic gonadotropin (hCG).

**Growth Factor**

A substance produced by normal cells during embryonic development, tissue growth, and wound healing that promotes the growth of cells. Growth factors include epidermal growth factor (EGF), fibroblast growth factor (FGF), erythropoietin (EPO), hematopoietic cell growth factor (HCGF), platelet-derived growth factor (PDGF), stem cell factors, and neurotrophins. Tumors produce large amounts of growth factors.

**Guanine (G)**

The purine nitrogenous base that makes up one member of the base pair GC (guanine and cytosine) in DNA.

# H

**Haploid**

The single set of chromosomes (half the full set of genetic material) found in the egg and sperm cells of animals and in the egg and pollen cells of plants. Human beings have 23 chromosomes in their reproductive cells.

**Hazard**

A potential source of harm.

**Hazard Assessment**

The process of determining whether exposure to an agent can cause an increase in the incidence of a particular adverse health effect (e.g., cancer, birth defect) and whether the adverse health effect is likely to occur in humans.

**Hazard Characterization**

A description of the potential adverse health effects attributable to a specific environmental agent, the mechanisms by which agents exert their toxic effects, and the associated dose, route, duration, and timing of exposure.

**Hazard Communication Standard**

An OSHA standard established in 1983 that required all employers to inform employees of the hazard of chemicals in the workplace and the steps necessary to avoid harm.

**Hazard Identification**

Risk assessment of the innate adverse toxic effects of an agent.

**Hazard Quotient**

The ratio of the potential chemical exposure level and the level at which no adverse effects are expected. This represents an estimate of hazard for a single chemical.

**HEENT**

The standard abbreviation for **H**ead, **E**yes, **E**ars, **N**ose, and **T**hroat.

**Hematocrit**

Hematocrit is the percentage of the volume of a blood sample occupied by erythrocytes, as determined by a centrifuge or device that separates the cells and other particulate elements of the blood from the plasma. The remaining fraction of the blood sample is called plasmocrit (blood plasma volume).

### Hematological
Referring to blood or to hematology.

### Hematopoiesis
The generation of blood or blood cells in the living body.

### Heparin
An anticoagulant (a substance that inhibits clot formation) drug injected directly into a vein to thin the blood when there is a danger of clotting.

### Hepatic Cancer
Cancer of the liver. Most forms originate in other locations and travel to the liver.

### Hepatic Necrosis
The death of liver cells (hepatocytes).

### Hepatitis
Inflammation of the liver caused by disease, viruses, or toxins. Several forms have been characterized.

### Hepatotoxicant
A systemic toxicant targeting the liver.

### Hepatotoxicity
Poisonous to the liver and associated bile duct and gall bladder.

### Heritable Translocation Assay
An *in vivo* mammalian mutation test. A test for mutagenicity in which exposed male fruit flies (*Drosophila*) or mice are bred to nonexposed females. The offspring males ($F_1$ generation) are then bred to detect the presence of chromosomal translocations indicating this specific type of mutation.

### Heterozygote
Individual with different alleles on homologous chromosomes.

### Highly Conserved Sequence
A length of DNA that is very similar across several different types of organisms.

### Histamine
Histamine is a biologically active chemical present in cells throughout the body that is released during an allergic reaction. Histamine is one of the substances responsible for the symptoms on inflammation and is the major reason for running of the nose, sneezing, and itching in allergic rhinitis. It also stimulates production of acid by the stomach and narrows the bronchi or airways in the lungs.

### Homologous Chromosome
One of a pair of chromosomes containing the same linear gene sequences as another, each derived from one parent.

### Homozygous
The state of having two identical alleles of a gene.

### Human Dose Equivalent
An estimation of the dose in humans needed to produces a specific effect based on the dose that produces the effect in animals. A conversion formula comparing animal to human body weight or animal to human body surface is used.

### Human Equivalent Concentration (HEC) or Dose (HED)
The human concentration (for inhalation exposure) or dose (for other routes of exposure) of an agent that is believed to induce the same magnitude of toxic effect as the experimental animal species concentration or

dose. This adjustment may incorporate toxi-cokinetic information on the particular agent, if available, or use a default procedure, such as assuming that daily oral doses experienced for a lifetime are proportional to body weight raised to the 0.75 power.

### Human Gene Therapy
An attempt to correct genetic errors by inserting normal DNA into cells.

### Human Genome Initiative
Collective name for several projects begun in 1986 by DOE attempting to create an ordered set of DNA segments from known chromosomal locations, develop new computational methods for analyzing genetic map and DNA sequence data, and develop new techniques and instruments for detecting and analyzing DNA. The DOE initiative is now referred to as the Human Genome Program. The joint national effort, led by DOE and NIH, is known as the Human Genome Project.

### Human Genome Project (HGP)
Previously titled Human Genome Initiative.

### Hybrid
The offspring of genetically dissimilar parents.

### Hypersensitivity
Describes an exaggerated response to a foreign agent due to state of altered immune reactivity in the body.

### Hypoxia
A reduction in the oxygen concentration supplied to cells or tissues.

### I

### Idiosyncrasy
An abnormal sensitivity of an individual to some drug or other substance.

### Immediately Dangerous to Life and Health (IDLH)
IDLH is a limit for personal exposure to a substance defined by the U.S. National Institute for Occupational Safety and Health (NIOSH), normally expressed in parts per million (ppm). This concentration is considered to be the limit beyond which an individual is not capable of escaping death or permanent injury without help in less than 30 minutes.

### Immune System
The complex system of cellular and molecular components with the primary function of distinguishing self from not self and defense against foreign organisms or substances. The primary cellular components are lymphocytes and macrophages and the primary molecular components are antibodies and lymphokines. Though involved in immune response, granulocytes and the complement are not always considered as part of the immune system per se.

### Immunoglobulin
An antibody or, more generally, antibodies that provide protection against infectious agents. Immunoglobulins are produced by lymphocytes of the B lymphocytes and plasma cells in response to the stimulation of infectious agents or the contents of vaccines (antigens). Immunoglobulins are soluble proteins present in blood serum and other body fluids. Temporary protection via immunoglobulins can be transferred to another person through injection of a purified portion of a donor's serum.

### Immunosuppression
A state in which the body's ability to respond to antigenic stimulation is diminished through infection, congenital defect, or drug

therapy. The artificial suppression of the immune response, usually through drugs, so that the body will not reject a transplanted organ or tissue. Drugs commonly used to suppress the immune system after transplant include prednisone, azathioprine (Imuran), cyclosporin, OKT3, and ALG.

### Immunotherapy

Exploiting the immune system to treat disease, for example, in the development of vaccines. May also refer to the therapy of diseases caused by the immune system.

### Immunotoxicity

Adverse effects on the functioning of the immune system. Can take several forms: hypersensitivity (allergy and autoimmunity), immunodeficiency, and uncontrolled proliferation (leukemia and lymphoma).

### Incidence

The number of new cases of a disease that develop within a specified population over a specified period of time.

### Informatics

The collection and organization of information using computers and statistical methods.

### Interactions

Measure of simultaneous exposure to two or more substances. The four types include additivity, antagonistism, potentiation, or synergism.

### Interphase

The interval in the cell cycle when DNA is replicated in the nucleus; followed by mitosis.

### Intron

A region of DNA that interrupts the protein-coding sequence of a gene; an intron is transcribed into RNA but is cut out of the message before it is translated into protein.

### Investigational New Drug Application (IND)

Dual purpose application submitted to the FDA by a pharmaceutical company to both provide preliminary evidence of safety in humans or animals and to allow for the interstate transport of the aforementioned unapproved drug for testing purposes.

### In Vitro

Studies performed in an environment outside a living organism, such as in a laboratory.

### In Vivo

Studies carried out within living organisms.

### Ionizing Radiation

Corpuscular (e.g., neutrons, electrons) or electromagnetic (e.g., gamma) radiation of sufficient energy to strip electrons from the irradiated material.

### Irritation

Local tissue reaction independent of an immunologic mechanism. It is a reversible inflammation.

### Islets of Langerhans

Also called *Islands of Langerhans*, irregularly shaped patches of endocrine tissue that secrete insulin and other hormones located within the pancreas of most vertebrates. The normal human pancreas contains about 1,000,000 islets. They are named for the German physician Paul Langerhans, who first described them in 1869.

### Isoenzyme

A chemically distinct enzyme performing the same biochemical function as another enzyme. The two enzymes may function at different speeds.

### Isomer
Chemicals with the same components in the same proportions with different structural arrangement and properties.

### Isotope
One of the several forms of an element possessing the same number of protons but differing numbers of neutrons in the nucleus. An isotope can be stable or radioactive, depending on the composition of its nucleus.

# K

### Karyotype
A photomicrograph of an individual's chromosomes arranged in a standard format to show the number, size, and shape of each chromosome type. It is used in low-resolution physical mapping in an attempt to correlate gross chromosomal abnormalities with the characteristics of specific diseases.

### Kilogram
A unit of weight equal to 1,000 grams ($10^3$ g).

### Knockout
Targeted deactivation of specific genes; used in laboratory organisms to study gene function.

# L

### Lamina Propria
A highly vascular layer of loose connective tissue under the basement membrane lining a layer of epithelium.

### Latency Period
The period of time between a stimulus and response as in an exposure and onset of toxicity.

### $LC_0$
Lethal Concentration 0%. The calculated concentration of an air contaminant at which none of the population is expected to die.

### $LC_{10}$
Lethal Concentration 10%. The calculated concentration of an air contaminant at which 10% of the population is expected to die.

### $LC_{50}$
Lethal Concentration 50%. The calculated concentration of an air contaminant at which 50% of the population is expected to die.

### $LC_{90}$
Lethal Concentration 90%. The calculated concentration of an air contaminant at which 90% of the population is expected to die.

### $LD_0$
Lethal Dose 0%. The estimated dose of a toxicant at which none of the population is expected to die.

### $LD_{10}$
Lethal Dose 10%. The estimated dose of a toxicant at which 10% of the population is expected to die.

### $LD_{50}$
Lethal Dose 50%. The estimated dose of a toxicant at which 50% of the population is expected to die.

### $LD_{90}$
Lethal Dose 90%. The estimated dose of a toxicant at which 90% of the population is expected to die.

### Leiomyosarcoma
A rare malignant tumor consisting of smooth muscle cells and small cell sarcoma tumor most commonly found in the uterus, abdomen, or pelvis.

### Lesion
A nonspecific term referring to an abnormal change in structure of an organ or part due

to injury or disease, especially one that is circumscribed and well defined.

### Leukemia

General term used to describe malignancies of either lymphoid or hematopoietic origin. Malignant proliferation of hematopoietic cells, characterized by replacement of bone marrow by neoplastic cells. The leukemic cells usually are present in peripheral blood and may infiltrate other organs of the reticuloendothelial system, such as liver, spleen, and lymph nodes. Leukemia is broadly classified into acute and chronic leukemia, with multiple distinct clinicopathologic entities subclassified in each.

### Linear Dose Response

A pattern of frequency or severity of biological response that varies directly with the amount of dose of an agent. This linear relationship holds only at low doses in the range of extrapolation.

### Linearized Multistage Model

A cancer assessment model used by the EPA to conservatively quantify progression. It assumes linear extrapolation with a zero dose threshold from the upper confidence level of the lowest dose that produced cancer in an animal test or in a human epidemiology study.

### Linearized Multistage Procedure

A modification of the multistage model used for estimating carcinogenic risk that incorporates a linear upper bound on extra risk for exposures below the experimental range.

### Lipid Soluble

Describes something that is capable of being dissolved in fat or in solvents that dissolve fat. Usually refers to non-ionized compounds.

### Liposarcoma

The soft tissue sarcomas are a group of cancers that develop from a number of different supportive tissues in the body, including fibrous tissue, muscle, ligaments, tendons, and fat. The most common form of soft tissue carcinoma.

### Lowest Observed Adverse Effect Level (LOAEL)

The lowest exposure level at which there are biologically significant increases in frequency or severity of adverse effects between the exposed population and its appropriate control group.

### Lumen

Refers to a cavity or channel within a tube or tubular organ.

### Lye

Generally synonymous with sodium hydroxide. May also refer to the potash lye, a strong caustic alkaline solution of potassium salts, obtained by leaching wood ashes. It is used in making soap.

### Lymphocyte

Any of the colorless weakly motile cells originating from stem cells and differentiating in lymphoid tissue into T lymphocytes and B lymphocytes (as of the thymus or bone marrow) that are the typical cellular elements of lymph, include the cellular mediators of immunity, and constitute 20–30% of the white blood cells of normal human blood.

### Lymphoid

Cells derived from stem cells of the lymphoid lineage—large and small lymphocytes, plasma cells. Referring to lymphocytes and the tissues from which they arise.

### Lysosome

A sac-like cellular organelle that contains various hydrolytic enzymes. Sometimes called the digestive system of the cell.

# M

**Macrophage**
A phagocytic tissue cell of the reticuloendothelial system that may be fixed or freely motile, is derived from a monocyte, and functions in the protection of the body against infection and noxious substances—called also histiocyte—by ingesting anything considered non-self.

**Magnetic Resonance Imaging (MRI)**
A diagnostic tool that uses magnetic fields of hydrogen atoms to generate three-dimensional pictures of internal organs.

**Malignant Cell**
A cancer cell with the potential to invade surrounding tissues and spread to other areas of the body (metastasis).

**Malignant Tumor**
A growth that can invade surrounding tissues or metastasize to distant sites with life-threatening consequences.

**Margin of Safety (MOS)**
The maximum exposure amount that produces no measurable effect in animals divided by the actual amount of human exposure. The ratio of the dose that is just within the lethal range ($LD_{01}$) to the dose that is 99% effective ($ED_{99}$), $LD_{01}/ED_{99}$. A ratio of greater than 1 gives comfort to the physician, whereas a ratio of less than 1 denotes caution.

**Mass Spectrometry**
A technique used to identify chemicals in a substance by their mass and charge.

**Mast Cell**
Cells that play an important role in the body's allergic response. Mast cells are present in most body tissues but are particularly numerous in connective tissue, such as the dermis (innermost layer) of skin. In an allergic response, an allergen stimulates the release of antibodies, which attach themselves to mast cells. After subsequent allergen exposure, the mast cells release substances such as histamine (a chemical responsible for allergic symptoms) into the tissue. Can also release heparin when they degranulate.

**Maximum Tolerated Dose (MTD)**
Refers to the highest dose used in an animal cancer test that can be tolerated without serious weight loss or other toxic effects.

**Mechanism of Action**
The specific manner by which a substance evokes its characteristic effect.

**Median Toxic Dose**
The level at which 50% of the population will experience toxic effects upon exposure.

**Megakaryocyte**
Very large bone marrow cells that release mature blood platelets by shedding cytoplasm.

**Meiosis**
The process of two consecutive cell divisions in the diploid progenitors of sex cells, resulting in four rather than two daughter cells (as in mitosis), each with a haploid set of chromosomes.

**Melanoma**
The most serious life-threatening form of skin cancer arising in the melanocytes.

**Melatonin**
A hormone produced by the pineal gland that boosts the immune system and helps people with jet lag or insomnia. It is linked to the control of circadian rhythms.

## Meningioma
Common benign brain tumors that arise from the pia-arachnoid cells of the meninges. Meningiomas tend to occur along the superior sagittal sinus, along the sphenoid ridge, or in the vicinity of the optic chiasm. These slow-growing tumors are easily treated with surgery or hydroxyurea.

## Mesentery
The membranes, or one of the membranes (consisting of a fold of the peritoneum and enclosed tissues), that connect the intestines and their appendages with the dorsal wall of the abdominal cavity. It contains the arteries, veins, nerves, and lymphatic ducts supplying the intestines. The mesentery proper is connected with the jejunum and ilium, the other mesenteries being called mesocecum, mesocolon, mesorectum, and so on.

## Mesothelioma
Mesothelioma is a rare form of cancer that invades mesothelial cells, specialized cells that make up the membranes lining the chest and abdominal cavity. Mesothelium, or the tissue formed by mesothelial cells, helps protect the organs by producing a lubricating fluid that allows the organs to move without irritating nerves. It is usually associated with asbestos exposure.

## Messenger RNA (mRNA)
The form of RNA responsible for carrying the genetic information from the nucleus to the ribosomes, where it acts as the template for protein synthesis.

## Metabolism
Metabolism is the uptake and digestion of food and the disposal of waste products. The sum of anabolic and catabolic processes in the body.

## Metabolite
The breakdown product resulting when a substance is metabolized by a biological organism.

## Metaphase
The stage in mitosis or meiosis when the chromosomes are aligned along the equatorial plane of the cell.

## Metastasis
Describes the movement of diseased cells, particularly cancer cells, from the site of origin to another location in the body.

## mg/kg
A commonly used term that stands for milligram of a substance per kilogram of body weight.

## mg/kg/day
A commonly used term that denotes milligram of a substance per kilogram of body weight on a daily basis.

## mg/m$^3$
A term for units of exposure used to express concentrations of particulates in the air, standing for milligrams of compound per cubic meter of air.

## Microarray
Semiconductor device with miniaturized chemical reaction areas that may also be used to test DNA fragments, antibodies, or proteins.

## Microgram (µg)
A commonly used unit of weight equal to one millionth ($1 \times 10^{-6}$) of a gram.

## Micronuclei
Chromosome fragments that remain unincorporated into the nucleus at cell division.

## Micronucleus Test
Examination of bone marrow or peripheral blood cells conducted in the presence of

micronuclei (broken pieces of chromosomes surrounded by a nuclear membrane) to test for mutagenicity.

## Milligram

The most commonly used unit of mass in medicine and toxicity equal to one thousandth of a gram ($1 \times 10^{-3}$ g).

## Minimal Risk Level (MRL)

An estimate of the daily human exposure to a hazardous substance that is likely to be without appreciable risk of adverse noncancer health effects over a specified duration of exposure.

## Mitochondrial DNA

The genetic material found in mitochondria that are the organelles that generate cellular energy. Not inherited in the same fashion as nucleic DNA.

## Mitochondrion

Any of various round or long cellular organelles of most eukaryotes that are found outside the nucleus, produce energy (in the form of ATP) for the cell through cellular respiration, and are rich in fats, proteins, and enzymes.

## Mitosis

Mitosis is a complex process that allows the cell to give identical copies of its DNA to each of the daughter cells produced by cellular cleavage.

## Model

A mathematical function with parameters that can be adjusted so the function closely describes a set of empirical data. A mechanistic model usually reflects observed or hypothesized biological or physical mechanisms and has model parameters with real world interpretation. In contrast, statistical or empirical models selected for particular numerical properties are fitted to data; model parame-

ters may or may not have real world interpretation. When data quality is otherwise equivalent, extrapolation using mechanistic models (e.g., biologically based dose–response models) often carries higher confidence than extrapolation using empirical models (e.g., logistic model).

## Model Organisms

An extensively studied laboratory animal or other organism useful for research.

## Modeling

The use of mathematical tools including statistical analysis, computer analysis, or model organisms to predict outcomes of research.

## Modifying Factor (MF)

A factor used in the derivation of a reference dose or reference concentration. The magnitude of the MF reflects the scientific uncertainties of the study and database not explicitly treated with standard uncertainty factors (e.g., the completeness of the overall database). An MF is greater than zero and less than or equal to 10, and the default value for the MF is 1.

## Molecular Biology

The study of the molecular basis of life including the structure, function, and makeup of biologically important molecules.

## Molecule

A unit of matter, the molecule is the smallest particle of a substance that retains all the physical and chemical properties of that substance, consisting of a single atom or a group of atoms bonded together.

## Morbidity

A diseased condition or state, the incidence of a disease, or of all diseases within a circumscribed population.

**Mucosa (pl. mucosae)**
A moist semipermeable layer of tissue that lines hollow organs (stomach, etc.) and body cavities and makes mucus.

**Multihit Model**
The least conservative quantitative risk assessment model. It operates on the assumption that several interactions are needed before a cell can be killed, damaged, or transformed into a cancerous cell.

**Murine**
Relating to organisms in the genus *Mus*. A rat or mouse.

**Muscularis Propria**
The major muscular layer of a hollow organ typically made up of two layers of smooth muscle, an inner circular layer and an outer longitudinal layer.

**Mutagen**
A substance that causes a permanent genetic change in a cell. Does not include changes occurring during normal genetic recombination. A substance that results in mutations (genetic damage).

**Mutagenicity**
The ability of a chemical or physical agent to generate permanent genetic alterations.

**Mutation**
DNA damage resulting in permanent genetic alterations with changes ranging from one or a few DNA base pairs (gene mutations) to gross changes in chromosomal structures (chromosome aberrations) or in chromosome number. Any heritable change in DNA sequence.

**Myelin**
The soft white somewhat fatty material that forms an insulating sheath about the protoplasmic core of a myelinated nerve fiber.

Facilitates rapid conduction of electrical impulses and insulates axons.

**Myeloid**
A collective term for the nonlymphocyte groups of white blood cells. It includes cells from the granulocyte, monocyte, and platelet lineages. Referring to or resembling bone marrow.

**Myometrium**
The muscular outer wall of the uterus.

# N

**Nanogram (ng)**
A unit of weight equal to one billionth of a gram ($1 \times 10^{-9}$ g).

**National Institute of Occupational Safety and Health (NIOSH)**
A federal agency in the Public Health Service that conducts research on health hazards in the workplace.

**Natural Killer (NK) Cells**
Natural killer cells are large lymphocytes that are part of nonspecific immune defense. They are the first line of defense against viruses and other invaders because they do not need to wait for an antibody response to identify foreign cells and invaders. They attack infected cells and cells that appear as though they might cause cancer rather than directly attack the microorganism.

**Necrosis**
The sum of the morphological changes indicative of unprogrammed cell death and caused by the progressive degradative action of enzymes; it may affect groups of cells or part of a structure or an organ. Usually produces an inflammatory response.

**Neonates**
Newborn animals; newborn humans younger than 4 weeks.

**Neoplasia**
Refers to new and abnormal growth of tissue (neoplasm), benign or cancerous, serving no purpose.

**Neoplasm**
Refers to any new and abnormal growth; specifically a new tissue growth that is disorganized, uncontrolled, and progressive. Malignant neoplasms differ from benign in that the former show a greater degree of anaplasia and have the properties of invasion and metastasis. Also called tumor.

**Neoplastic**
Related to or like a neoplasm or neoplasia (tumor).

**Nephron**
The nephron is the microscopic functional unit of the kidney, responsible for the actual purification and filtration of the blood. The cortex of each kidney contains approximately 1 million nephrons; each nephron consists of a renal corpuscle and a renal tubule.

**Nephrotoxicant**
A systemic toxicant whose target organ is the kidney.

**Neurilemma**
Sometimes called the sheath of Schwann, this is the plasma membrane surrounding a Schwann cell of a myelinated nerve fiber and separating layers of myelin.

**Neuroblastoma**
A highly malignant fast-growing childhood tumor that arises in the adrenal gland or in tissue in the nervous system that is related to the adrenal gland.

**Neuroendocrine**
Interactions between the nervous and endocrine systems. Term for cells that release a hormone into the circulating blood in response to a neural stimulus. Such cells may comprise a peripheral endocrine gland (e.g., the insulin-secreting beta cells of the islets of Langerhans in the pancreas and the adrenaline-secreting chromaffin cells of the adrenal medulla); others are neurons in the brain (e.g., the neurons of the supraoptic nucleus that release antidiuretic hormone from their axon terminals in the posterior lobe of the hypophysis).

**Neuroglia**
Supporting tissue intermingled with the essential elements of nervous tissue especially in the brain, spinal cord, and ganglia. Refers to the microglial and macroglial cells.

**Neuromuscular**
Relating to both the nervous and muscular systems.

**Neuron**
A grayish or reddish granular cell with specialized processes, capable of receiving and transmitting electrical signals, that is the fundamental functional unit of the nervous tissue.

**Neurotoxicant**
A chemical, not of biological origin, whose target organ is the nervous system. The term *neurotoxin* is used to describe neurotoxicants of biological origin.

**Neurotoxicity**
Exerting a toxic effect on cells of the central nervous system (brain and spinal cord) and the peripheral nervous system (nerves outside the central nervous system).

**Neutron**
A neutron is a subatomic particle, approximately the same size as a proton, found in

the nucleus of every atom except that of simple hydrogen. The particle derives its name from the fact that it has no electrical charge; it is neutral.

## New Drug Application (NDA)

The process by which a manufacturer of a new drug applies to the Food and Drug Administration for formal approval to market the drug upon the completion of clinical trials.

## Nitrogenous Base

A nitrogen-containing purine or pyrimidine molecule having the chemical properties of a base. DNA contains the nitrogenous bases adenine (A), guanine (G), cytosine (C), and thymine (T).

## No Effect Level (NEL)

The quantity of a substance that is below the threshold on the dose–response curve.

## Nonclinical Laboratory Study

An investigational study of a pharmaceutical performed with laboratory animals designed to provide the basis for human clinical investigations.

## No Observed Adverse Effect Level (NOAEL)

The highest exposure level at which there are no biologically significant increases in the frequency or severity of adverse effect between the exposed population and its appropriate control; some effects may be produced at this level, but they are not considered adverse or precursors of adverse effects.

## No Observed Effect Level (NOEL)

An exposure level at which there are no statistically or biologically significant increases in the frequency or severity of any effect between the exposed population and its appropriate control.

## Northern Blot

Laboratory procedure that locates mRNA sequences on a gel (cellulose or nylon membrane) that are complementary to a piece of DNA used as a probe.

## Nucleic Acid

A large molecule consisting of nucleotide subunits.

## Nucleotide

A subunit of DNA or RNA composed of a phosphate molecule, a sugar molecule (deoxyribose in DNA and ribose in RNA), and a nitrogenous base (adenine, guanine, thymine, or cytosine in DNA; adenine, guanine, uracil, or cytosine in RNA). Thousands of nucleotides are linked to form a single DNA or RNA molecule.

## Nucleus

The cellular organelle in eukaryotes that contains the majority of the genetic material.

# O

## Occupational Exposure Limits (OELs)

Values set by government agencies or other relevant organizations as limits for concentrations of hazardous compounds in workplace air. An OEL is the maximum average air concentration that most workers can be exposed to for an 8-hour workday, 40-hour workweek for a working lifetime (40 years) without experiencing significant adverse health effects. A very small percentage of individuals experience some discomfort or adverse health effects at or below the exposure limit because of a wide variation in individual sensitivities or pre-existing conditions.

**Occupational Safety and Health Administration (OSHA)**
The division of the Department of Labor responsible for ensuring safe working conditions.

**Octanol-to-Water Partition Coefficient**
The ratio of the amount of a substance that dissolves in octanol versus the amount that dissolves in water. Octanol is used as a surrogate for natural organic matter and the ratio is useful in determining environmental fate. The higher the octanol-to-water partition coefficient, the greater the tendency of substance to be stored in fatty tissues.

**Oligonucleotide**
A short string of nucleotides, usually composed of 25 or fewer, used as a DNA synthesis primer.

**Oncogene**
A gene (one or more forms) associated with the development of cancer. Many oncogenes are involved, directly or indirectly, in controlling the rate of cell growth.

**Oncologist**
A physician who specializes in the diagnosis and treatment of various types of cancer.

**One-Hit Model**
This is the most conservative quantitative cancer assessment model. It assumes that a single catastrophic intracellular event can induce a cell transformation that leads to cancer.

**Operon**
A set of functionally related genes (an operator, a promoter, and one or more structural genes) transcribed under the control of an operator gene.

**Organogenesis**
The period of fetal development when the cells of the embryo differentiate and specific organs develop.

**Osmosis**
Movement of a solvent through a semipermeable membrane (as of a living cell) from a solution of lower solute concentration into a solution of higher solute concentration with a tendency to equalize the concentrations of solute on the two sides of the membrane.

**Osmotic**
Referring to or of the nature of osmosis.

**Oxidation**
A change in a chemical characterized by the addition of oxygen, the loss of hydrogen, or the loss of electrons. Opposes reduction.

# P

**Parenchyma**
The essential elements of an organ or gland, used in anatomical nomenclature as a general term to designate the functional elements of an organ or gland, as distinguished from its framework or stroma.

**Parietal Peritoneum**
The peritoneum is a thin bilayer membrane that lines the abdominal and pelvic cavities and covers most abdominal viscera. The parietal peritoneum is the outer layer that lines the abdominal and pelvic cavities. It is composed of a layer of mesothelium supported by a thin layer of connective tissue.

**Partition Coefficient**
General term for the log ratio of the concentration of the solute in the solvent.

**Passive Transfer**

The movement across a membrane by simple diffusion along a concentration gradient.

**Pathology**

The branch of medicine that studies the functional and structural changes in tissues and organs resulting from disease.

**Penetrance**

The probability of a phenotypic trait being expressed among individuals with a specific genotype. "Complete" penetrance means the gene or genes for a trait are expressed in all the population who have the genes. "Incomplete" penetrance means the genetic trait is expressed in only part of the population. The percent penetrance also may change with the age range of the population.

**Peptide**

Natural or synthetic compound of two or more amino acids joined by a peptide bond.

**Percutaneous**

Passage through the skin. Also transcutaneous.

**Permissible Exposure Level (PEL)**

The standard defined by OSHA as the highest safe level of exposure to a chemical in the workplace. The maximum permitted 8-hour time-weighted average concentration of an airborne contaminant.

**pH**

A measure of acidity and alkalinity of a solution using a scale where 7 is the equivalent of neutral. Numbers lower than 6.5 are indicative of acidic solutions, whereas numbers above 7.5 are indicative of alkaline solutions. On the scale, each unit of change represents a 10-fold change in acidity or alkalinity.

**Pharmacogenomics**

The study of the genetic basis for individual response to drugs.

**Pharmacokinetics**

Quantitation of the time course of the chemical absorption, distribution, metabolism, and elimination of a drug.

**Pharmacology**

The science that deals with the development, mechanisms, and actions of drugs.

**Phenotype**

A set of observable physical characteristics (the observed manifestation of a genotype) expressed physically, biochemically, or physiologically by an individual organism. The traits are not necessarily genetic. A single characteristic can be referred to as a "trait," although a single trait is sometimes also called a phenotype. For example, blond hair could be called a trait or a phenotype, as could obesity. A phenotype can be the result of many factors, including an individual's genotype, environment, and lifestyle, and the interactions among these factors.

**Phototoxic**

Heightened toxicity of a substance in or on the skin due to exposure to light (usually ultraviolet light).

**Physiologically Based Pharmacokinetic (PBPK) Model**

A model that estimates the dose to a target tissue or organ by taking into account the rate of absorption into the body, distribution among target organs and tissues, metabolism, and excretion.

**Picogram (pg)**

A unit of mass equal to one quadrillionth of a gram ($1 \times 10^{-12}$ g).

**Placenta**

The temporary vascular organ in mammals, except monotremes and marsupials, that unites the fetus to the maternal uterus and mediates its metabolic exchanges through a more or less intimate association of uterine mucosal with chorionic and usually allantoic tissues.

**Plasma**

The noncellular liquid component of blood, lymph, or milk as distinguished from suspended material.

**Plasmid**

Self-replicating extrachromosomal circular DNA molecules, distinct from the normal bacterial genome and nonessential for cell survival under nonselective conditions. Some plasmids are capable of integrating into the host genome. A number of artificially constructed plasmids are used as cloning vectors and are the principal tools for inserting new genetic information into microorganisms.

**Platelets**

A particle found in the bloodstream that binds at the site of a wound to begin the blood clotting process. Platelets are formed in bone marrow by the shedding of megakaryocytes.

**Pleura**

The delicate double-layered serous membrane that lines each half of the thorax of mammals and is folded back over the surface of the lung of the same side. The visceral pleura lines the outside of the lungs and the parietal pleura lines the inside of the chest wall.

**Poison**

A toxic substance capable of causing injury, illness, or death when absorbed into the body in a relatively small quantity.

**Polymerase Chain Reaction (PCR)**

A method for rapidly synthesizing DNA sequences by amplifying a DNA base sequence using a heat-stable polymerase and two 20-base primers, one complementary to the (+) strand at one end of the sequence to be amplified and one complementary to the (−) strand at the other end. Because the newly synthesized DNA strands can subsequently serve as additional templates for the same primer sequences, successive rounds of primer annealing, strand elongation, and dissociation produce rapid and highly specific amplification of the desired sequence. The method is used to detect minute concentrations of specific DNA or RNA in a specimen and is useful in measuring things like viral load.

**Polymerase, DNA or RNA**

The enzyme that catalyzes the synthesis of nucleic acids on preexisting nucleic acid templates, assembling RNA from ribonucleotides and DNA from deoxyribonucleotides.

**Polymorphism**

Differences in DNA sequence among individuals that may be tied to differences in health. Genetic variations occurring in more than 1% of a population are considered useful polymorphisms for genetic linkage analysis.

**Polypeptide**

A protein or portion of a protein composed of a chain of amino acids joined by a peptide bond.

**Polyploidy**

Having more than the normal number of chromosomes.

**Population Genetics**

The study of genetic variation and evolution among a group of individuals.

**ppb**

A unit of measure expressed as parts per billion. Equivalent to $1 \times 10^{-9}$.

**ppm**

A unit of measure expressed as parts per million. Equivalent to the number of units of a substance in a million units. ppm is a common concentration unit for dilute samples of dissolved substances or airborne substances.

**Primary Dermal Irritation Test**

A test with laboratory animals (usually rabbits) that determines dermal toxicity of a substance when applied to the skin. Results assessed primarily by the manifestation of erythema, edema, and eschars.

**Primary Site**

The anatomical site where the original tumor is located. Primary cancer is usually named after the organ in which it starts. For example, cancer that begins in the breast is always breast cancer even if it spreads (metastasizes) to other organs such as bones or lungs.

**Probit Model**

A risk assessment model that assumes log normal distribution for tolerances of an exposed population and utilizes binary regression. It is generally considered inappropriate for the assessment of cancer risk.

**Progesterone ($C_{21}H_{30}O_2$)**

A female steroid sex hormone that is secreted by the corpus luteum to prepare the endometrium for implantation and later by the placenta during pregnancy to prevent rejection of the developing embryo or fetus. Has an antiestrogen effect.

**Prognosis**

A prediction of a patient's potential clinical outlook based on the status and probable course of his or her disease.

**Prokaryote**

Cell or organism from the kingdom *Monera* (or Prokaryotae) that lacks a membrane-bound, structurally discrete nucleus and other subcellular compartments. Bacteria are examples of prokaryotes.

**Prolactin**

Produced from the anterior pituitary gland and found in the serum of normal females and males, the principal physiological action of prolactin is to initiate and sustain lactation after parturition.

**Proliferation**

The continuous reproduction or multiplication of similar forms, especially of cells and morbid cysts.

**Protein**

Any of the numerous naturally occurring complex macromolecules comprised of amino acid residues joined by peptide bonds. Contain the elements carbon, hydrogen, nitrogen, oxygen, usually sulfur, and occasionally other elements such as phosphorus or iron. Examples include many essential biological compounds (as enzymes, hormones, or immunoglobulins).

**Proteomics**

The study of the full set of proteins expressed by a genome.

**Proton**

A proton is a subatomic particle found in the nucleus of every atom. It carries a positive electrical charge, equal and opposite to that of the electron, and is approximately the same size as a neutron.

**Pseudogene**

A sequence of nonfunctional DNA that is similar to a gene; it is probably the remnant of a once-functional gene that accumulated mutations.

**Purine**
A nitrogenous, double-ring, organic compound that occurs in nucleic acids. The purines in DNA and RNA are adenine and guanine.

**Pyrimidine**
A nitrogenous, single-ring, organic compound that occurs in nucleic acids. The pyrimidines in DNA are cytosine and thymine; in RNA, cytosine, and uracil.

# Q

**Quantitative Structure–Activity Relationship (QSAR)**
Quantitative structure–activity relationships use a mathematical relationship to link chemical structure and pharmacological activity in a quantitative manner for a series of compounds.

# R

**Radioactive Isotope**
Isotope refers to one of two or more atoms of the same element that have the same number of protons in their nucleus but different numbers of neutrons. A radioactive isotope is a natural or artificially created isotope of a chemical element having an unstable nucleus that decays, emitting alpha, beta, or gamma rays until stability is reached. Isotopes of a given element have identical chemical properties but slightly different physical properties and very different half-lives, if they are radioactive.

**Recessive Gene**
A gene expressed only if there are two identical copies.

**Recombinant DNA Molecules**
A type of DNA molecule comprised of DNA from different origins joined using recombinant DNA technologies.

**Recombinant DNA Technology**
Procedure used to combine DNA segments in an environment outside a cell or organism. Under appropriate conditions, a recombinant DNA molecule can enter a cell and replicate there, either autonomously or after it has become integrated into a cellular chromosome.

**Reduction**
A change in a chemical characterized by the gain of electrons by removing oxygen or adding hydrogen.

**Reference Concentration (RfC)**
An estimate (with uncertainty spanning perhaps an order of magnitude) of a continuous inhalation exposure to the human population (including sensitive subgroups) that is likely to be without an appreciable risk of deleterious effects during a lifetime. It can be derived from a NOAEL, LOAEL, or benchmark concentration, with uncertainty factors generally applied to reflect limitations of the data used. Generally used in EPA's noncancer health assessments.

**Reference Dose (RfD)**
An estimate (with uncertainty spanning perhaps an order of magnitude) of a daily oral exposure to the human population (including sensitive subgroups) that is likely to be without an appreciable risk of deleterious effects during a lifetime. It can be derived from a NOAEL, LOAEL, or benchmark dose, with uncertainty factors generally applied to reflect limitations of the data used. Generally used in EPA's noncancer health assessments.

**Reference Exposure Level (REL)**
The concentration level at or below which no adverse health effects are anticipated for a specified exposure duration.

**Reference Value (ReV)**
An estimation of an exposure for a given duration to the human population (including susceptible subgroups) that is likely to be without an appreciable risk of adverse effects over a lifetime. It is derived from a BMDL, a NOAEL, a LOAEL, or another suitable POD, with uncertainty/variability factors applied to reflect limitations of the data used.

**Relative Potency/Relative Toxicity**
The dose of a reference compound required to cause a particular incidence of a specific toxic response divided by the dose of a test compound needed to cause an equal incidence of that same effect.

**Relative Risk (RR)**
A statistical calculation of the ratio of incidence of disease in an exposed population to that of an unexposed population.

**Reporter Gene**
A gene whose activity is easily determined.

**Reproductive Toxicity**
Toxicity of the male or female reproductive system; toxic effects can include damage to the reproductive organs or offspring.

**Respiratory Toxicity**
Toxicity in the upper (nose, pharynx, larynx, and trachea) or lower (bronchi, bronchioles, and lung alveoli) respiratory system manifested by symptoms that can include acute and chronic pulmonary conditions, including local irritation, bronchitis, pulmonary edema, emphysema, and cancer.

**Restriction Enzyme, Endonuclease**
A protein that recognizes specific short nucleotide sequences and cuts the phosphodiester bonds at those sites. Bacteria contain over 400 such enzymes that recognize and cut more than 100 different DNA sequences.

**Reticuloendothelial System**
A group of cells having the ability to take up and sequester inert particles and vital dyes; includes macrophages or macrophage precursors, specialized endothelial cells lining the sinusoids of the liver, spleen, and bone marrow, and reticular cells of lymphatic tissue (macrophages) and of bone marrow (fibroblasts). All phagocytic cells in the body save granulocytes.

**Retinoblastoma**
A malignant ocular neoplasm of the retina. Usually arising in the first 2 years of life, it is the most common form of intraocular malignancy in children.

**Retrospective Cohort Study**
An epidemiology study that identifies and follows cohorts according to past exposure to track the subsequent development of symptoms.

**Reverse Transcriptase**
Retroviral enzyme used to form a complementary DNA sequence (cDNA) from their RNA. The resultant DNA is subsequently inserted into the chromosome of the host cell.

**Ribose ($C_5H_{10}O_5$)**
The five-carbon sugar that serves as a component of RNA, nucleotides, and nucleic acids.

**Ribosomal RNA (rRNA)**
A type of RNA that is a structural component of the ribosomes of cells.

**Ribosome**

RNA-rich cytoplasmic organelles synthesized in the nucleolus; these sites of protein synthesis can be found free in the cytoplasm or bound to the endoplasmic reticulum.

**Risk**

The probability of adverse effects resulting from exposure to an environmental agent or mixture of agents.

**Risk Assessment**

The evaluation of scientific information on the hazardous properties of environmental agents (hazard characterization), the dose–response relationship (dose–response assessment), and the extent of human exposure to those agents (exposure assessment). The product of the risk assessment is a statement regarding the probability that populations or individuals so exposed will be harmed and to what degree (risk characterization).

**Risk Characterization**

The integration of information on hazard, exposure, and dose–response to provide an estimate of the likelihood that any of the identified adverse effects will occur in exposed people.

**Risk Communication**

In genetics, a process in which a genetic counselor or other medical professional interprets genetic test results for patients and counsels them on the ramifications for them and their offspring.

**Risk Management**

A decision-making process that accounts for risk-related information together with political, social, economic, and engineering implications to develop, analyze, and compare management options and select the appropriate managerial response to a potential chronic health hazard.

**RNA (Ribonucleic Acid)**

A polymeric constituent found in the nucleus and cytoplasm of cells that plays an important role in protein synthesis and other chemical activities of the cell. It is structurally similar to DNA. There are several classes of RNA molecules, including messenger RNA, transfer RNA, ribosomal RNA, and other small RNAs, each serving a different purpose.

**Roentgen**

The international unit of x- or gamma-radiation exposure, abbreviated r or R; named after the German physicist, Wilhelm Roentgen, who discovered the roentgen ray in 1895.

# S

**Safety Factor**

Criteria used in the calculation of acceptable humans or environmental exposures. They are applied to data from laboratory experiments or epidemiology studies. An example would be the reductive factor by which a NOAEL dose is divided to obtain a safe standard. Factors of 10 are normally used to account for such uncertainties in the data on which risk assessments are made. Similar to uncertainty factors.

**Sarcoma**

A malignant neoplasm arising in tissue of mesodermal origin (as connective tissue, bone, cartilage, or striated muscle). One of the four major types of cancer.

**Sensitization**

An immune capability developed following an individual's exposure to a specific antigen that can lead to heightened response. Subsequent exposure results in an immune reaction.

**Sensitizer**

A substance that provokes an allergic immune response.

**Sequencing Technology**

The tools and methods used to determine the order of nucleotides in DNA.

**Serum**

The noncellular clear liquid that separates from the blood when it is allowed to clot. This fluid retains any antibodies that were present in the whole blood.

**Sex Chromosome**

The X or Y chromosome in human cells that determines the gender of an individual. Females have two X chromosomes in diploid cells; males have an X and a Y chromosome. The sex chromosomes comprise the 23rd chromosome pair in a karyotype.

**Sex Linked**

Traits or diseases associated with the X or Y chromosome; most often seen in males.

**Short-Term Exposure Limit (STEL)**

A 15-minute time-weighted average exposure that is not to be exceeded at any time during a workday even if the 8-hour time-weighted average is below the PEL; an occupational exposure value.

**Sinoatrial Node**

The sinoatrial (SA) node is a section of nodal tissue that is located in the upper wall of the right atrium. This impulse-generating tissue is also referred to as the pacemaker of the heart.

**Sister Chromatid Exchange Assay (SCE)**

A mutation test in which bone marrow cells or lymphocytes of exposed individuals are microscopically examined for evidence of complete chromosome breakage and chromatid fragment rejoining errors. Error detection is accomplished by demonstrating that there has been an exchange in the sister chromatids during the rejoining process.

**Solubility**

Refers to the ability of a substance to be dissolved in a particular solvent. It is expressed according to the solvent (e.g., water solubility, solubility in acetone, etc.).

**Somatic Cell**

Every cell in the body except gametes and their precursors.

**Southern Blotting**

Transfer by absorption of electrophoretically separated DNA fragments to membrane filters for the detection of specific base sequences by radio-labeled complementary probes.

**Sphincter**

A ring-like band of muscle fibers that constricts a passage or closes a natural orifice to regulate the passage of substances; also called musculus sphincter.

**Squamous Cell Carcinoma**

A malignant neoplasm of squamous cells. In the white population, squamous cell carcinoma of the skin is associated with prolonged exposure to ultraviolet light, and these neoplasms are slow to metastasis even after becoming invasive. Can occur in all the free surfaces, cutaneous, mucous, and serous, including the glands.

**Staging**

A term used to define the size and physical extent of a cancer; staging is the process of assigning a stage to a particular cancer in a specific patient in light of all the available information. For example, TMN staging is staging of tumors according to three basic components: primary tumor (T), regional nodes (N), and metastasis (M) from 0 (undetectable) to 4.

**Standard Deviation**

The statistical calculation measuring the variability of the responses to an exposure and can be thought of as a measure of uncertainty. One standard deviation encompasses 68% of the responses, whereas two standard deviations encompass 95% of the responses.

**Steatosis**

Lipid accumulation in hepatocytes as a result of a variety of stresses. It is a marker for sublethal cellular injury.

**Stem Cell**

"Master cells" that have the capacity to differentiate into many distinct cell types. Each tissue within the body contains a unique type of stem cells that renew and replace that tissue (e.g., nerve, brain, cartilage, blood) when required by damage or wear. Hematopoietic stem cells (stem cells of the blood) generate all other blood cells in the human body, including erythrocytes, platelets, and leukocytes. Sources of hematopoietic stem cells include umbilical cord blood, bone marrow, peripheral blood, and embryos.

**Stenosis**

A stricture of any opening, as in aortic stenosis (narrowing of the aortic valve in the heart), pulmonary stenosis (narrowing of the pulmonary valve in the heart), pyloric stenosis (narrowing of the outlet of the stomach), spinal stenosis (narrowing of the vertebral canal, often with impingement upon the spinal cord). From the Greek *stenos*, meaning narrow.

**Steroid**

Large family of structurally similar lipids whose basic skeleton consists of four interconnected carbon rings. The class includes hormones, corticosteroids, and anabolics. All hormones affecting the development and growth of sex organs, like testosterone and estrogen, are steroids. Synthetic steroids are useful cancer treatments, but they might have undesirable side effects.

**Stromal Cells**

Nonblood cells derived from blood organs. Connective tissue cells of an organ found in the loose connective tissue. These are most often associated with the uterine mucosa and the ovary as well as the hematopoietic system and elsewhere.

**Structure–Activity Relationship (SAR)**

Structure–activity relationships can be described as the relationship of the molecular structure of a chemical with a physicochemical property, environmental fate attribute, and/or specific effect on human health or an environmental species.

**Subacute Exposure**

Repeated or continuous exposure to a chemical for 1 month or less.

**Subchronic Exposure**

Exposure to a substance spanning approximately 10% of the lifetime of an organism.

**Subchronic Toxicity**

The adverse effects exerted by a toxic agent on an organism with repeated exposure over a period of several weeks or months.

**Sufficient Evidence**

A term used in evaluating study data for the classification of a carcinogen under the 1986 U.S. EPA guidelines for carcinogen risk assessment. This classification indicates that there is a causal relationship between the agent or agents and human cancer.

**Superfund**
Federal authority established by the Comprehensive Environmental Response, Compensation, and Liability Act (CERCLA) in 1980 to respond directly to releases or threatened releases of hazardous substances that may endanger health or welfare.

**Suppressor Gene**
A gene that reverses the effect of another gene.

**Susceptibility**
Increased likelihood of an adverse effect, often discussed in terms of relationship to a factor that can be used to describe a human subpopulation (e.g., life stage, demographic feature, or genetic characteristic).

**Susceptible Subgroups**
May refer to life stages, for example, children or the elderly, or to other segments of the population, for example, asthmatics or the immune compromised, but are likely to be somewhat chemical specific and may not be consistently defined in all cases.

**Synaptic**
Referring to the junction across which a nerve impulse passes from an axon terminal to a neuron, muscle cell, or gland cell.

**Syndrome**
The group of symptoms that collectively characterize a disease or disorder.

**Systemic Effects or Systemic Toxicity**
Toxic effects as a result of absorption and distribution of a toxicant to a site distant from its entry point.

**Systemic Toxicant**
A toxicant that adversely impacts the entire organism or a specific system(s).

# T

**Target Organ**
The biological organ(s) most adversely affected by exposure to a chemical, physical, or biological agent.

**T Cells**
T cells are thymus-derived lymphocytes that either orchestrate the immune response or directly attack the infected/invading cells. They are the major component of cell-mediated immunity. There are several types of T cells: Cytotoxic T cells destroy cancer cells and foreign invaders; helper T cells work in conjunction with white blood cells; and suppressor T cells play a role in controlling white blood cell function.

**$TD_0$ (Toxic Dose 0%)**
The estimated dose at which none of the population is expected to exhibit toxic effects.

**$TD_{50}$ (Toxic Dose 50%)**
The estimated dose required to produce toxic effects in 50% of the population.

**$TD_{90}$ (Toxic Dose 90%)**
The estimated dose required to produce toxic effects in 90% of the population.

**Teratogen**
An agent that produces birth defects in a developing fetus.

**Teratogenesis**
The process by which a substance disrupts the normal development of tissues or organs in a growing fetus.

**Teratogenic**
Substances such as chemicals or radiation that exert a deleterious effect on the development of an embryo.

**Teratogenicity**
Birth defects that arise as a consequence of exposure to a teratogenic toxicant.

**Teratoma**
A benign tumor of germ cell origin, composed of nonproliferating somatic tissues with cells from all three embryonic cell layers: ectoderm, mesoderm, and endoderm. In the testis, teratomas are rare and usually found in prepubertal children.

**Testosterone**
A hormone produced especially by the testes or made synthetically and that is responsible for inducing and maintaining male secondary sex characteristics.

**Therapeutic Index (TI)**
The ratio of the dose required to produce the desired therapeutic response to the dose producing adverse effects.

**Threshold**
The dose or exposure below which no deleterious effect is expected to occur.

**Threshold Limit Value (TLV)**
Recommended guidelines for occupational exposure to airborne contaminants published by the ACGIH. TLVs represent the average concentration in $mg/m^3$ for an 8-hour workday and a 40-hour workweek to which nearly all workers may be repeatedly exposed, day after day, without adverse effect.

**Thymine (T)**
One of the pyrimidine nitrogenous bases in DNA, one-half of the base pair AT (adenine-thymine).

**Thyroxine ($C_{15}H_{11}I_4NO_4$)**
An iodine-containing hormone that is an amino acid produced by the thyroid gland as a product of the cleavage of thyroglobulin.

Thyroxine increases metabolic rate, affects protein synthesis, and is used to treat thyroid disorders.

**Tolerance**
The ability of an organism to endure unusually large doses of a substance without ill effect. Toxic effects are decreased with continued exposure to the substance.

**Toxicant**
Any chemical that has the potential to produce an adverse effect from an exposure.

**Toxicity**
Deleterious or adverse biological effects elicited by a chemical agent.

**Toxicogenomics**
An emerging field of study that uses genomics and bioinformatics to study how genomes respond to environmental stressors or toxicants. Combines genome-wide mRNA expression profiling with protein expression patterns using bioinformatics to understand the role of gene–environment interactions in disease and dysfunction.

**Toxicokinetics**
The determination and quantification of the time course of absorption, distribution, biotransformation, and excretion of chemicals (sometimes referred to as pharmacokinetics).

**Toxicologist**
A person who studies harmful effects of chemicals, including the mechanisms responsible for those effects, and the probability that the effects will occur under specific exposure conditions.

**Toxicology**
The study of harmful interactions between chemical agents and biological systems.

**Toxic Substance**
A chemical agent that may cause an adverse effect or effects to biological systems.

**Toxin**
A substance of biological origin, produced by certain plants, animals, and microorganisms, that is highly toxic to other organisms (snake venom).

**Transcription**
The synthesis of a complementary strand of RNA from a sequence of DNA (a gene); the first step in gene expression.

**Transcription Factor**
A protein that binds to regulatory regions and helps initiate, enhance, or inhibit gene expression.

**Transfer RNA (tRNA)**
A class of RNA having structures with triplet nucleotide sequences that are complementary to the triplet nucleotide coding sequences of mRNA. tRNA carries amino acids to ribosomes, where they are assembled into proteins according to the genetic code carried by mRNA.

**Transgenic**
An experimentally produced organism whose genome has been altered by the introduction of exogenous DNA into the organism's genome.

**Translation**
The process following transcription in which the genetic code carried by mRNA to the ribosomes directs the synthesis of proteins from amino acids. Has three phases—initiation, elongation, and termination.

**Tumor**
An abnormal uncontrolled growth of cells. Synonym: neoplasm

**Tumor Markers**
Tumor markers are measurable biochemicals associated with a malignancy. They are either produced by tumor cells (tumor-derived) or by the body in response to tumor cells (tumor-associated). Their presence in serum is indicative of the presence of the tumor. There are a few exceptions to this, such as tissue-bound receptors that must be measured in a biopsy from the solid tumor or proteins that are secreted into the urine.

# U

**Uncertainty Factor (UF)**
One of several, generally 10-fold, default factors used in operationally deriving the RfD and RfC from experimental data. The factors are intended to account for (1) variation in susceptibility among the members of the human population (i.e., interindividual or intraspecies variability); (2) uncertainty in extrapolating animal data to humans (i.e., interspecies uncertainty); (3) uncertainty in extrapolating from data obtained in a study with less-than-lifetime exposure (i.e., extrapolating from subchronic to chronic exposure); (4) uncertainty in extrapolating from a LOAEL rather than from a NOAEL; and (5) uncertainty associated with an incomplete database.

**Unscheduled DNA Synthesis (UDS)**
Synthesis of DNA that occurs outside the normal mitotic process. It is considered a sign of DNA damage and the first step in mutagenesis. The most commonly used test for UDS measures the uptake of tritium-labeled thymidine into the DNA of rat hepatocytes or human fibroblasts.

### Uracil

A nitrogenous pyrimidine base normally found in RNA but not DNA; uracil is capable of forming a base pair with adenine.

## V

### Vapor Pressure

The pressure exerted by a vapor in equilibrium with its liquid or solid phase. The higher the vapor pressure, the higher the volatility.

### Variability

Variability refers to true heterogeneity or diversity. For example, among a population that drinks water from the same source and with the same contaminant concentration, the risks from consuming the water may vary. This may be due to differences in exposure (i.e., different people drinking different amounts of water and having different body weights, different exposure frequencies, and different exposure durations) as well as differences in response (e.g., genetic differences in resistance to a chemical dose). Those inherent differences are referred to as variability. Differences among individuals in a population are referred to as interindividual variability, whereas differences for one individual over time are referred to as intraindividual variability.

### Volatility

Refers to the ease with which a material forms a vapor at ordinary temperature. The higher the vapor pressure, the more volatile the substance.

## W

### Weight of Evidence (WOE) for Carcinogenicity

A system used by the EPA for characterizing the extent to which the available data support the hypothesis that an agent causes cancer in humans. Under EPA's 1986 risk assessment guidelines, the WOE was described by categories "A through E," where group A is for known human carcinogens and group E is for agents with evidence of noncarcinogenicity. The approach, outlined in EPA's *Guidelines for Carcinogen Risk Assessment* (2005), considers all scientific information in determining whether and under what conditions an agent may cause cancer in humans and provides a narrative approach to characterize carcinogenicity rather than categories.

### Western Blot

A technique that quantifies the amount of a protein in a cell extract by first separating the cell proteins using gel electrophoresis and then "blotting" the resultant spots onto a thin nitrocellulose or nylon membrane.

## X

### Xenobiotic

A chemical substance foreign to the body.

# Index

# R

Ramazzini, Bernardino, 8

RAS transfected BALB 3T3 (Bhas 42) cells, 327

Reabsorption, 134–135

Reactive airways dysfunction syndrome (RADS), 249

Recognition and Management of Pesticide Poisonings (National Pesticide Telecommunications Network), 22

Recommended exposure limits (RELs), 296

Red tide, 66, 240

Reference dose (RfD), 379, 380, 389

Registry of Toxic Effects of Chemical Substances (RTECS) number, 16

Regulatory agencies. *See also specific agencies*
    function of, 279–280
    occupational, 294–296
    websites for, 301–302

Regulatory issues
    Agency for Toxic Substances and Disease Registry and, 298–299
    Consumer Product Safety Commission and, 300
    Environmental Protection Agency and, 290–294
    federal legislation and, 280
    Food and Drug Administration and, 283–290
    industrial vs. environmental standards and, 296–297
    National Toxicology Program and, 299–300
    public awareness and, 281–283
    standards vs. guidelines and, 279
    on toxicity testing, 330–331
    websites for, 301–302

Regulatory toxicologists, 273

Relative density, 18

Relative molecular mass, 17

Relative potency factor (RPF), 388

Relative vapor density, 18

Renal excretion, 133–135

Renal secretion, 135

*Report on Carcinogens* (National Toxicology Program), 188–190, 300

Reproductive/developmental toxicity, 385–386

Reproductive toxicity tests, 321–322, 329

Reptiles, 73–74

Reptile venom
    explanation of, 74–75
    methods to treat, 76

Resource Conservation and Recovery Act (RCRA), 292

Respiratory system
    airborne toxicants and, 241
    air pollutant exposure and, 244–246

defense strategies of, 246–248

functional divisions of, 241–243

function of, 240

injury to, 243–244, 248–250

overview of, 239–240

toxicant absorption in, 115, 121–122

Respiratory toxicity tests, 329

Response, 105. *See also* Dose-response relationship

Restricted use pesticides, 355, 356

Right to Know Hazardous Substance Fact Sheets (New Jersey Department of Health & Senior Services), 22

Risk
    explanation of, 375–376
    websites on, 391

Risk assessment
    cancer, 381–383
    dose-response assessment component of, 378
    ecological, 385–386
    explanation of, 376–377
    exposure assessment component of, 378–379
    in federal government, 394–396
    hazard identification component of, 377–378
    interaction types and, 387–388
    noncancer, 379–381
    pesticide, 354
    in response to public concerns, 389–391
    risk characterization component of, 383–384
    toxicant interaction and, 386–389

*Risk Assessment in the Federal Government: Managing the Pocess* (National Research Council), 394–395

Risk characterization
    deterministic, 386
    explanation of, 383–384

Risk management, 384

RNA
    comparison of DNA and, 158, 159
    explanation of, 157, 160

Rodent chromosomal assay, 313

Rumsfeld, Donald, 393

# S

S. E. Massengill Company, 282–283

Safe Drinking Water Act (SDWA), 280, 382, 388

*Salmonella* mutagenicity test. *See* Ames mutagenicity assay

*Salmonella typhimurium*, 162, 327

Sarcomas, 175

Sarcoplasmic reticular function, 231